Water and Sanitation for Disabled People and Other Vulnerable Groups

Water and Sanitation for Disabled People

and Other Vulnerable Groups

Designing services to improve accessibility

Hazel Jones & Bob Reed

Water, Engineering and Development Centre
Loughborough University
2005

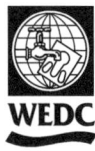

Water, Engineering and Development Centre
Loughborough University
Leicestershire
LE11 3TU UK

A reference copy of this publication is also available online at:
http://www.lboro.ac.uk/wedc/publications/

Jones, H.E. and Reed, R.A. (2005)
Water and Sanitation for Disabled People and Other Vulnerable Groups
– Designing services to improve accessibility
WEDC, Loughborough University, UK.

ISBN Paperback 1 84380 079 9

This document is an output from a project funded by the UK
Department for International Development (DFID)
for the benefit of low-income countries.
The views expressed are not necessarily those of DFID.

Photographs taken by Hazel Jones, illustrations by Rod Shaw and Ken Chatterton
at WEDC, unless stated otherwise.

Designed and produced at WEDC by Glenda McMahon, Sue Plummer and Rod Shaw

Printed by MWL Print Group

About the authors

Hazel Jones is an Assistant Programme Manager at Loughborough University. She is a specialist in community approaches to the inclusion of disabled people, and is the principal researcher for the DFID-funded Knowledge and Research (KaR) project which has culminated in this book.

Bob Reed is Senior Programme Manager at Loughborough University with over 30 years' experience of public health engineering. He has a particular interest in water supply and sanitation for low-income communities and in emergencies.

Collaborators

The research project 'Water supply and sanitation access and use by physically disabled people' was funded by the Department for International Development (DFID) of the British Government.

The following organisations have acted as peer reviewers for this research. They have given advice on project design and implementation, provided information, reviewed draft documents, and have been involved in and provided support for field research. This project would not have been possible without their support and encouragement.

Opinions contained in this document are solely those of the authors and do not necessarily represent those of DFID or collaborators.

Action to Positive Change on People with Disabilities, Uganda.

British Council of Disabled People.

Centre for Disability Studies, Leeds University, UK.

Centre for the Rehabilitation of the Paralysed (CRP), Bangladesh.

Disability Action Council (DAC), Cambodia.

Healthlink Worldwide.

World Federation of Occupational Therapists.

Further contributions by Sudha Lahman.

Acknowledgements

The authors would like to thank the following people for their contribution to the research, and production of this document. The opinions contained in this book are those of the authors, although every effort has been made to incorporate the views and advice of contributors from a wide range of personal and professional perspectives.

Advisory panel members:

Emi Aizawa, Assistant Resident Representative, Japan International Cooperation Agency (JICA) Cambodia Office;

Carolyn Baylies, Senior Lecturer in Sociology, Centre for Disability Studies (sadly now deceased);

Dr Julie Fisher, Assistant Programme Manager, WEDC;

Dr Sam Kayaga, Assistant Programme Manager, WEDC;

Dr Elly Macha, Executive Director, Tanzania Disabled Women Development Network Programme;

Dr AKM Momin, previously Director, Centre for the Rehabilitation of the Paralysed, Bangladesh (CRP);

Joy Morgan, Freelance Hygiene and Sanitation Consultant;

Elijah Musenyente, Chairman, Uganda Society of Hidden Talents (HITS);

Heather Payne, previously Disability Adviser, Healthlink Worldwide;

Adam Platt, previously Director of Programmes, HelpAge International;

Dr Avizit Reaz Quazi, Chief, Research Cell, NGO Forum for DWSS, Bangladesh;

Samantha Shann, Lecturer in Occupational Therapy, Northumbria University, UK delegate to World Federation of Occupational Therapists.

Mohammed Mushfiqul Wara, previously Research Officer, Centre for the Rehabilitation of the Paralysed, Bangladesh (CRP).

Co-researchers:

Dr. Kenneth J. Parker FCIBSE, Senior Research Fellow, Robert Gordon University, Aberdeen, U.K.;

Sarah House, Water / Public Health Engineer, freelance consultant.

Reviewers:

Bill Albert, Consultant, chair of the International Committee of the British Council of Disabled People (BCODP), Director of International Disability Equality Agency (IDEA);

Herve Bernard, Head of Social Inclusion, Handicap International;

Elizabeth Carrington, International Development Adviser, Chartered Society of Physiotherapy;

Idrissa Doucoure, West Africa Regional Manager, and colleagues, WaterAid;

Jacqui Christy James, International representative of the International Committee of the BCODP; Co Director of IDEA,

Roger Drew, Health and Development Consultant;

Steve Harknett, Adviser, Disability Development Services Pursat (DDSP), Cambodia;

Dominic Haslam, Public Funding Manager, WaterAid;

Ray Heslop, engineering adviser, WaterAid;

Julius Kamwesiga, Principal, Occupational Therapy Training School, Uganda;

Liz Mackinlay, Gender and Diversity Adviser, World Vision Cambodia;

Kerry Anne McKenzie, Senior Operations Manager, World Vision Cambodia;

Karen Reiff, International Department, and colleagues from The Danish Council of Organizations of Disabled People (DSI);

Jan-Willem Rosenboom, Country Team Leader, Water & Sanitation Programme (WSP), Cambodia;

Rebecca Scott, Assistant Programme Manager, WEDC;

Lorraine Wapling, Advocacy Officer, Action on Disability and Development (ADD), UK;

David Werner, HealthWrights;

Vince Whitehead, Technical Adviser, Development Technology Workshop (DTW), Cambodia;

Advice on issues of gender, diversity, participation and concrete:

Rose Lidonde, Assistant Programme Manager, WEDC;

Brian Reed, Assistant Programme Manager, WEDC.

Illustrations

Reproduced with kind permission from the Indian Institute of Cerebral Palsy, Kolkata.

David Werner, Healthwrights, US,

Gerry van der Hulst, and

Handicap International.

Contents

Chapter 9. Case studies **153**

Bangladesh

Cambodia

Uganda

Tibet

List of boxes

List of tables

List of figures

xvi

xvii

Glossary of terms and abbreviations

CBR	community-based rehabilitation
DPO	disabled people's organisation
DRA	Demand Responsive Approach
g.i.	galvanised iron
MDGs	Millennium Development Goals
NGO	non-governmental organisation
PRA	Participatory rural appraisal, or participatory reflection and action
PRSP	poverty reduction strategy paper/process
WATSAN	water and sanitation
PVC	polyvinyl chloride, a type of plastic from which water pipes are made
VIP latrine	ventilated improved pit latrine

Organisations

APCPD	Action to Positive Change on People with Disabilities
BPKS	Bangladesh Protibandhi Kallyan Somity
BCODP	The British Council of Disabled People
CABDIC	Capacity building of people with disabilities in the community
CRP	Centre for the Rehabilitation of the Paralysed
CSID	Centre for Services & Information on Disability
DFID	Department for International Development, UK
HI-B	Handicap International Belgium
HITS	Uganda Society of Hidden Talents
IICP	Indian Institute of Cerebral Palsy
SCI Centre	Spinal Cord Injury Centre
UN	United Nations
UNICEF	United Nations Children's Fund
WEDC	Water Engineering and Development Centre
WSP	World Bank Water and Sanitation Program

Language of disability

disabled people's organisation	An organisation run by and for disabled people themselves
disability sector	Refers in this book to disabled people's organisations and disability service providers (government and non-government) with a focus and interest in disability and development.
disability	The outcome of the interaction between a person with an impairment and the environmental and attitudinal barriers he or she may face.

impairment	Problems in an individual's body structure or function (including psychological function) as a significant deviation or loss.
impairment and disability	It is most accurate to refer to people with impairments, or disabled people, not 'people with disabilities'. But the term 'disability' is often used interchangeably with the less common 'impairment', particularly outside the UK. This document therefore includes direct quotes that use the term disabilities to refer to impairments.
environmental factors	Make up of the physical, social and attitudinal environment in which people live and conduct their lives.
social model of disability	Recognises that disability is caused not by a person's impairment, but by the disadvantage or restriction of activity caused by a society which takes little or no account of people who have impairments.

Language of infrastructure

accessible facility	Facilities with features – whether designed and constructed to be accessible, or with changes or additions that make them more comfortable, less hard work, or simply possible to use by a disabled or frail elderly person, with or without the support of a family member or piece of equipment.
adapted facilities	Facilities with additions, or changes which are fixed to the structure in order to increase accessibility.
assistive device	Aid or equipment used by a disabled person, often designed specifically to meet their individual needs, which enables him or her to carry out an activity more easily or more independently.
cement mortar	A mixture of sand, cement and water.
cement screed	A thin layer of cement and water to give a hard, smooth finish.
gradient	Way of measuring how steep a slope is.
inclusive design	Aims to create beautiful and functional environments that can be used equally by everyone, irrespective of age, gender or disability. It extends from inception, through the planning process, design, construction, occupation, management and operation. Each of these stages should be fully inclusive involving disabled people and other potential consumers in their development and evaluation. Disabled people are not a homogenous group with identical needs, and when the principles of 'inclusive design' are applied, the built environment will also become accessible to other users who are excluded through poor design or discriminatory attitudes.

inclusive environment	An inclusive environment does not attempt to meet every single need, but, by considering people's diversity, inclusive environments can break down barriers and exclusion and will often achieve superior solutions that benefit everyone. [2]
kerb	A low raised edge along a path or ramp.
pointing	Cement mortar, sand or earth between bricks or blocks of a path to improve stability and drainage.
ramp	A slope constructed with an even surface, with a gradient of 1 in 20 or steeper, that makes it possible to pass from one level to another.
sarong/ wrapper	Large rectangular piece of cloth often with a variety of uses, including clothing (e.g. skirt, dress, shawl or headscarf) and for covering the body during and after bathing. Also known as a lunghi, sin, khrama, etc.
transfer	To move to and from a wheelchair, to the ground, or another seat, such as a toilet seat or bathing seat.

Units of measurement

Metric measurements have been used throughout, usually centimetres (cm). If more than 2 metres, given in metres. Occasionally millimetres have been used, where it is usual, e.g. for diameter of pipes, tap sizes, etc.

cm	centimetre
mm	millimetre
m	metre
L, W, D, H	length, width, depth, height
LH, RH	left-hand, right hand
L	litre
%	per cent
º e.g. 90º	degrees – e.g. 90 degrees
Ø or dia	diameter
~	approximately
>	more than
<	less than
1 : 20, 1 : 15, etc.	way of describing how steep a gradient or slope is, i.e. a 1 : 20 slope rises 1cm over a length of 20cm.

References

1. WHO (2001) The International Classification of Functioning, Disability and Health - ICF. World Health Organization: Geneva. http://www3.who.int/icf/icftemplate.cfm

2. Disability Rights Commission (2003) Creating an Inclusive Environment - a report on improving the Built Environment. http://www.drc-gb.org/publicationsandreports/publicationhtml.asp?id=157&docsect=0&section=0

Chapter 1

Introduction

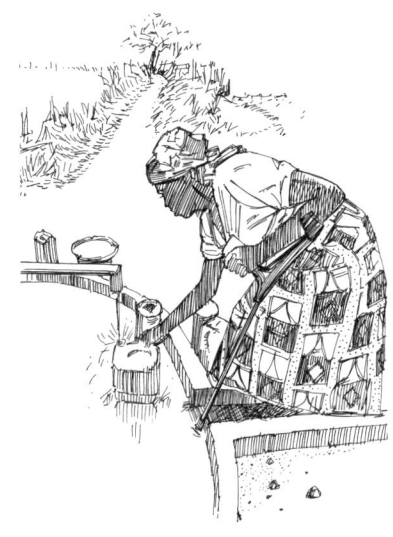

1.1 Why this book was written

Water supply and sanitation services and facilities are traditionally designed for the 'average' person, which ignores the fact that in real communities, people come with a wide range of shapes, sizes, abilities and needs. As a result, large numbers of these 'non-average' people are excluded from normal services and facilities. One such group is disabled people and others who have physical limitations.

This book has been written to raise awareness among the water and sanitation sector about the needs of disabled people and other vulnerable groups, and to provide practical information, ideas and guidance about how these needs could be addressed within normal water and sanitation programmes and services.

The book's main target audience is therefore planners and service providers in the water supply and sanitation sector. In addition, disabled people's organisations, and organisations that provide support to disabled people and their families, may find useful information for their work.

The research on which this book is based was funded by the UK DFID: KaR [Knowledge and Research] 8059: 'Water supply and sanitation access and use by physically disabled people'. (See Appendix 6 on page 285 for a description of the research). It is designed to contribute to DFID's commitment to poverty reduction of disabled people in low-income communities (DFID, 2000).

1.2 Focus of the book

The main focus of this resource book is on access to domestic water supply and sanitation, which may be at either household or communal level. Some of the ideas and suggestions can also be applied in institutional settings, such as schools and hospitals, and in some emergency situations, although the issues particular to those settings are not addressed in this book.

The focus is on the accessibility of the physical environment for children, women and men who experience limitations in carrying out activities related to water and sanitation. These may be disabled people, or other people who are not usually thought of as disabled, such as frail elderly people, pregnant women, small children, women and girls carrying babies, and people who are ill, including people with AIDS.

A disabled person may have difficulty squatting, for example, but so will a pregnant woman. A person with a paralysed arm may have difficulty grasping, but so might a person who is weak with fever, or a frail elderly person.

Because so little has been previously done in this area, it is recognised that the information in this book is far from comprehensive, and should be seen as a work in progress. We strongly encourage practitioners to try out some of these ideas and solutions in their own work, in such a way that we can all learn from them.

1.3 What you will not find in this book

- Standard designs for accessible public facilities. These are available in other publications and listed in Appendix 1.

- Details about specific impairments and medical conditions, or individual aids and equipment for disabled people, such as wheelchairs and crutches. These are covered comprehensively in other publications, some of which are listed in the relevant sections in Appendix 1.

- Issues of water and sanitation specifically related to institutions, such as health clinics and schools, although many of the ideas can be applied in institutional settings.

- Issues of water and sanitation in emergencies.

- Issues of water for productivity.

- Ways to address disability issues in health and hygiene promotion.

1.4 How to use the book

It is not necessary for every reader to read the whole book. Readers with different backgrounds and experience will find different sections useful.

Chapter 2 provides some answers to the question 'Why should the water and sanitation sector consider disabled people? It is mainly for readers who have had little previous contact with disabled people and disability issues. Readers from the disability sector may also find it provides information that they can use in their advocacy work.

Chapters 3 and 4 provide information to support communication and collaboration between the water supply and sanitation (WATSAN) and disability sectors. Chapter 3 is mainly for readers who have had little previous contact with the WATSAN sector, including disabled people, disability service providers, and agencies promoting social inclusion and advocacy on rights and access. Chapter 4 is mainly for readers who have had little previous contact with disabled people and disability issues, including WATSAN sector professionals, engineers, public health workers and community development workers.

Chapters 5 to 7 provide practical ideas for making physical facilities more accessible and inclusive. These will be useful for implementers of all backgrounds, including disabled people and their families.

Chapter 8 presents ideas for planning and implementing services that consider disabled people, and is divided into two main sections: section 8.2 presents issues that are mainly relevant to WATSAN service planners and providers, whilst section 8.3 is mainly relevant to the disability sector.

Chapter 9 provides a number of case-studies illustrating how disabled people and their families have benefited from improved access to water and sanitation facilities. These could be used in a number of ways: as advocacy material, as practical information for disabled people and their families, or as material for awareness-raising or problem-solving workshops.

The Appendices provide lists of further relevant information and resource material for which there is not enough room in the book.

Chapter 2

Why should the water and sanitation sector consider disabled people?

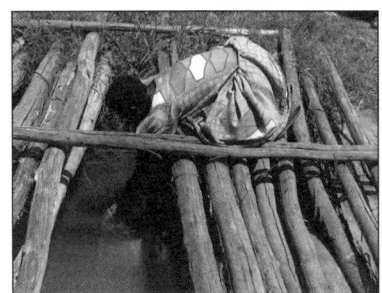

Figure 2.1. A typical back-breaking communal shallow well in Uganda.

This chapter is mainly for readers who have had little previous contact with disabled people and disability issues, and limited experience of including disability in their work. This is likely to include water and sanitation (WATSAN) sector professionals, community development workers and public health workers.

2.1 Disabled people are a part of every community

Disabled people are a part of every community, everywhere in the world. They are among the poorest, most marginalised and disadvantaged, and are often hidden. Sadly, disabled people have the least access to basic WATSAN services, which contributes to their continued isolation, poor health and poverty.

The aim of infrastructure and development, including WATSAN programmes, is to improve the well-being of everyone in a community, whether they are male or female, rich or poor, young or old, disabled or non-disabled. It follows therefore that all WATSAN programmes and activities are relevant to disabled people, so a disability perspective should always be included. For example, WATSAN activities targeted at poor people must consider poor disabled people, those targeting poor women must consider poor disabled women, and so on.

Increasingly, WATSAN service providers are recognising that in order to reduce poverty, there is a need to target the poorest, most disadvantaged and vulnerable sections of the population, to provide more equitable access to basic services. This must therefore include disabled people.

2.2 Inclusive facilities bring benefits for all

Improved access to water and sanitation facilities brings a range of benefits to disabled people and their families, including:

- Increased dignity and self-reliance for disabled people. Being able to carry out an activity independently, where they previously relied on others for support.

- Improved health and nutrition.

- Reduced poverty and improved well-being: disabled people and their families save time and effort, which releases time for other activities, such as income generation, household chores, or schooling.

Every community is made up of a variety of individuals with a wide range of needs. Women have different needs and concerns from men, elderly people have different needs from children, and so on. In the same way, disabled women, children and men have a range of needs, many of which are similar to those of other women, children and men.

All over the world, the traditional approach to service provision is to divide people and their needs into 'normal' and 'special', with so-called 'normal' services for the majority of the population, with 'special' facilities or services for disabled people sometimes as an added extra. These 'normal' services rarely consider the reality of the wide range of human needs, with the result that many people in the community are unable to or have difficulty using them.

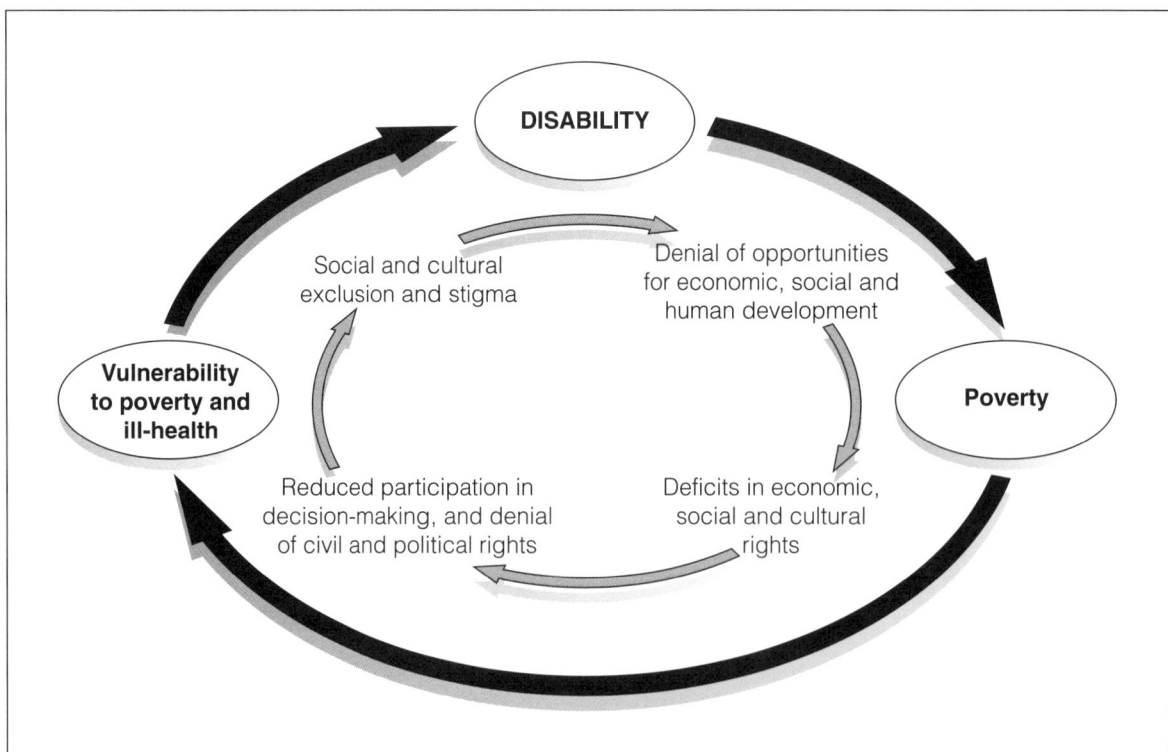

Figure 2.2. Poverty and disability – a vicious cycle (1).

Why consider disabled people?

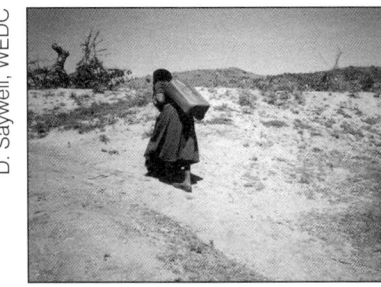

D. Saywell, WEDC

Figure 2.3. Carrying water uphill.

The majority of disabled people do not need 'special' facilities – their needs can be met by ordinary services with a little extra thought, and only minor adjustments. Making WATSAN facilities and services inclusive would therefore benefit the whole community. These might include frail elderly people, pregnant women, girls, parents with small children, and people who are injured or sick, including people with HIV/AIDS. Any of these people may have difficulty with their balance or co-ordination, with weak grip, limited flexibility, squatting or lifting, most of which are needed to access WATSAN facilities. Because of this they are likely to experience many of the same problems of exclusion as many disabled people, although they are not described in this way.

2.3 Disability is a poverty issue

Poverty is not only about low income, but also about limited opportunities, choices and social exclusion, all of which particularly apply to disabled people (2). Poverty is both a cause and a consequence of disability (Figure 2.2):

- Poor people are more likely to be disabled. Why? Poor nutrition, bad water, inadequate living conditions, poor hygiene and sanitation, limited health services, environmental pollution, war, conflict and disaster, lack of information, HIV/AIDS, and hazardous working conditions are all causes of impairment.

- Disabled people are more likely to be poor. Why? Inadequate treatment to reduce impairments, lack of suitable equipment such as crutches, lack of access to education or employment, isolation, discrimination. Disabled people are also at high risk of HIV/AIDS infection, as they lack access to health information and are least able to protect themselves (3).

The impact of disability is felt by the whole family, because of:

- Lost income of family members who support disabled people;

- Reduced health of disabled people, leading to increased costs of treatment and medicines, and increased family workload;

- Reduced health and well-being of the family, increased vulnerability and poverty.

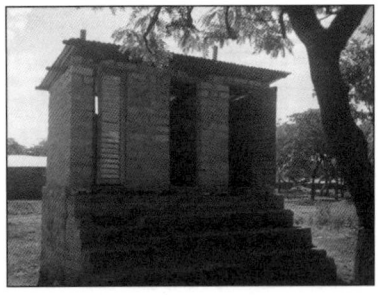

P. Harvey, WEDC

Figure 2.4. Latrine in Tanzania with steep steps and narrow doors.

Lack of clean water and sanitation are key factors in keeping people poor, unhealthy and unable to improve their livelihoods. For disabled poor people, its impact can be doubly difficult. For example, in communities where women go out to defecate at night, moving around in the dark can be extra hazardous for a disabled woman. In many rural areas, diarrhoea is a regular occurrence for everyone, but for a disabled person who needs support, this can place an extra workload on family members.

It is therefore clear that development targets such as the Millennium Development Goals (4) of poverty reduction, improved health, and access to safe water, will never be equitably met unless disabled people are included (5). (See Section 3.4. Millennium Development Goals).

2.4   Inclusive access is good economics

The economic costs of excluding disabled people far outweigh the costs of including them. The costs of exclusion are borne not only by the family, but also by the whole community, in terms of the lost economic and social contribution by the disabled person and their family to the community. On the service delivery side, the creation of 'special', often separate services and facilities is costly, and often a lack of funds means that only a small minority of disabled people benefit.

An inclusive approach to facilities and services is more cost-effective. If inclusion is planned from the beginning, the additional cost is minimal – often as little as 0.2 per cent (6, 7). Even where inclusion has not been planned from the outset, and existing facilities need to be adapted to make them more inclusive, this does not need to be highly technical or expensive.

2.5   Access to water and sanitation is a human right

'Access to safe water is a fundamental human need and therefore a basic right.' Kofi Annan (8)

'We … confirm our unswerving commitment to water, sanitation and hygiene as human rights and as vital components of sustainable human development.' (9)

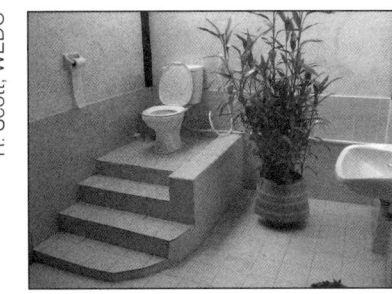

R. Scott, WEDC

Figure 2.5. Steps to the toilet.

The right to safe water is enshrined in Article 25 of the UN Declaration of Human Rights (10), and in Article 27 of the UN Convention on the Rights of the Child (11). A UN Convention on Disabled People's Rights is also currently under discussion, in which the current draft, Article 23 specifically mentions 'Access to clean water' as part of an adequate standard of living (12).

For the majority of disabled people in low-income communities, their human rights to life, food, water and shelter are a daily struggle. The only way they will access these basic needs and rights, and thus an acceptable quality of life, is through inclusion in mainstream services and programmes.

2.6 I'm an engineer, not a disability 'specialist' – what can I do?

As we have pointed out, disabled people have the same needs and rights as everyone else: to adequate living conditions, including sanitation and safe water, access to education and health services, decent roads and transport. The majority of people, including frail elderly people, parents with small children and disabled people, could get their basic needs met and their livelihoods improved through mainstream services and programmes, if a disability perspective was part of the usual way of looking at service provision.

Disabled people do not expect more or better facilities than other people, only to be included, so that they can have equal access. Equity, equal access, and equality of opportunity do not mean that everyone must be treated exactly the same. In order to access their same basic needs, some people may need something a bit different. For example, for a person with difficulty walking to have equal access to water (in other words, spend the same amount of time fetching water as her neighbours), the water point needs to be nearer to her home than to those of her neighbours. Services need to be flexible enough to be able to provide a range of options.

Some disabled people have healthcare needs, and require certain equipment to support them. However, for this individual support to be provided, but without accessible services being available, is often of little or no use to the disabled person concerned (Figure 2.6).

It is not possible for a mainstream WATSAN service to meet the individual needs and demands of all. Some needs are too challenging and beyond the scope of the public health engineer. But not all disabled people need a 'special' service.

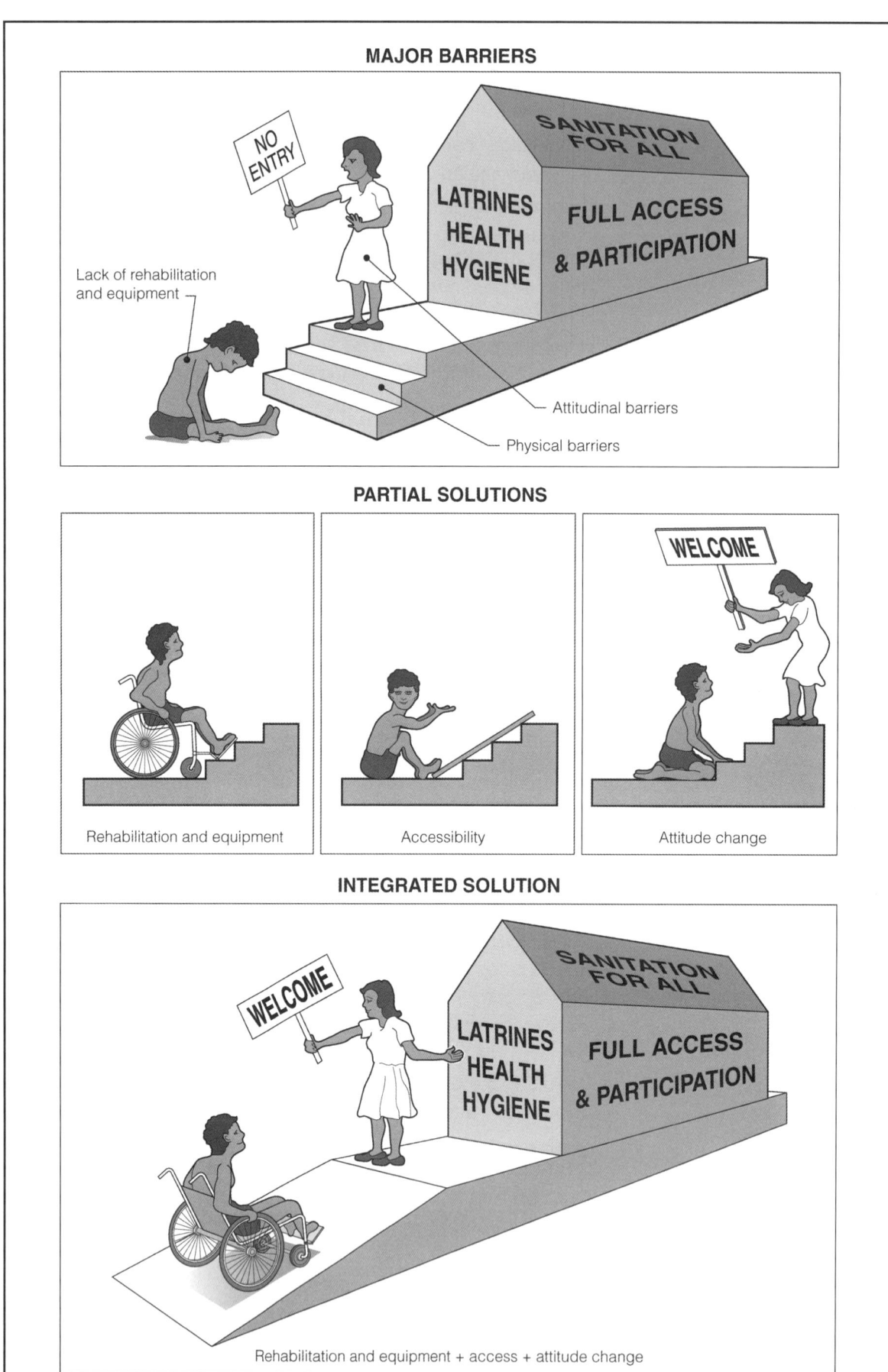

Figure 2.6. Holistic approach to including disabled people (adapted from Werner, 1987).

Why consider disabled people?

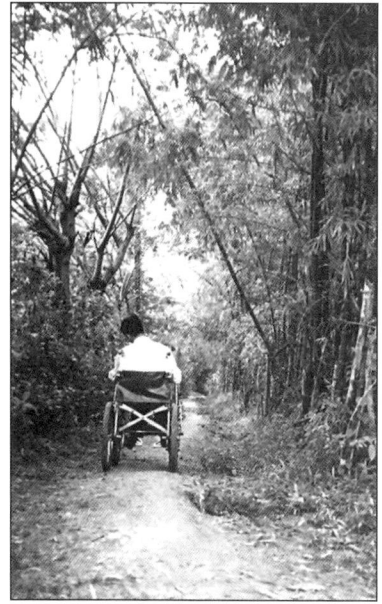

Figure 2.7. Many rural roads are a challenge for wheelchair users.

A little extra information, awareness and thought on the part of service providers can make the difference between a disabled person being included or excluded by a service.

This means that service providers cannot simply pass responsibility for disabled people to 'specialists'. Doing nothing is not acceptable. All service providers need to consider ways to ensure that disabled people are not excluded from their services and programmes.

Whilst engineers have design knowledge and skills, they are not always aware of the needs of disabled people. Disabled people, on the other hand, whilst not generally knowledgeable about engineering (although there are disabled engineers) do understand their own access needs. So, when planners and engineers start the process of designing a WATSAN project, they should consult local disabled people's organisations (DPOs), including disabled women's sections, to get their input.

2.7 Disabled people are only a small minority, we have to think of the majority first

There are more than 500 million disabled people in the world according to UN estimates. Approximately 80 per cent live in low-income countries (12, 13). Estimates vary from 4 to 10 per cent of the population (14), although a recent survey in Bangladesh found 14 per cent were disabled (15). These numbers are increasing, because of factors such as violent conflict, accidents, HIV/AIDS, environmental pollution and ageing populations. In low-income countries the proportion of older people is predicted to rise from 8 to 19 per cent by 2050 (16).

However, among the poorest of the poor in low-income countries, as many as 1 in 5 are likely to be disabled (17). This means that almost every chronically poor family is affected in some way by disability.

2.8 We don't discriminate – everyone is included

The WATSAN sector is developing strategies and approaches to understand and respond to the different perspectives and needs of communities, as part of the process of planning and project design. Unfortunately, without intending to, the service delivery process often excludes many disabled people, so their concerns and needs remain hidden.

Sometimes exclusion is deliberate, direct and explicit; for example, by specifying certain groups that are not allowed to participate. But most exclusion is indirect, and arises through a lack of awareness or thought (see Box 2.1). For example, holding meetings in locations where only men are allowed will exclude women. In the same way, holding a meeting on the second floor of a building with no lift or ramp will exclude people who have difficulty walking. Social factors can also lead to exclusion. Where it is the norm for powerless groups such as women, elderly women, disabled people and people of low caste to only speak when asked a direct question, their participation in a meeting will be limited.

The effect of exclusion is the same whether or not exclusion is intended. All the more reason why including a disability perspective has to become the accepted way of thinking about benefiting the whole community, because this is the best way to make buildings and services more accessible for everyone.

Box 2.1. Indirect exclusion

An HIV/AIDS education and awareness project aimed at teenagers and young people in Indonesia welcomed all young people without exception – or so they thought. The organisers admitted that of 5,000 young people using the service in the past year, they knew of not one who was a disabled person. On further questioning, it turned out that the main route to young people, using posters, outreach workers and peer counsellors, was through secondary schools. When it was pointed out that no disabled young people attended mainstream secondary schools in that province, the organisers recognised that they had to find alternative ways to reach disabled young people, such as through a local vocational training centre. *(Author's own experience)*

Box 2.2. Hazardous facilities

A 60 year-old man with physical impairment had a simple toilet of bamboo pieces placed over a ditch. The toilet was very old, and could not protect his privacy. But he could not afford to mend it, so he only used the toilet at night. One night he went to the toilet. When he sat on the bamboo it broke, and he fell into the ditch full of stinky, dirty refuse. No one heard him shouting for help. He was only discovered the next morning, when a person saw some hair of the old man in the ditch. He had died in the night (18).

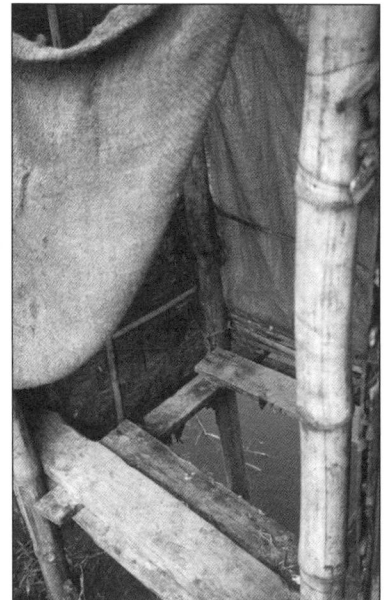

Figure 2.8. Hanging latrine in Bangladesh – a challenge for all but the very agile.

2.9 So how do disabled people manage?

Some disabled people manage, some do not. Some develop their own solutions, by using and adapting local materials to make equipment that suits them. Others receive support from disability services, which may provide special equipment and advice. However, because water and sanitation are personal private issues, these solutions are often not shared with others who could benefit, so most disabled people must search for solutions in isolation.

Many disabled people do not find solutions, and are forced to use unhygienic practices, like defecating in the bushes, waiting to use the latrine at night (Box 2.2), or using unclean water sources, all of which are damaging to their health and that of their family.

Box 2.3. No more cleaning bed-pans

Mr Mofizuddin could not get into the family's old pit latrine in his wheelchair, so he had to use a bed-pan. His wife had to empty and clean it every day, which she found dirty and unpleasant. Now a local DPO has provided the family with their own latrine, designed so that Mr Mofizuddin can use it independently. The whole family likes using the latrine: it is light, well ventilated, and there is no bad smell, which makes it pleasant to use. But best of all for his wife, the smooth concrete finish makes it easy to keep clean. It is less work and much more pleasant than emptying and cleaning a bed-pan. *(Case-study 9.2, page 161)*

Box 2.4. Reducing a mother's workload

Mrs Kabiito has four disabled children who are unable to walk or speak. She is a teacher, and leaves them each day in the care of their sister, playing and crawling around the family compound. During the day, they urinate and defecate in their shorts. When she comes home from work, Mrs Kabiito has the task of washing all four children and their shorts.

Now Mrs Kabiito has been given a commode stool, which she is gradually training her children to use. She puts the stool with a container under it in a convenient place, so she can keep an eye on the child and continue with other jobs at the same time. As the children gradually learn to defecate into the container, instead of their shorts, she has less clothes washing to do, and already her workload has begun to reduce (19).

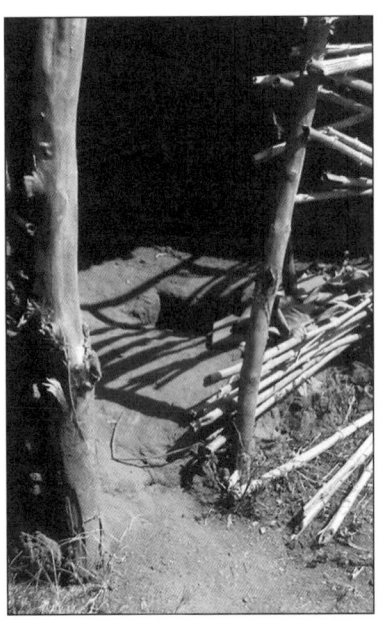

Figure 2.9. A family latrine in Uganda.

Family support – a gender dimension

In many communities, particularly where traditional family ties are strong, families consider it their duty and responsibility to support each other. This includes support to disabled people and frail elderly relatives, young children and people who are sick. For the family, this support can become a problem when the workload becomes heavy. Finding ways to make support tasks easier, more pleasant, quicker and more hygienic is helpful to the whole family.

There is an important gender dimension to improving access. Improvements for the disabled person often bring improvements for women and children, since support tasks frequently fall most heavily on them (Box 2.3). Support is often provided by a child in the family (usually a girl) who is likely to be taken out of school as a result (Box 2.4).

2.10 Why didn't we know?

Firstly, the right questions were probably not asked, because personal hygiene issues are not subjects for public discussion in most cultures. Most people are unaware that alternative options are possible and so don't raise the issue. And thirdly, many disabled people are isolated and hidden because of misunderstanding and ignorance in their community (see Section 4.3).

Disabled people are not present: many people find it difficult to move far from their home to access services or attend meetings, including people with difficulty moving, frail elderly people and blind people, among others. Family members who provide support to a disabled person, usually women, may be unable to leave them unattended to come to the meeting on their behalf, and they may be too difficult to carry.

Keeping it in the family: traditionally, it is the family's responsibility to support a disabled member, so they may feel guilty about raising the problems, for fear of being accused of avoiding their responsibility.

References

1. DFID (2000) *Disability, Poverty and Development*. Issues Paper. Department for International Development: UK. http://www.dfid.gov.uk/Pubs/files/disability.pdf

2. DFID (2001) *Poverty: Bridging the Gap. Guidance Notes*. Issues. Department for International Development: UK.

3. de Vries, C. (2004) *Disabled Persons are more vulnerable to HIV*. Dutch Coalition on Disability and Development: Utrecht, Netherlands. http://www.dcdd.nl

4. World Bank (2003) *Millennium Development Goals*. http://www.developmentgoals.org/Hiv_Aids.htm

5. European Disability Forum (2002) *Development Cooperation and Disability*. European Disability Forum: Brussels. http://www.edf-feph.org

6. Metts, R.L. (2000) *Disability Issues, Trends and Recommendations for the World Bank*. World Bank: New York.

7. Office of the Deputy President (1997) *Integrated National Disability Strategy White Paper*. Government of South Africa: http://www.gov.za/whitepaper/1997/disability.htm

8. WaterAid and Rights and Humanity (2004) *The Right to Water*. http://www.righttowater.org.uk.

9. Water Supply and Sanitation Collaborative Council (WSSCC) (2004) Global WASH Forum. Dakar Statement. http://www.wsscc.org/dataweb.cfm?code=516.

10. United Nations (1948) *Universal Declaration of Human Rights*. United Nations: Geneva. http://www.un.org/Overview/rights.html

11. United Nations (1989) *Convention on the Rights of the Child*. United Nations: New York. http://www.crin.org/docs/resources/treaties/uncrc.htm

12. Working Group of the Ad Hoc Committee on International Convention on the Rights of Persons with Disabilities. New York, 5 - 16 January 2004. Report of the Working Group to the Ad Hoc Committee. A/AC.265/2004/WG/1 United Nations. http://www.un.org/esa/socdev/enable/

13. WHO DAR (2003) *Disability and Rehabilitation*. http://www.who.int/ncd/disability/index.htm

14. Helander, E. (1999) *Prejudice and Dignity: an Introduction to Community-Based Rehabilitation. Second edition*. UNDP: New York.

15. Actionaid Bangladesh (1996) *Four Baseline Surveys on Prevalence of Disability*. Disability & AIDS Coordination Unit. Actionaid: Dhaka, Bangladesh.

16. HAI (2002) *State of the world's older people 2002*. HelpAge International: London, UK. http://www.helpage.org

17. Elwan, A. (1999) *Poverty and Disability: a survey of the literature*. World Bank: Washington, USA.

18. Lewis, I., Jones, H. & Reed, R. (eds.) (2002) *Water supply and sanitation access and use by physically disabled people: e-conference synthesis report*. WEDC, Loughborough University and DFID: UK.

19. Jones, H.E. and Reed, R.A. (2003) *Water Supply and Sanitation Access and Use by Physically Disabled People*. Report of field-work in Uganda. WEDC, Loughborough University and DFID: UK.

Chapter 3

Understanding the water supply and sanitation sector

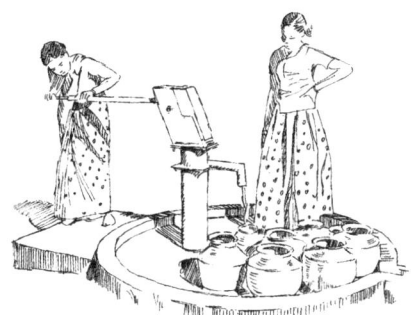

This chapter is mainly for readers who have had little previous contact with the water supply and sanitation (WATSAN) sector, including disabled people, disability service providers, and agencies promoting social inclusion and advocacy on rights and access.

Policymakers, donors and international organisations are now starting to address the issue of disability in development programmes. However, in terms of implementation, it is often not clear what each sector needs to do in practice. In the WATSAN sector there is some recognition among professionals that they should, in principle, be addressing the needs of disabled people, but most have never considered the issue. It has never been part of their training and most would not know where to start. There is very little information on the issue that is relevant to engineers.

The disability sector, and DPOs in particular, have a key role to play in advocating for the inclusion of a disability perspective in the WATSAN sector. But it is an unfamiliar area to most people in the disability sector, with different perspectives and a different language, that can hinder communication between the sectors. The risk is that engineers see disability as irrelevant to them, or as yet another 'cross-cutting issue' to be mainstreamed, adding to 'issues overload'.

The information in this chapter is designed to help the disability sector understand more about the WATSAN sector, and to think more strategically about effective ways to get practical change.

3.1 Water supply and sanitation – the great divide

Water supply and sanitation are grouped together for historical reasons more than practical ones. In most rural and peri-urban communities they have little or nothing in common, require completely different skills and are implemented by different organisations in different ways. The only time there is a close link between water supply and sanitation is when a sewerage system (underground pipes connected to individual houses to carry away liquid wastes) is in place. This is rare in most countries, and restricted to the centres of major towns and cities.

For most organisations, water supply is an institutional issue driven by technology and founded on the needs of the community. Engineers work in a variety of ways with different partners to provide and manage water supplies for communities. Decisions on what to build and where are based primarily on technical and political criteria, founded on general considerations of demand and usually with little thought for the needs of the individual.

In contrast, domestic sanitation is viewed as a social issue founded on the needs of the family, with minimal involvement of institutions. Technical inputs are small, with the major focus being on raising demand from users. The role of institutions is usually limited to setting standards and monitoring uptake and quality.

3.2 Who's who in the water supply and sanitation sector

Government

Government generally plays a major role in water supply. A ministry or government department usually takes responsibility for national policy and strategy, and setting and monitoring standards. They are also often responsible for constructing large water systems such as those covering large areas or major urban communities.

Smaller systems are usually the responsibility of local government. Local government is also commonly responsible for operating and maintaining water supplies, although in some larger towns a separate water organisation may be established to carry out that role.

Government's role in sanitation provision is often weak and diverse. It is common for the Ministry of Health to take overall responsibility, but this is usually interpreted as setting standards and monitoring. Sometimes a water authority may take partial responsibility for sanitation, but this usually only covers people who are connected to public sewers. The biggest government partner in sanitation is normally local government. They are usually responsible for solid waste collection, keeping drainage channels clean, and the provision and operation of communal toilets. In most countries government sees domestic excreta disposal as the responsibility of the family.

Non-governmental organisations

Non-governmental organisations (NGOs) play a major role in the provision of water supply and sanitation, particularly to poor rural and urban communities. They tend to work more closely with the communities they wish to serve and often develop close working relationships with the local government.

Private sector

The private sector plays two roles in WATSAN. It is commonly the sector that actually builds the systems. They provide the raw materials, deliver them to the area, drill the boreholes, construct the pipelines and dig the pit latrines. It is also common for the private sector to take responsibility for the detailed design and supervision of construction of major systems. The companies that do this are usually called consultants.

Donors

A large proportion of new WATSAN schemes are funded by external organisations, such as international banks and rich countries. These donors have a large impact on what and how things are done. Since they provide a large part of the money, they can specify how it is spent and where.

Communities

The role of communities in rural water supply provision has increased dramatically in recent years. They now play a major role in planning, design, operation and maintenance of systems.

They play a lesser role in sanitation, but are still often involved in mobilising community members, persuading households to comply and subsidising the poorest.

3.3 Communicating with the water supply and sanitation sector

Communication between the disability sector and the WATSAN sector can be hampered by different perspectives, different ways of working and ways of using language. It may take time and patience to understand each other and to work out how to capitalise on the strengths of each. The onus is on the disability sector to communicate in a way that will be heard, understood and acted on by the target audience.

Box 3.1. New Bubajjwe Primary School accessible latrine

Save the Children in Uganda were involved in installing toilets in a Primary School in Kampala. The school insisted that one toilet be accessible to a student who used a wheelchair. The project engineer wanted to do something, but had never seen accessible facilities, and had no information, so initially he felt helpless. Fortunately an occupational therapist from a local disability NGO brought miniature 3D models of accessible latrines to show the teachers and engineer. When the preferred option was agreed, he drew up detailed measurements which the engineer felt confident to implement.

The design was not perfect and the engineer can now see its drawbacks. Next time he says he will have the confidence to adapt the specifications and try something different. *(Case-study 9.29, page 242)*

Concepts versus designs

For disabled people, the achievement of rights only makes sense if these are turned into relevant solutions that produce practical improvements in their lives. However, a non-technical person may lack the knowledge or confidence to explain in concrete terms what form those solutions might take. As a result, the discussion tends to remain abstract and conceptual.

By contrast, the experience, skills and strengths of engineers are in working out what needs to be done, the best way of doing it, and then getting it done. While DPOs are presenting an argument about access for disabled people, the engineer is likely to be three steps ahead, enjoying the idea of a new challenge and sketching some designs on the back of an envelope.

In other words, each sector has a similar goal in mind, which is to develop services and facilities that meet the needs of all in the community. Each sector has a different set of perspectives, experiences and skills, and a different contribution to make (Box 3.1).

Decision-making processes

Engineers tend to make decisions in different ways from people working in the social sector. Traditionally, the engineering decision-making process is linear: a factual analysis is followed by a professional conclusion on the solution and design of a facility. This may be checked by a line manager for accuracy, but will not usually look at the issue from a different perspective.

Engineers in general tend to prefer logical argument: this is the problem, so this is what we would like you to do about it.

Many engineers are used to working as individuals rather than in teams, and may find it unusual to work in a multi-disciplinary way, with a range of perspectives and opinions, which is the norm in the social sector.

The language divide

In all communication between people, there is a gap between what the speaker means and says, and what the listener hears and understands. Many of us spend our time trying to bridge that gap, to find quicker and more effective ways of communicating with others. We do this by developing short-cuts: we use acronyms like MDG and DPO; we give words a particular meaning in a specific context, such as 'access', or 'process' (Table 3.1), and we develop a common understanding about the background of a particular activity or approach, which saves us having to discuss and explain every time.

The result is that much of our communication is unspoken, the context is understood, and the words have become a short-cut to conveying a much wider meaning. When we know the listener well, or have similar experiences and background, this makes communication more effective.

The problems arise when we need to communicate with people we do not know well, who have a different background and experiences. Our efficient, technically precise language is heard and perceived by others as impenetrable jargon, with the result that they stop listening. We may not realise that differences in understanding even exist, so we do not

---

This section draws on linguistic theory as applied to the issues of communication (and miscommunication) between gender 'specialists' and engineers (1).

Table 3.1. Examples of words given different meanings by different sectors

	Watsan sector	Disability sector
Access	Available to a household, as in: '24% of households in rural areas have access to safe water'.	The possibility to reach, enter, and use a facility, as in: 'The communal toilets do not provide access for wheelchair users'.
Stress	A force acting within a section of steel or concrete	Psychological pressure
Process	a) Project design and implementation from start to finish (b) Water treatment process	Discussion, negotiation towards project implementation

---

Table 3.2. Potential areas for miscommunication

Speaker	Listener	Result
Uses unfamiliar words, acronyms, jargon, e.g. DPO, CBR, impairment, social model.	Doesn't understand.	Listener switches off
Uses familiar words with understood specific meaning, e.g. disabled people.	Ascribes different meaning, e.g. 'people in wheelchairs' 'ex-soldiers with an amputation', so misunderstands.	Listener switches off
Uses words with assumed understood context, e.g. equal opportunities, right to participation, inclusion	Substitutes different context, e.g. this is the responsibility of politicians, social welfare officials, social development sector, so assumes irrelevant.	Listener switches off
Format of presentation unfamiliar, e.g. emphasis on abstract conceptual reasoning, flow-charts	Feels intimidated. Doesn't understand	Listener switches off

recognise the need to decode short-cuts, clarify and correct mistaken assumptions. As a result, the listener hears the words, but may understand a completely different meaning from what is intended.

Even if all the pitfalls in Table 3.2 are avoided, the content of the message must be perceived as relevant by listeners. If they cannot make a link with their own area of work and responsibilities, it will be perceived as irrelevant. The disability sector must start by making the relevance of their message absolutely clear from the very beginning.

3.4 Relevant trends and concerns in the water supply and sanitation sector

It is useful to identify and understand the issues and challenges that currently face the WATSAN sector, and to demonstrate that addressing the issue of disability will contribute to, rather than detract from, other issues of major concern.

Coverage

Numerous challenges face the WATSAN sector in most low-income countries. At least 1.1 billion people in the world do not have access to safe water, whilst 2.6 billion people lack access to basic sanitation. Every day, 6,000 children die from a lack of clean water and sanitation (2).

In relation to water, access means 'available to the household'*. Access is therefore not only an issue for disabled people. In Cambodia, for example, less than 10 per cent of the rural population has access to sanitary latrines, and only 24 per cent to clean drinking water (3). For many service providers, their top priority is to maximise coverage using their inadequate available resources, with a focus more on quantity than equity.

The disability sector needs to demonstrate that:

- Providing inclusive services costs very little extra;

- Services that meet the needs of all people can help to increase coverage;

- Including a disability perspective is therefore great added value.

Millennium Development Goals

The Millennium Development Goals (MDGs) are international development goals that aim to reduce poverty and promote human development in all countries. They are accepted by the UN and international agencies as a framework for measuring development progress (4). There are eight MDGs:

1. Eradicate extreme poverty and hunger.

2. Achieve universal primary education.

3. Promote gender equality and empower women.

4. Reduce child mortality.

5. Improve maternal health.

6. Combat HIV/AIDS, malaria and other diseases.

7. Ensure environmental sustainability.

8. Develop a global partnership for development.

Each MDG is sub-divided into several targets. Under Goal 7, Ensure environmental sustainability, there are three sub-targets, one if which is concerned with water and sanitation:

- Target 10 – Halve by 2015 the proportion of people without sustainable access to safe drinking water and basic sanitation.

* Some guidelines specify a distance, e.g. within 500m, others specify the time required, taking into consideration hilly terrain, time spent queuing and other factors.

The majority of low-income countries now use this target as a starting point for developing water-related policies and strategies.

The MDGs have been criticised for their focus on numbers and coverage, with no mention of equitable development. More importantly, disabled people are not mentioned at all, which has led some people to assume that the MDGs do not apply to disabled people, which of course is untrue. Even if disabled people as a specific group are not mentioned, there are references to target groups within which disabled people are significantly represented.

The disability sector needs to:

- Emphasise that disabled people are among the poorest of the poor; and

- Show that where WATSAN strategies focus on 'marginalised', 'underserved', or 'most vulnerable' target populations, these clearly include disabled people.

Poverty reduction strategy processes and water supply and sanitation

An increasing number of low-income countries now produce poverty reduction strategy papers (PRSPs). These describe the country's policies and programmes, and allocate budget to promote growth and reduce poverty. PRSPs are prepared by governments through a participatory process involving civil society, private sector and funding agencies, including the World Bank and bilateral donors (5). Funding for WATSAN has historically been a low priority for most governments, so PRSPs present an opportunity to identify clear links between improved access to WATSAN and poverty reduction (6).

In theory, PRSPs emphasise participatory, country-owned national development strategies for reducing poverty. In reality, economic and structural reform policies are often developed outside the country, with 'participation' merely formulaic (7). Needless to say, disabled people are largely absent from both the PRSP process and the resulting strategies (8).

The disability sector needs to:

- Ensure that DPOs and disability agencies are represented on all PRSP task groups, including the WATSAN task group.

Sustainable livelihoods approach

The sustainable livelihoods approach is a way of putting

people at the centre of development, with the aim of assessing and improving the effectiveness of poverty reduction efforts. The use of a sustainable livelihoods framework and objectives helps those involved to understand, analyse and increase the sustainability of poor people's livelihoods.

A sustainable livelihoods analysis of WATSAN at household level can help to understand more clearly the links between water and poverty reduction. It can show how water not only brings health benefits, but also improves the overall well-being and livelihood of the household (9). For example, water can also provide a resource for household production, and increase the family income.

- **For the disability sector**, a sustainable livelihoods framework can provide a useful tool to analyse the constraints that disabled people face, that reduce their opportunities, and increase the poverty and dependency of the family as a whole. It can also be used to show that improving access to WATSAN for a disabled person can contribute to improving the livelihood of the whole family.

People-centred approaches

Traditionally, the WATSAN sector has followed a 'supply-led' approach. This means that services have been based on the equipment and designs available, rather than what communities and households need. For example, many WATSAN agencies provide one standard design of latrine or handpump throughout the country, because it is simpler and cheaper to mass-produce one design than to manufacture a range of designs from which local people can choose. However, this approach tends to reflect the needs of the majority (or the most powerful), and does not meet the needs of all communities, or all groups, especially the poorest, within a community.

The increased focus on MDGs and poverty alleviation has resulted in a range of approaches that aim to put people and their lives, rather than technologies, at the centre of WATSAN service planning and delivery (10, 11).

Demand responsive approach

The key feature of the Demand Responsive Approach (DRA) is that community members are given choices. These include:

- Whether to participate in the project;

- The level of technology and service they require, based on how much they are prepared to pay (based on the principle that more expensive systems cost more);

- When and how their services are delivered;

- How funds are managed and accounted for; and

- How their services are operated and maintained.

As governments struggle to meet the costs of providing water, they look for alternative sources of funding, through the use of the private sector and user contributions. Users are often willing to pay more for options that meet their priorities, such as privacy and convenience. A crucial aspect of DRA is to provide adequate information to the community, including the available technology options, to enable them to make choices. The project design includes procedures for providing information, and facilitating decision-making at community level.

In principle, DRA offers the possibility of providing inclusive design options as part of a range of technology options. However, the effectiveness of DRA depends on how demand is assessed. If the voices of only the most powerful are heard, then those in most need of improved services, such as women, the poorest, disabled people and many others, are very likely to be further marginalised and could be worse off than before (11). If people don't demand, service providers won't provide. But if disabled people don't know that accessible designs are possible, how can they know to demand them?

Box 3.2. NGO discovers why there's no demand

A representative of the NGO Forum for Drinking Water and Sanitation in Bangladesh attended a meeting where the issue of WATSAN for disabled people was discussed. As the organisation's research officer, he realised that his organisation had no information about disability in the areas where it worked. He saw an opportunity to do something about this. The following month a community baseline survey was planned for a new WATSAN programme. It was not difficult to add several questions about disability in the survey.

The results from the survey helped the organisation start to think more clearly what it needed to do about the issue of disability. A significant result was the finding that disabled people and their families do not demand accessible facilities, because they are unaware that the possibility exists. Messages about accessibility and its benefits are therefore essential, as well as the hardware. (12)

Understanding the water and sanitation sector

For further information about participatory approaches, see Appendix A1.2 on page 256.

Approaches to participatory consultation

Participatory approaches can be used to ensure the participation of the poor in consultations carried out within DRA. Community groups are helped to collect and analyse information about aspects of their lives, in a way that helps them make decisions. A number of frameworks draw on participatory approaches that have been specifically adapted for use in the WATSAN sector, such as Methodology for Participatory Assessments (13), and Participatory Hygiene and Sanitation Transformation (14).

The focus on listening to disadvantaged groups could provide an opportunity for poor disabled people to make their voice heard. However, the effectiveness of all participatory approaches depends on the skills of the community facilitators. The danger is that if disabled people do not have the information they need to make choices, and are unable to make their views known, they are likely to remain marginalised by more powerful voices in the community.

The challenge for the disability sector is to:

- Gain an understanding of the 'people-centred' approaches being used in the WATSAN sector;

- Identify how disabled people's concerns can be considered alongside those of other poor and marginalised groups, as an integral part of existing processes;

- Show that additional, separate 'disability' approaches are not necessary;

- Create demand by disseminating information to disabled community members about accessibility options;

- Strengthen the capacity of national and local DPOs to participate in consultations and to make their demands known; to engage with WATSAN agencies on the best ways to assess the demands of disabled people;

- Be kind: look at the intentions behind the words, which may appear insensitive. Most are interested to learn, and to do their job properly.

References

1. Reed, B.J., Christie, C. and Fisher, J. (draft) *Did I Phrase that Correctly?* WEDC: Loughborough, UK. http://wedc.lboro.ac.uk/projects/new_projects3.php?id=19

2. Lenton, R. and Wright, A. (2004) *Interim Report of Task Force 7 on Water and Sanitation. Executive Summary.* Millennium Project, UNDP: http://www.unmillenniumproject.org/documents/tf7interimexecsum.pdf

3. Jones, H.E., Reed, R.A. and House, S.J. (2003) *Water supply and sanitation access and use by physically disabled people.* Report of field-work in Cambodia. WEDC, Loughborough University and DFID: UK.

4. World Bank (2003) *Millennium Development Goals.* http://www.developmentgoals.org/Hiv_Aids.htm

5. World Bank (2004) *Poverty Reduction Strategies.* http://www.worldbank.org/poverty/strategies/

6. WaterAid (2004) *Poverty Reduction Strategy Papers.* http://www.wateraid.org.uk/in_depth/policy_and_research/poverty_reduction_strategy_papers/default.asp.

7. Eurodad (2004) *PRSP: Eurodad's work on Poverty Reduction Strategy Papers.* http://www.eurodad.org/workareas/default.aspx?id=92.

8. Handicap International and NFOWD (2003) *Disability and the PRSP in Bangladesh.* A position document. HI-Bangladesh: Dhaka.

9. Nicol, A. (2000) *Adopting A Sustainable Livelihoods Approach to Water Projects: Implications for Policy and Practice.* Sustainable Livelihoods Working Paper Series. Overseas Development Institute: London. http://www.odi.org.uk/publications/wp133.pdf

10. DFID and WELL (1998) *Guidance Manual on Water Supply and Sanitation Programmes.* Water Engineering and Development Centre: Loughborough University, UK.

11. Deverill, P. et al. (2002) *Designing water supply and sanitation projects to meet demand in rural and peri-urban communities. Book 3: Ensuring the participation of the poor.* WEDC, Loughborough University: UK. http://wedc.lboro.ac.uk/publications/pdfs/dwss/dwss3.pdf

12. Jones, H.E. and Reed, R.A. (2004) *Water supply and sanitation access and use by physically disabled people: report of second field-work in Bangladesh.* WEDC, Loughborough University and DFID: UK.

13. Mukherjee, N. and van Wijk, Christine (eds) (2003) *Planning and Monitoring in Community Water Supply and Sanitation. A Guide on the Methodology for Participatory Assessment (MPA) for Community-Driven Development Programs.* World Bank Water and Sanitation Programme; International Water and Sanitation Centre: Washington. http://www.wsp.org/pdfs/mpa%202003.pdf

14. Sawyer, R., Simpson-Hébert, M. and Wood, S. (1998) *PHAST step-by-step guide: A participatory approach for the control of diarrhoeal diseases.* WHO: http://www.who.int/water_sanitation_health/hygiene/envsan/phastep/en/

Chapter 4

Understanding the disability sector

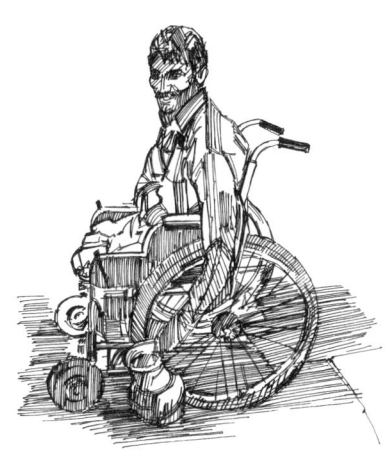

This chapter is mainly for readers who have had little previous contact with disabled people and disability issues, including WATSAN sector professionals, engineers, public health workers and community development workers.

4.1　Who's who in the disability sector

A range of agencies are involved in the disability sector, but can be divided into two main groups – disabled people's organisations (DPOs) and disability service providers.
It is important to recognise the difference, as they have fundamentally different views, experience and interests and different roles to play in the development of WATSAN for disabled people.

Disabled people's organisations
These are organisations OF disabled people, run BY and FOR disabled people themselves. Disabled people control and make the decisions, although they may employ non-disabled people within their organisation.

Some organisations are for people with the same impairments, such as physical impairments only, or visual impairments only. Others have cross-impairment membership, which means that they include members with all types of impairment.

DPOs generally focus on advocacy for rights and access to services, creating networks of local disabled people's groups, and capacity building of members to promote their rights. Their projects are based on the priorities of members, such as savings and credit, or income generation. Some DPOs provide services to their members, and a few provide services to the wider community, including non-disabled people.

Many DPOs have a women's wing or committee; some DPOs are run by and for disabled women themselves.

For the WATSAN sector: any consultation with the disability sector should start wherever possible with DPOs, and wherever possible with disabled women in their own right.

This is because DPOs are in the best position to represent the views of their disabled members.

Disability service providers
These are agencies, whether government departments or NGOs, that provide services FOR disabled people, usually run by non-disabled professionals. Services may be provided either in institutions, such as a hospital or residential centre, or in the community, often called 'community-based rehabilitation' (CBR). Sometimes a combination of both approaches is used.

Some organisations have a medical focus, such as operations or physiotherapy, some provide charitable handouts, whilst others focus on education or social issues, such as attitudes and behaviour of communities.

For the WATSAN sector: When identifying relevant agencies to consult on WATSAN issues, those with a more social or community focus are likely to have more relevant experience to offer, and are more likely to be interested in collaboration.

4.2 Who do we mean by disabled people?

Disabled people are people who have an **impairment**. An **impairment** is a loss or limitation of functioning, whether physical, sensory (vision or hearing), intellectual (learning and understanding) or mental health. People who have impairments are disabled by **external factors**, which reduce their opportunities to participate in family and community activities on an equal basis with others. These external factors may be barriers in the physical environment, or to do with social exclusion and discrimination (Box 4.1). This view of disability is called the **social model of disability**, because it sees society as a whole as responsible for disability.

For example, Rita has weak legs, which cannot support her weight - a **physical impairment**.

This means she cannot walk, and moves around by shuffling using her hands – **activity limitation**.

What **disables** her most, however, are the external factors: the fact that she has no wheelchair, the latrine is too far away, the path is muddy, and her family don't like her using the same latrine as the rest of the family, because she crawls and makes it dirty. So she uses the bushes, but always waits until dark, so her health suffers.

Box 4.1. Disabled by poverty and inaccessible toilets

Daniel is 15 and has weak legs – **a physical impairment**.

He has difficulty moving around – **activity limitation**, but he wears calipers and uses crutches, which help.

He is **disabled** by his poor quality calipers, which often break, and by poverty - there is never the money to repair them. So he often has to crawl around, which makes his hands dirty. His father refuses to eat with him because of this.

He is **disabled** by inaccessible toilets, both at home and at school, which he cannot get into with his crutches. At home, his mother gives him her plastic shoes to wear on his hands, to protect them when he crawls in. At school, however, he says he never uses the toilets because he has nothing to wear on his hands there, and there is urine all over the toilet floor. (1)

This contrasts with the traditional medical way of thinking about disability, in which the disabled person is seen as the problem, for which the solution is to provide treatment and therapy to enable him to fit into 'normal' society.

Many people who have impairments may choose not to identify themselves as disabled – elderly people, or people living with HIV/AIDS, for example. But as they become more frail, they may experience similar limitations to disabled people. Many of the ideas in this book will therefore be helpful for them.

4.3   Barriers and obstacles faced by disabled people

It is not always possible to do anything about the individual impairment of a disabled person. However, most problems for disabled people in accessing WATSAN facilities are caused by external factors, such as barriers in the natural environment or the physical infrastructure, institutional or organisational factors, and social barriers. Examples of different external factors are detailed in Table 4.1.

It is often very possible to make changes in the external environment. This is where the knowledge and skills of the engineer are indispensable.

Table 4.1. Examples of obstacles faced by disabled people

External factors	Examples
Barriers in the natural environment	Unmade, steep, or flooded roads and paths; Muddy and slippery banks of ponds and rivers; Water sources too far away; Non-existent sanitation.
Physical infrastructure	High concrete platforms; Steps; narrow entrances, slippery floors, handles too high, too low, too heavy; High well walls, containers without handles, etc.
Institutional factors	WATSAN policies and strategies that do not mention disabled people; Community WATSAN consultation without representation of disabled people's concerns; Lack of staff knowledge, information or skills on disability issues; Disability seen as a 'specialist' or welfare issue.
Social barriers	Lack of knowledge and understanding, negative behaviour of family and community; prejudice, pity, overprotection; isolation. The whole family may be ostracised or isolated for having a disabled family member, so the family may hide them at home. For example, disabled and elderly people may be prevented from sharing family or community facilities, for fear that they will contaminate water, or make a facility dirty for other people.

4.4 Approaches to addressing disability

Different strategies and programmes address the issue of disability in different ways. They fall broadly into the following types:

Disability-focused projects/services
These provide services or interventions which focus on disabled people, such as mobility aids, operations, physiotherapy, artificial limbs, vocational training, capacity building. They may be stand-alone or a sub-component of a wider programme, e.g. Primary education programme + Project on education for disabled children with learning difficulties.

As with projects that focus on women, disability-focused projects are appropriate under certain conditions. The risk is that they increase the isolation of disabled people, if they are seen as an end in themselves, rather than as a necessary basis for improving social inclusion.

Including a disability perspective

Also called 'integration' or 'mainstreaming', this is where the project/ programme recognises that disability, elderly infirmity, and ill-health are experienced by all communities, and explicitly considers and responds to this diversity and range of needs in its service provision. There is no expectation that disabled people should be 'cured' or 'rehabilitated' first before they can be included.

Twin-track approach

This recognises that 'including a disability perspective' and 'disability-focused projects' are both needed (2). Disability-focused projects aim to maximise the skills and abilities of disabled people, which are an essential prerequisite to enabling them to access inclusive services.

Prevention of impairments/disability prevention

Examples of strategies for prevention of impairments include immunisation to prevent polio, Vitamin A to prevent night blindness, and accident prevention campaigns. These are necessary components of any public health programme, but cannot be considered as development approaches to disability, as they do not benefit disabled people who are part of every community.

For the WATSAN sector: The key approach is the second, i.e. including a disability perspective. This means that every WATSAN project, programme and service should consider the needs of disabled people from the beginning and throughout, as the usual way of doing things. This is the most important contribution that the WATSAN sector can make, and is an essential component of a twin-track approach to disability.

4.5 Different approaches to problem-solving

Disability organisations often use approaches to solve issues of disabled and other vulnerable people that are different from the approaches that most engineers are used to. The disability sector tends to focus on the needs of individual disabled people and their families, rather than on whole communities, so the focus is usually at an individual household level, rather than a community level.

A meeting between the disabled person and their family and relevant community/ health workers is a common approach to problem-solving. The purpose should ideally be to listen to what the disabled person has to say, and how they see

Box 4.2. Not the perfect solution – Maya and her family

Maya is a 22-year-old wheelchair user, living with her family in a rural area of Bangladesh. Her arms and legs are stiff and she needs help with many everyday tasks, which is the responsibility of her sister-in-law.

The family is poor, and as there was no latrine, they all used the surrounding fields to defecate. This was impossible for Maya, who would squat behind the house, and her sister-in-law swept the faeces into the bushes.

An NGO provided the family with a brick-built latrine, with a concrete ramp that was accessible for Maya's wheelchair. The idea was that the whole family, including Maya, would benefit from using the sanitary latrine.

A few years later, this had not happened. An older brother had got married and built his house in front of the latrine, so it was no longer possible to get into it in a wheelchair. And anyway the toilet was blocked. The family had gone back to defecating in the fields, and Maya was squatting behind the house. It was not clear whether the house came first or the toilet was blocked first.

The solution had appeared fine in theory, but what was the practical reality? Even at first, Maya needed her sister-in-law's help to use the latrine. It was a distance from the house, up a slope, so she needed her to push her wheelchair. She needed help to move from wheelchair to the toilet. The toilet seat was narrow so her sister-in-law had to stay with her while she used the toilet, otherwise she might fall off. For the sister-in-law, this took up a lot of time and effort, and increased her workload. It was quicker and easier to let Maya squat behind the house.

The failure of the solution provided indicates that one solution does not fit all. It is important to consider the disabled person not in isolation but in the context of the family. The views of the sister-in-law and her workload needed to be considered. It did not consider alternative solutions that would enable Maya to do more for herself, rather than rely more on others. (4)

the solution to the difficulties they face. It is common to find several different opinions on the causes and solutions to a problem, and to negotiate the solution that most suits the disabled person. Any solution imposed by an 'expert' is likely to meet resistance or lack of interest, if it is not seen as achieving the desired outcome (Box 4.2).

For the WATSAN sector: The engineer can be a valuable resource, by:

- Providing information about possible options (where the disabled person has no opinion);

- Working out the strengths and weaknesses of different solutions; and

- Helping to turn an idea into reality.

The final choices and decisions should still be made by the disabled person and their family.

Issues of difference

Disabled people are women, men and children, of all ages, with different impairments, needs, lifestyles and views. They may be doubly marginalised for other reasons, e.g. disabled elderly people, disabled people from ethnic minority communities, disabled girls, disabled people living with HIV/AIDS. One solution does not suit all. For example, an ex-soldier with an amputated leg is unlikely to have the same concerns and needs as a mother with a disabled child, and it should not be assumed that he can represent her views. It is therefore important to consult, not only articulate men with a physical impairment, but also those who are rarely consulted – poor disabled women, people with communication difficulties, people unable to leave the house, and their family carers.

4.6   Introduction to working with disabled people

The majority of DPOs in low-income countries have formed only within the last ten to twenty years. For many, their main struggle is to make their voices heard, and to be granted the same human rights as everyone else, instead of being seen as objects of pity and charity.

Because of this, some disabled people may not be immediately convinced that it is worth spending time discussing the issue of WATSAN, and that it will lead to practical results. Most disabled people have not reached the stage of systematically working out practical solutions to the problems of access and inclusion.

This does not mean that they don't have ideas and solutions; they do, but they may find it difficult to explain the issues in a way that engineers can immediately relate to. It may take a while to develop trust and an understanding of how to work together.

Meeting disabled people

Non-disabled people do not always understand the practical difficulties that disabled people face. We may not recognise how our own behaviour can enable or disable, help or hinder someone who is different and may have an impairment. Understanding our own reactions and behaviour towards people who are different may take some time. Basic common sense, and courtesy that we normally show other people, can do a lot to help overcome barriers. Just act as you would with anyone else and be open and honest.

For a list of further resources on working with disabled people, see Appendix A1.6 on page 262.

The following advice may also help. It does not include the full range of impairments, which is why the first point is particularly important.

- Everyone is unique. Try not to make assumptions about a person's capacity or needs. Listen to what they have to say and respect what they tell you.

- Try not to make assumptions about who is and is not disabled as some impairments are hidden, e.g. diabetes.

- Offer help, but be careful not to take over. Don't be upset if help is rejected. Sometimes it will be welcome, but sometimes it won't be needed, or may hinder the person doing an activity in his or her own, maybe slower, way.

- Speak directly to the disabled person, not at or to their helper or interpreter.

- Look at the disabled person, not at their impairment, or the wheelchair/trolley.

- When talking to a wheelchair/trolley user, try to sit down at a similar height, or stand with a suitable space to allow direct eye contact. It can be very exhausting having to look up all the time. Don't lean on the chair, you may tip it over! This can also be intimidating and an invasion of personal space.

- When communicating with a person with a speech impairment, give them time to express themselves, concentrate and don't be afraid to ask for something to be repeated if you don't understand an answer.

- Disabled people often have a lack of self-esteem and confidence – be encouraging and sensitive to their needs. Be patient, show trust and respect confidentiality.

- When communicating with someone who is deaf or has a hearing impairment, find out how they choose to communicate. If they lip read, face the person and speak slowly and clearly, with the light on your face. Don't shout or cover your mouth. Be patient because lip reading involves a high level of concentration and it can be exhausting.

- You may need to use an interpreter, particularly if someone uses a sign language or communication system you do not understand.

- When talking to a blind or visually impaired person, make sure they know who you are – they may not recognise your voice. And remember to say when you are leaving them, so that they do not end up speaking to the air.

- When talking to people with difficulty understanding, speak simply, using short words and sentences.

- Find out more from national level DPOs who can provide locally appropriate information and advice.

Language

The language we use when describing or speaking to other people can convey respect or disrespect. This is the same for disabled people. Words that seem straightforward at first glance may have a negative or offensive meaning for disabled people. They may be acceptable in one language or country, but unacceptable when translated into another language. Users should also be aware of who decides whether a term is acceptable: a word used by a doctor, for example, may not be acceptable to disabled people, or parents with a disabled child.

Table 4.2 contains some guidelines reproduced from materials that reflect current thinking in the UK. These are for guidance only, they are not exhaustive and are likely to change over time. They will need to be adapted for use in other languages. If in doubt, ask disabled people which words they find acceptable, and reject words that they find unacceptable.

This book also frequently refers to disabled adults and children, disabled girls and boys, or women and men with disabilities, to keep in focus the gender and age differences of disabled people.

4

Table 4.2. Appropriate language

Avoid	Use
Cripple, defective Invalid *(this literally means 'not valid')* Retarded, subnormal	Disabled person, disabled child Person who uses/walks with crutches Person with an impairment or Children with disabilities, people with disabilities
Handicapped *This is derived from 'cap in hand' and implies begging, which reinforces negative stereotypes.*	
'The disabled', 'The blind', 'The deaf', etc. Phrases like these are dehumanising.	Disabled people Blind people, people with visual impairments Deaf people, people with hearing impairments
An epileptic, a cleft lip girl, a CP case, etc. It is offensive to label people with their impairment.	Person with epilepsy Girl with a cleft lip Person with cerebral palsy (CP)
Victim of … Crippled by … Suffering from … Afflicted by....	Person who has … Person with … Person who experienced …
Wheelchair bound Confined to a wheelchair	Wheelchair user, wheelchair rider *For many disabled people, a wheelchair is a liberation, not a confinement.*
Normal and abnormal: describing people who are not disabled as 'normal', implies that disabled people are abnormal. In fact disabled people are a normal part of every society. Sick: implies that disabled people are all unhealthy. Everyone is sick from time to time. For example, a woman with difficulty walking as a result of polio may fall sick with diarrhoea like anyone else, but having weak legs does not mean that she is sick.	Non-disabled people and disabled people

References

1. Teachers from Mpika, Zambia (2003) *Researching our Experience*. Enabling Education Network (EENET): Manchester, UK. http://www.eenet.org.uk/

2. DFID (2000) *Disability, Poverty and Development*. Issues Paper. Department for International Development: UK. http://www.dfid.gov.uk/Pubs/files/disability.pdf

3. Werner, D. (1995) *Strengthening the Role of Disabled People in Community Based Rehabilitation Programmes*. Innovations In Developing Countries For People With Disabilities. Lisieux Hall Publications: UK. http://www.eenet.org.uk/parents/book/bookcontents.shtml

4. Jones, H.E. and Reed, R.A. (2003) *Water supply and sanitation access and use by physically disabled people: report of field-work in Bangladesh*. WEDC, Loughborough University and DFID: UK.

4

4

Chapter 5

Accessibility – general issues

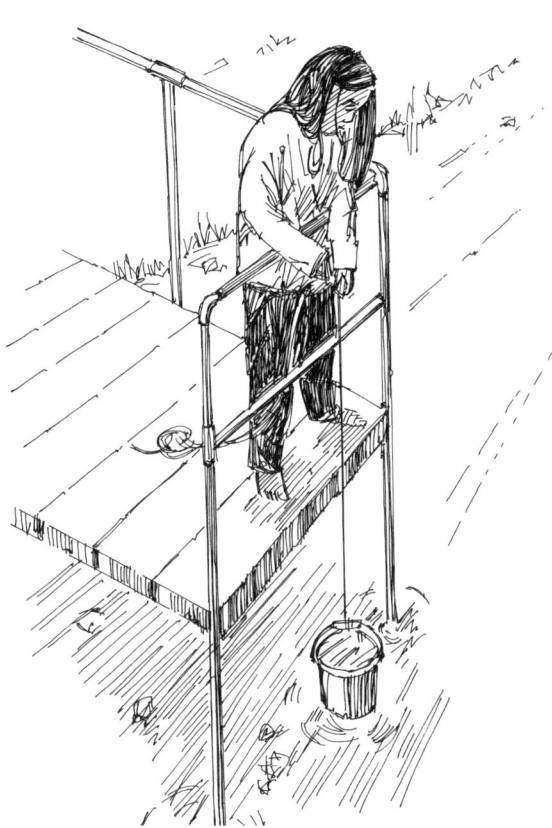

This chapter identifies some general issues of access for all people with a range of needs, including disabled people, frail elderly people, pregnant women, parents with young children, people who are injured or sick, including people living with HIV/AIDS. A range of possible solutions is then presented. Some disabled people may have already identified their own solutions, while others may have no idea of what is possible. The ideas in chapters 5 to 7 can provide starting points for discussion, reinforced by case-studies in Chapter 9 that illustrate the benefits of accessible facilities to the whole family.

5.1 Contrasting approaches – inclusive facilities or individual equipment?

The focus of this document is on water and sanitation facilities for household use. As described in Section 3.2 on page 18, toilets are commonly installed by individual families according to their available resources, for use by a specific group of people. In this situation, only the current and short-term needs of the household are likely to be considered in the design or choice of facility.

Nevertheless, many households all over the world use communal facilities, especially water points, which are used by a larger number of people with a much wider range of needs. In this situation, where communal facilities are being designed and built from scratch, it is more appropriate to apply the principles of **inclusive design**, rather than to choose a design based on the needs of one or two individuals.

5

Thus two apparently conflicting approaches to improving access can be taken:

1. An inclusive design approach, which aims to create functional environments to accommodate a diverse range of users and can be used equally by everyone, irrespective of age, gender or disability (1). This is the approach used in the UK and Europe, reinforced by Disability Rights legislation.

2. An individual approach, which provides an aid or equipment for the use of a disabled person based on their individual needs, to enable them to access an existing facility or environment.

A combination of the two approaches is often needed (Figure 2.6).

The authors propose that inclusive design be the ultimate goal of WATSAN providers, but also acknowledge that a pragmatic approach is needed to cope with the current reality of disabled people's lives. This document therefore incorporates ideas from both approaches.

5.2 Principles of inclusive design

The principles of inclusive design are to provide:

- Ease of use by as many people as possible without undue effort, special treatment or separation;

- Freedom of choice and access to mainstream activities, to allow people to participate equally in all activities. Users should be able to choose whether to use a support person or not, and whether to use the same or separate facilities;

- Diversity and difference: facilities should provide for a range of user needs;

- Safety;

- Legibility and predictability: facilities should be organised and laid out in a logical and ordered way, that is easy for the user to 'read' or understand.

Comprehensive recommendations for inclusive design of public facilities will not be repeated here, as they are available in other publications (see Appendix A1.1, page 255). It is also recognised that these may not always be immediately applicable in rural and peri-urban areas of low-income countries, where infrastructure is poor, and resources are scarce.

A range of access solutions is presented in the following chapters. These vary from high-cost, durable solutions, which draw on the principles of inclusive design, to low-cost short-term solutions, which may be based on the needs of an individual. The choice of solution will depend on whether the facility is communal or domestic, on available resources, and on the situation and aspirations of disabled people and their families.

5.3   User dimensions

Trying to accommodate all disabled people's needs is not always straightforward. Where a facility is for the use of one family, or a limited group of households, it is important to talk to all users to identify the range of needs and preferred solutions (see the section 8.3 on working with disabled people and their families on page 147).

The design and space requirements will depend on the kind of support users need for mobility (Figures 5.1 and 5.2). Dimensions of users and their equipment will vary from one person to another and from one country to another (Table 5.1).

If a variety of people with different needs use the facility, design for the biggest dimensions. The space suggestions in this document are for guidance only, and are not intended to be inclusive design recommendations.

For suggested dimensions see Table 5.1.

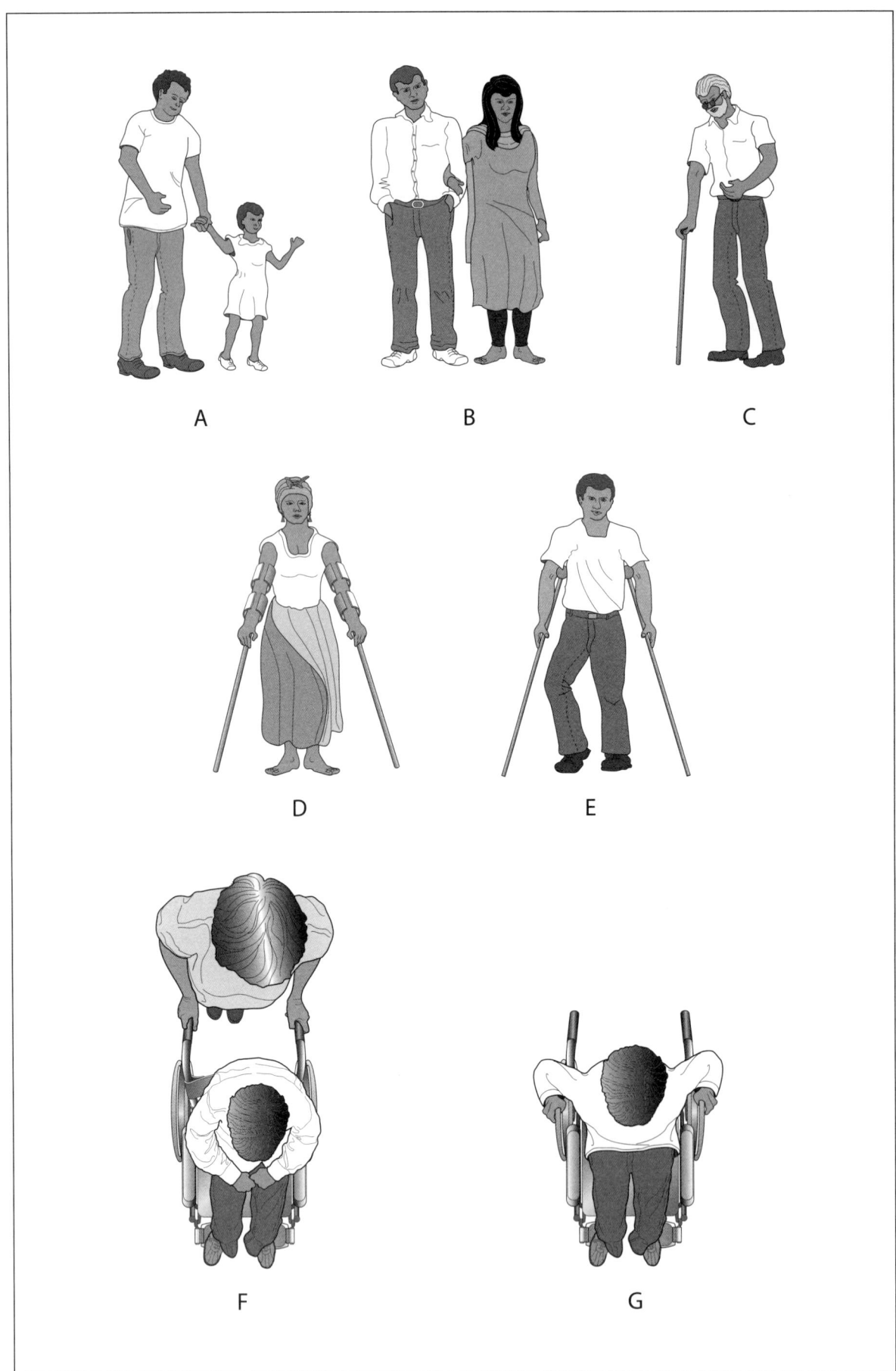

Figure 5.1. Disabled people and aids and support for mobility.

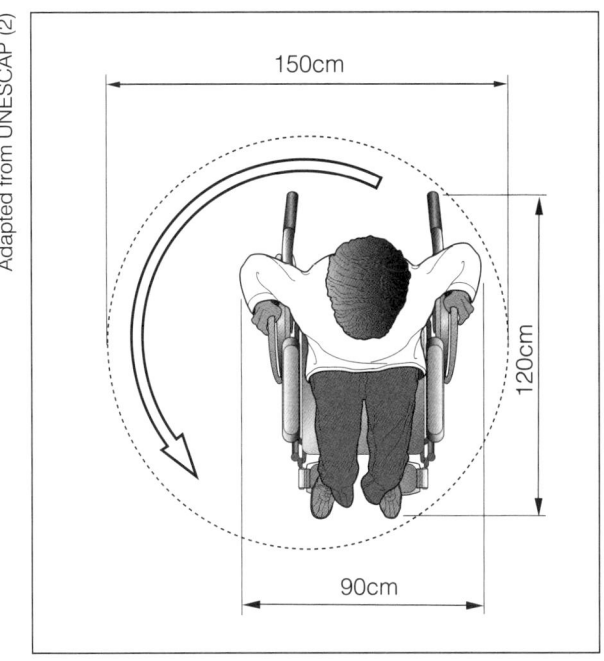

Figure 5.2. Space allowance for wheelchair users.

Wheelchair dimensions
Dimensions of wheelchairs depend on the design, and will affect the width of paths and doorways needed, the internal dimensions of bathrooms and toilets, and the location of handrails, etc.

5.4   Aspects of accessibility

Getting there
It does not matter how well the facility is adapted if the disabled user cannot get to it in the first place.

Proximity (how near it is)
A major factor in being able to reach a facility is how near it is. One of the simplest ways to achieve this is to locate a facility as near as

		Dimensions (in cm)				
		Bangladesh	India	UN/ ESCAP	Uganda	UK
A	Width of adult + child walking side by side					110
B	Width of 2 adults walking side by side					120
C	Width of adult walking with a stick					75
D & E	Width of person walking with crutches			92		90
F	Length of wheelchair + helper					175
G	Length of wheelchair and user	112	130	120	110	114
G	Width of wheelchair + self-propelling user	90	88		87	90

Table 5.1 Dimensions of disabled people and their support for mobility

Letters in the left-hand column refer to the drawings in Figure 5.1.
Data from this research and various sources (1, 2, 3, 4, 5, 6, 7).

possible to the disabled or elderly user. This can be done in a number of ways, depending on local factors such as available space, technology, culture and preference:

- Providing piped water into or next to the house;

- Installing a rainwater tank or storage jar near the house;

- Installing a household well in the compound of the disabled person's home;

- Installing a communal well near the disabled person's home;

- Providing a toilet inside or close to the disabled person's house.

Specific benefits of proximity include:

- Water can be drawn as it is needed, so the need for storage is reduced, and the difficulties in accessing stored water avoided;

- Carrying time is reduced, therefore smaller quantities of water are drawn each time, e.g. up to 5 litres. Carrying small quantities is possible for many disabled people who cannot carry larger quantities.

An alternative way of reducing the distance between water source and place of use is to take the water-related activity to the water source. Bathing and washing clothes at the water source, for example, will reduce the quantity of water that needs transporting and storing.

For a list of further resources on transport and mobility, see Appendix A1.1, under Transport on page 256.

For a list of further resources on rainwater harvesting, see Appendix A1.2, under Techincal Infomation on page 257-8.

Box 5.1. Proximity alone is not enough

For one Ugandan wheelchair user, proximity is not enough to enable him to fetch water. His nearest handpump is too difficult to get to in his wheelchair, along a narrow, steep and bumpy path. He prefers to travel a whole mile to a different pump along a wider, smoother path which is accessible to his wheelchair *(Case-study 9.23, page 223)*.

If the facility cannot be nearby, many people can be helped by the provision of a place to rest on the way. The maximum distance that frail or elderly people can walk without a rest depends on many factors, including the slope and evenness of the ground. Some maximum walking distances are given in Table 5.2.

Width of path, slope or step
In addition to proximity, the width, smoothness and gradient of the approach path are important (Box 5.1).

The width of the path will depend on who will use it and what support they use (see Figures 5.1 and 5.2). A public path should ideally be 180cm wide to accommodate all types of non-vehicular traffic without passing places. The absolute minimum width is 120cm wide, with places provided to allow people to pass each other (6). At a household level, the path width should take account of the widest user. For example, using the dimensions in Table 5.1, a wheelchair user needs a path of at least 90cm wide. But if an elderly grandmother in the same household needs the support of a family member when walking, the path should be wide enough for two people side by side, i.e. 120cm wide.

Path gradient
Where the path is not level, steps or a slope will be needed. The steepness of the slope (gradient) is important. The aim should be

5

Table 5.2 Maximum walking distances (2)	
Group	**Recommended distance limit without a rest**
People who are blind or with a visual impairment.	150m
Wheelchair users.	150m
People with mobility impairment who do not require or use a walking aid.	100m
People with mobility impairment who use a walking aid.	50m

Adapted from Werner, 1987

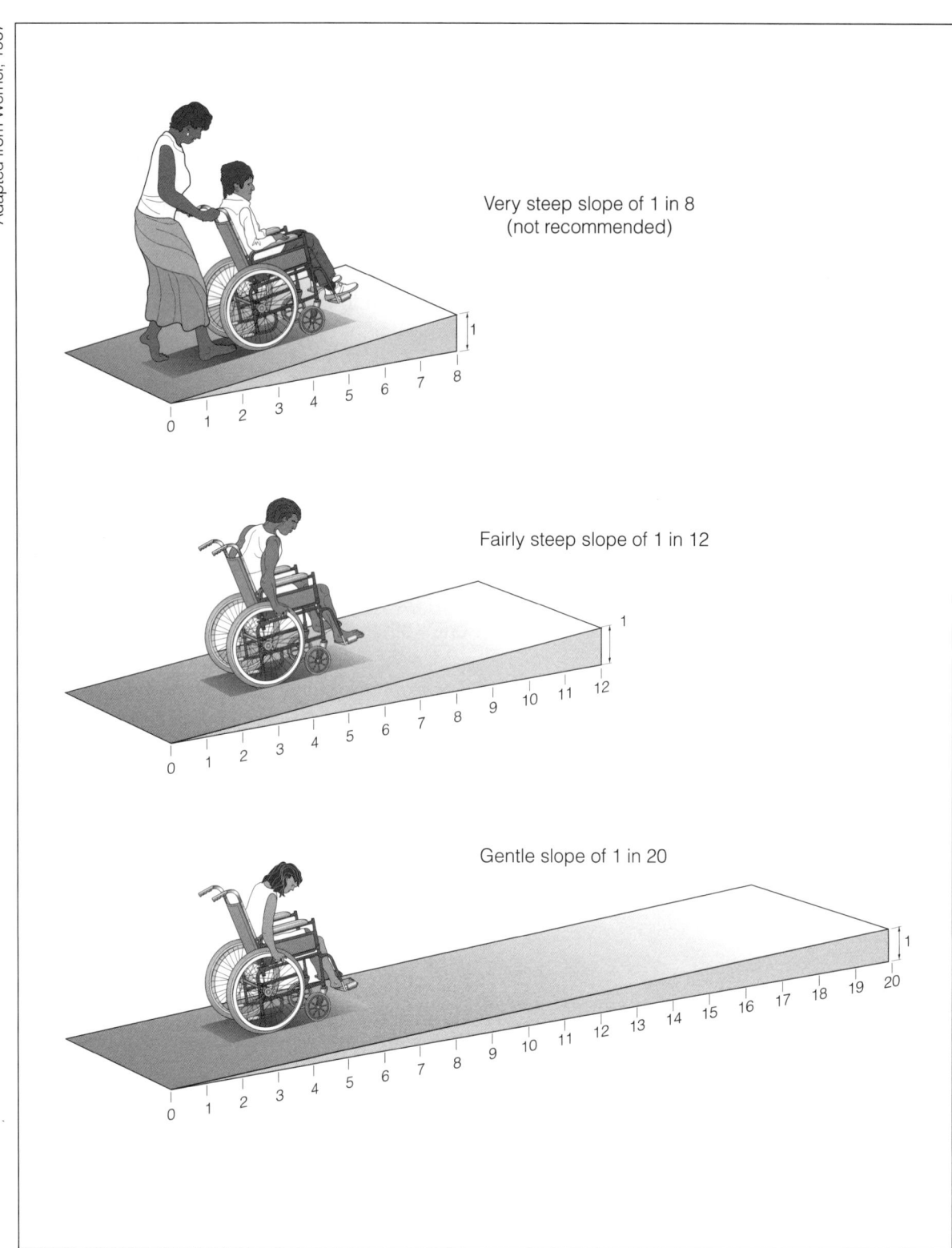

Very steep slope of 1 in 8
(not recommended)

Fairly steep slope of 1 in 12

Gentle slope of 1 in 20

Figure 5.3. Slope gradients.

for independent mobility, i.e. for the disabled person to reach their destination without help. Slopes should be as gentle as possible – a gradient of 1 in 15 or gentler is ideal. Steep slopes (more than 1:12) may be dangerous for many wheelchair users, who lack the strength to push themselves up a slope, and have difficulty in slowing down or stopping when descending. A steep gradient can cause the wheelchair to tip backwards when ascending.

Where space permits, both steps and a ramp should be provided. If only one option is possible, this should be a ramp.

If the slope is long, a level platform is needed at regular intervals where the user can rest (see Figures 5.4 and 5.5).

In some situations, for example where space is limited, it may be necessary to use a short steep slope of 1 in 10 or steeper. In this case the slope should be no longer than 1 metre. This is not a recommended option. A steep slope is only useful for very strong users, or if there is always someone available to push the wheelchair. Table 5.3 suggests maximum gradients for slopes.

5

Table 5.3 Slopes and recommended lengths for independent mobility

Type	Gradient	Maximum length of slope	Comments
Very gentle slope	1:20 (5%)	10m	Ideal gradient.
Gentle slope	1:15 (6.6%)	5m	Possible for average wheelchair users. 1:15 or gentler is the recommended slope for public buildings.
Fairly steep slope	1:12 (8%)	3m	Possible for riders with strong arms. Maximum recommended gradient for independent mobility.
Very steep slope	1:10 or less (12% or more)	1m	Not recommended for independent mobility. May be dangerous, as wheelchair may tip backwards.

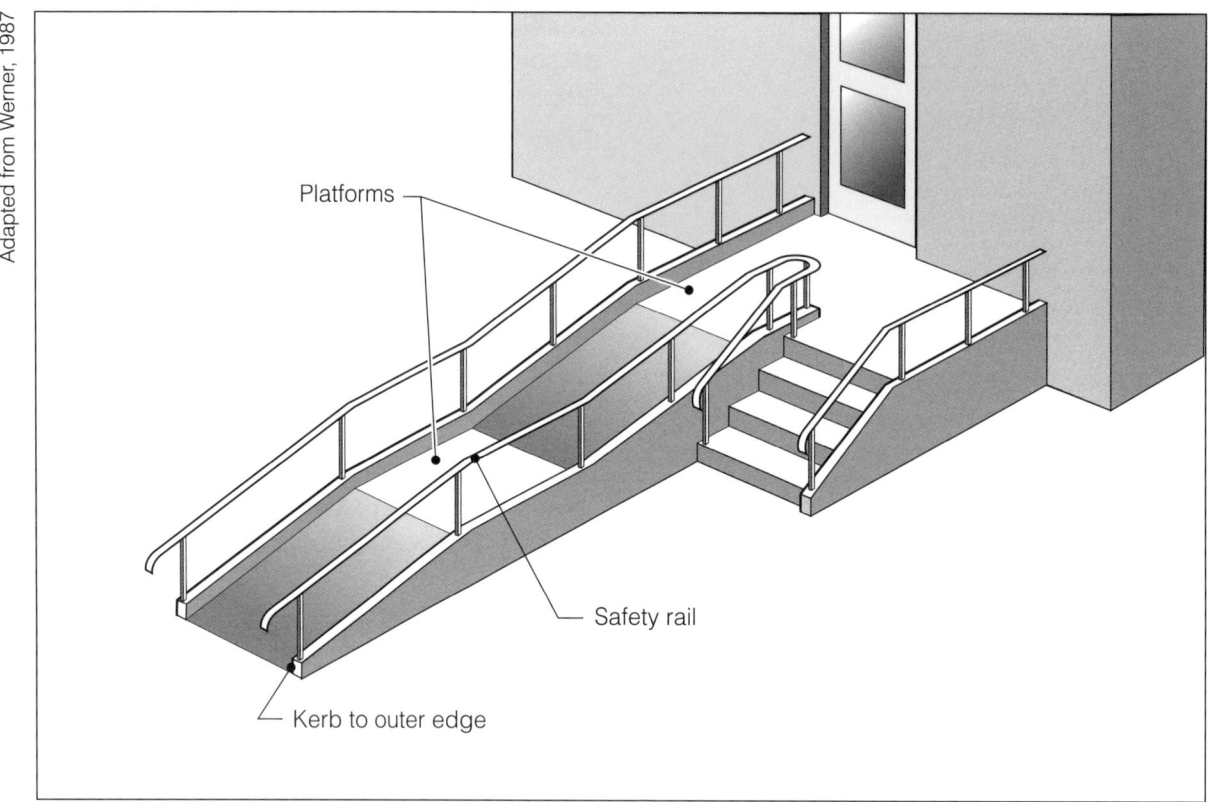

Figure 5.4. Ramp with mid-level resting platform.

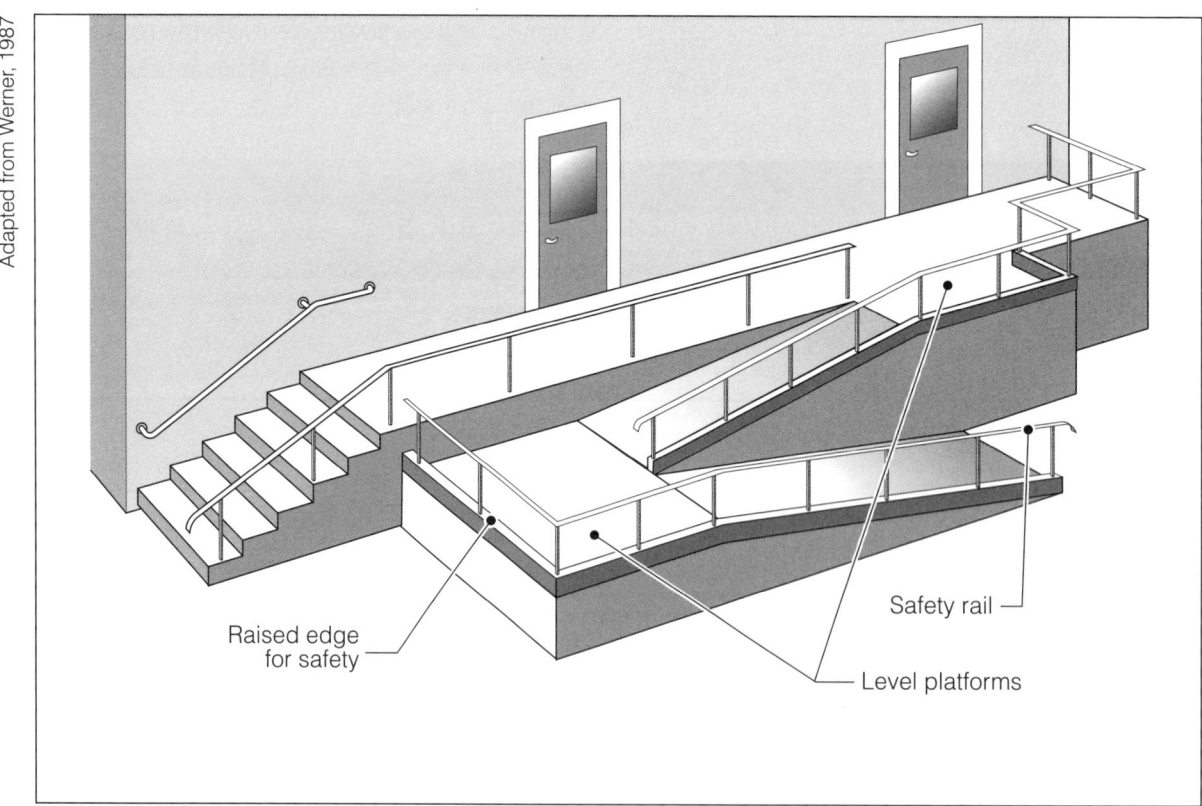

Figure 5.5. Alternative layout for ramp, with mid-level resting platform.

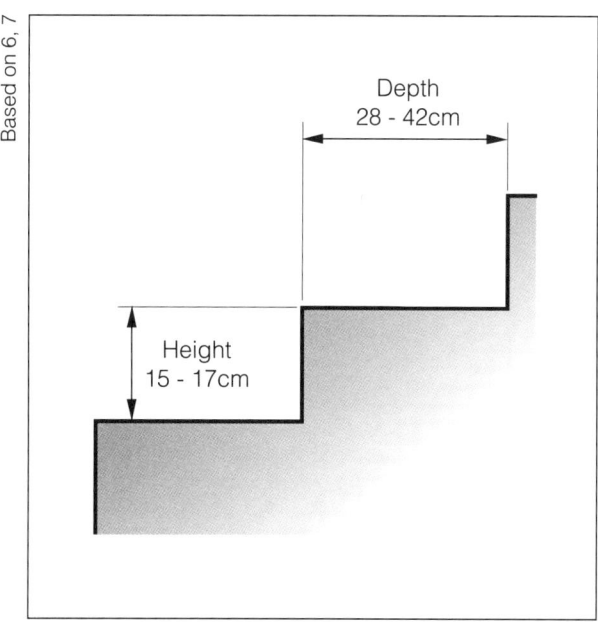

Figure 5.6. Suggested step dimensions.

Steps

Do not assume that a ramp suits everyone. Some disabled and older people, pregnant women and mothers with young children who are able to walk, may prefer to use steps rather than a long or steep slope. Where there is enough space, a choice of both steps and ramp should be provided, especially in communal facilities. A handrail should always be provided with steps.

All the steps in a flight should be of similar height and depth, with a maximum of 12 steps if the depth is 35cm or less; if more than 35cm, a maximum of 18 steps (Figure 5.6).

If the steps will be used by a person or people who crawl, it is recommended to reduce the step height to 10 – 15cm.

For people with difficulty seeing, the edge of each step should be highlighted with coloured paint or tape.

Surface of paths and steps

A firm, even, non-slip surface benefits everyone, not only wheelchair and crutch users. It reduces accidents, and is particularly helpful for people with poor balance or co-ordination such as frail elderly people, blind people and children. The surface can be made of wood, earth, bricks or concrete.

Concrete is most durable, but costly. Locally available materials such as brick or stone are cheaper than concrete, and when laid as a path can provide a firm surface, and prevent it becoming muddy and slippery in the rainy season. Bricks or stones should be evenly laid: an uneven or unstable surface is difficult for a wheelchair user, and can cause other users to trip and injure themselves.

An earth path has no material cost, and can be made smooth, but will become muddy and slippery when wet. It may get washed away by rain and need to be replaced regularly.

A slippery surface can be dangerous for a person using crutches, which can easily skid

Examples of approach paths

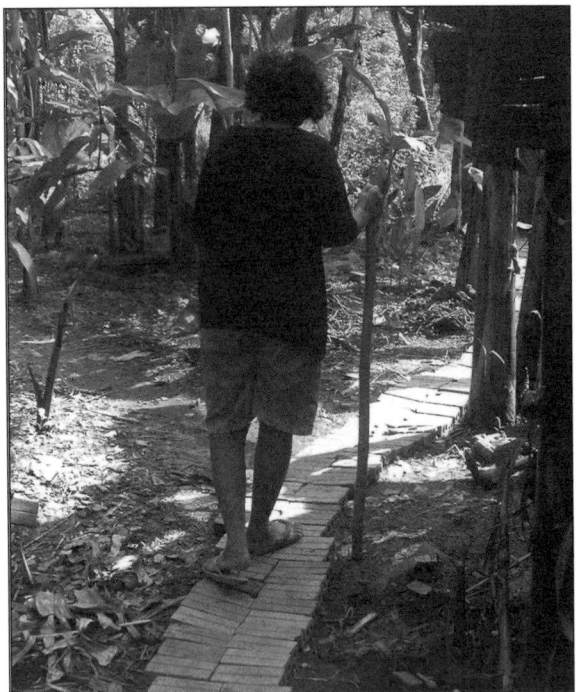

Figure 5.7. Narrow brick path.

Description	Path made of clay bricks laid in a double row. No mortar or earth used to fix them in place.
Dimensions	Width: ~ 40cm;
Gradient	level.
User	Person who uses a stick to walk.
Key features	Provides a flat, firm surface, so the user does not have to walk in mud in rainy season. Materials available free at nearby brick factory.
Drawbacks and comments	The bricks could be made more stable and therefore safer by fixing them in place with sand, cement mortar or earth pointing. A wider path (at least 85cm) would allow the user's stick to land on the firm path, providing a more stable support, instead of on the slippery ground beside the path.

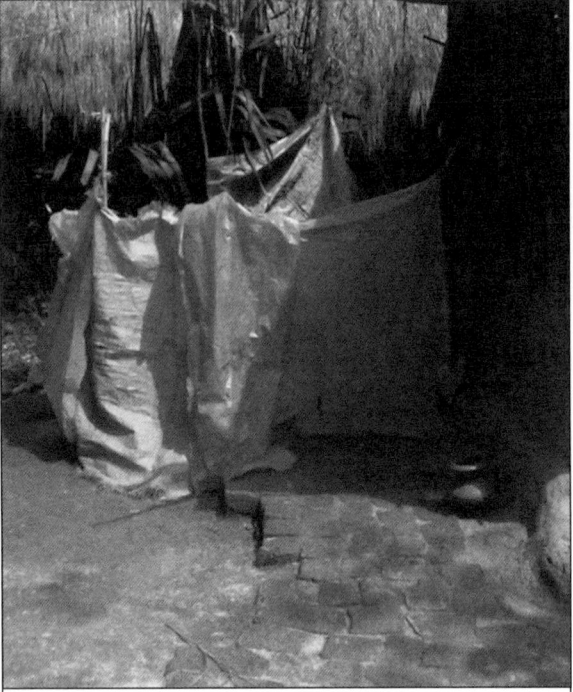

Figure 5.8. Brick path with earth and sand pointing leading to a bathing area.

Description	Clay brick path laid with earth pointing between the bricks for stability.
Dimensions	Width: ~ 1 metre.
Gradient	1 in 20 for 5 metres, then 1 in 10 for 1 metre.
User	Man with a low trolley for mobility.
Key features	Provides a firm surface so the user does not have to go through mud in the rainy season. Wide enough for the wheels of the trolley.
Drawbacks and comments	The surface of the bricks is uneven, which could cause problems for the trolley. Rain could wash the earth away, causing the bricks to become loose and more uneven. A 1 in 10 slope would be unsuitable for many wheelchair users. This could be avoided by making the entire slope slightly steeper, i.e. 1 in 17 for 6m.

Examples of approach ramps

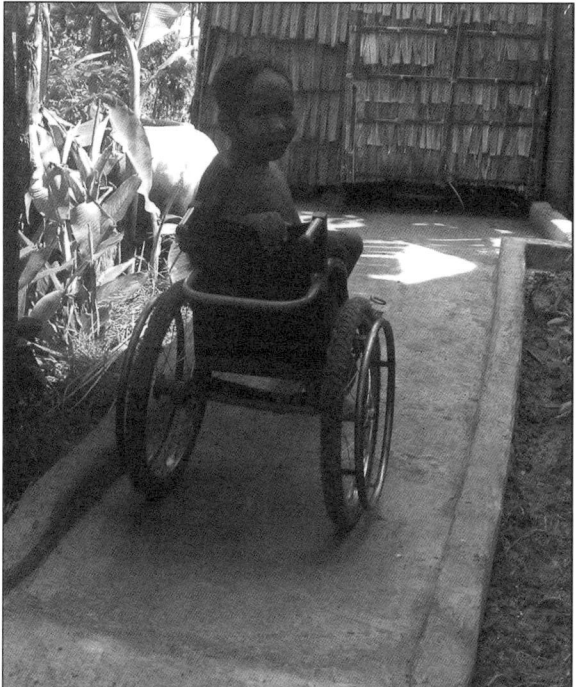

Figure 5.9. Concrete ramp from house to bathing area and toilet.

Description	Concrete ramp with kerb both sides; level platform midway and at top in front of the toilet door.
Dimensions	Ramp W: 75cm (to suit child's wheelchair). Ramp kerb: H: 6cm x W: 6cm. Flat platform: 134cm x 100cm.
Gradient	1 in 15, level platform midway.
User	Child using a wheelchair independently.
Key features	Smooth, firm, durable surface. Gradient gentle enough for child to propel himself up slope, and to make a controlled descent. Kerb on each side prevents wheelchair falling off. Flat platform in front of toilet door enables user to open door without risk of rolling backwards.
Drawbacks and comments	High cost. For little extra cost, the ramp and flat platform could have been made wider, making it suitable for when the child has an adult sized wheelchair, i.e. 90cm. (Recommended width of ramp for communal use: 150cm.)

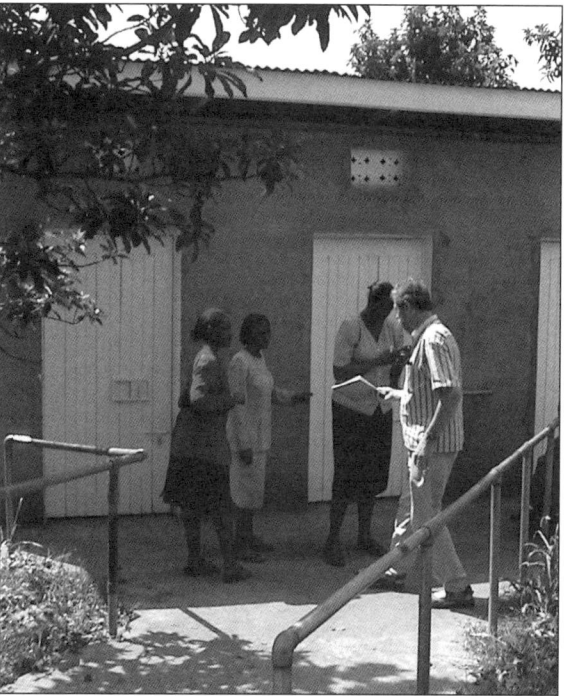

Figure 5.10. Wide concrete ramp with handrails both sides.

Description	Wide concrete ramp with handrails on both sides, leading to communal toilets.
Dimensions	Ramp W: 2 metres. Handrails: 5cm dia g.i. pipe; H: 90 – 100cm.
Key features	Wide ramp allows two wheelchair users to pass each other easily, essential where there are a number of users. Handrail provides support to users with poor balance, also prevents wheelchairs running over the edge.
Suitable for	Institutional setting. Child and adult wheelchair users, children with poor balance.
Drawbacks and comments	High cost.

5

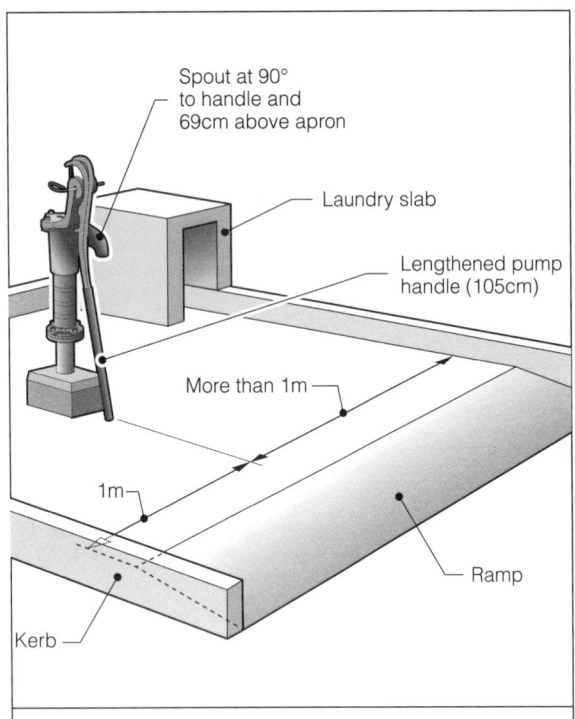

Figure 5.11. Ramp access to a handpump apron.

Labels on Figure 5.11:
Spout at 90° to handle and 69cm above apron
Laundry slab
Lengthened pump handle (105cm)
More than 1m
1m
Ramp
Kerb

Description	Wide concrete ramp leading onto a wide concrete apron around a handpump. The drainage slope is in the opposite direction to the approach ramp.
Dimensions	More than 1 metre wide.
Key features	The concrete ramp onto the apron makes wheelchair access easy. The ramp stays dry, because the water drains in the opposite direction.
Suitable for	All, especially wheelchair users. Institutional setting.
Drawbacks	The large area of concrete is expensive.

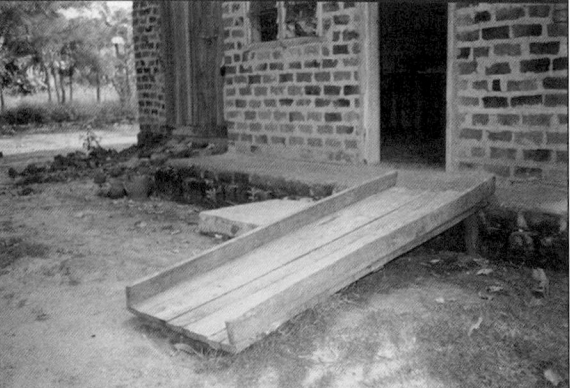

HITS, Uganda

Figure 5.12. Movable wooden ramp.

Description	Movable wooden ramp for wheelchair access to facilities with steps. Raised kerb on both sides.
Dimensions	W: 80cm; L: 3 metres.
Key features	Flexible - can be placed wherever needed. Cheaper than concrete. Kerb on each side prevents wheelchair rolling over the edge.
Suitable for	Wheelchair users with helpers available only. Temporary use. Crossing open drains or ditches.
Drawbacks	Less durable than concrete. User needs helpers to move ramp as needed.

5

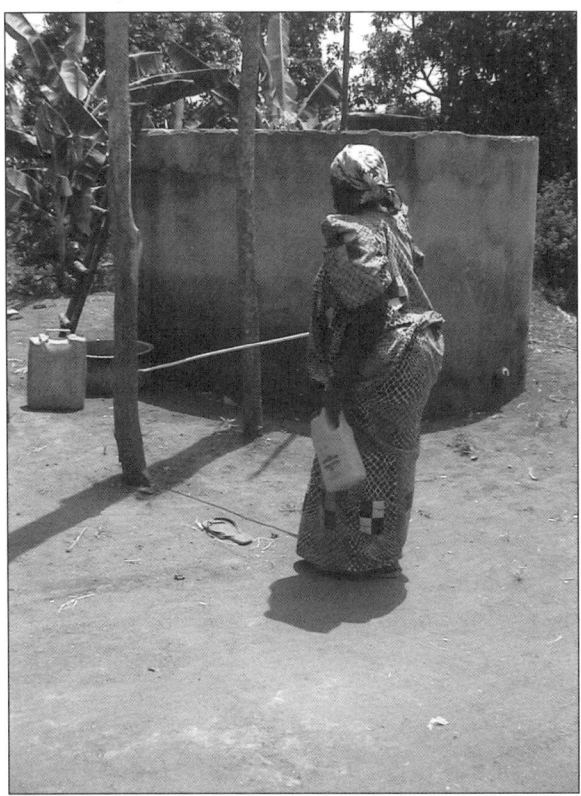

Figure 5.13. Two fixed wooden posts act as landmarks for a blind woman to find her way to and from the water tank or toilet. For a user with some vision, posts could be painted/marked a bright colour.
(Case-study 9.21, page 219)

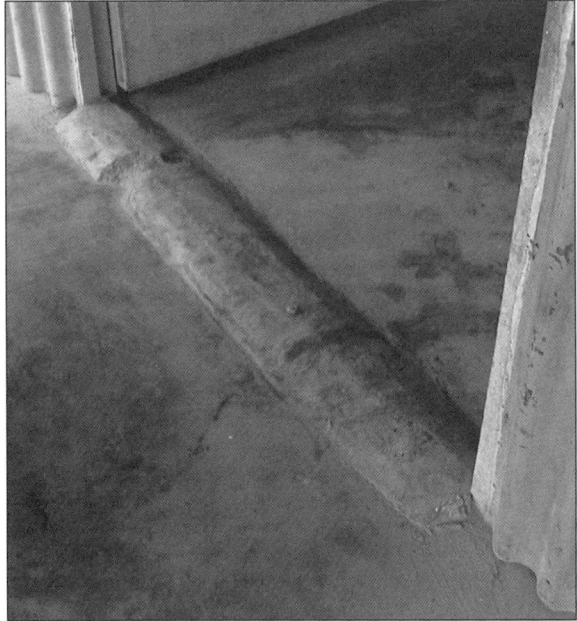

Figure 5.14. Low threshold for flood prevention, rounded for easy wheelchair access.
(Case-study 9.4, page 169)

on a slippery floor and cause the user to fall. The surface should be slightly rough to reduce this risk. The path should finish level with the floor of the facility to which it leads, so that there is no step between the two.

In the case of a slope or ramp, regular maintenance is important. If the ramp is made of earth, it will need to be replaced when it is washed away by rain. Where the slope is made of concrete or other durable materials, the point where the slope meets the surrounding earth should be as smooth and level as possible. This also needs to be replaced regularly. If the surrounding grass grows long, it should be cut.

Protected sides
Where there is a drop to one or both sides of a slope or path, a kerb is needed to prevent people falling over the edge. This is a low wall along the edge of the path or ramp, 7.5 – 10cm high. The addition of a safety rail warns the user where the edge of the ramp is, and provides support.

Support
For those with poor balance or co-ordination, or who crawl, some form of support is helpful, especially for a ramp or steps. This could be a rail of galvanised iron (g.i.) pipe, wood, bamboo or rope, or similar locally available materials. For more details, see the section on Types of support rails on page 102.

Issues for blind and visually impaired people
Blind and visually impaired people need to be able to find their way around using their remaining vision, or by touch, using a stick, white cane, or their hands, to feel for familiar objects.

To help them do this, they need familiar **'landmarks'** – permanent structures wherever possible, such as gate-posts, trees or large rocks. These existing features cost nothing. Additional landmarks can also be put in place, such as vertical poles or horizontal guide-rails,

5

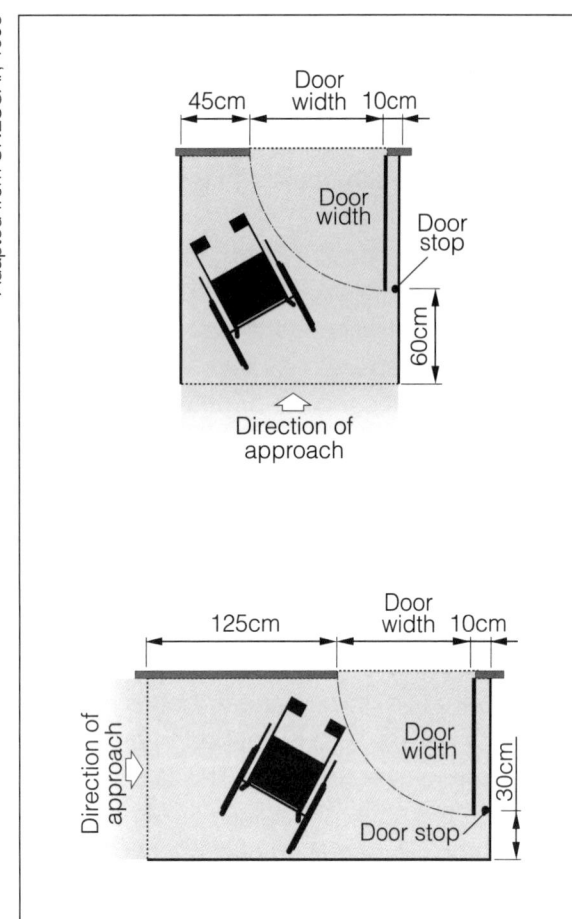

Figure 5.15. Minimum dimensions of flat platform for opening a door.

which should be fixed so that they cannot easily be moved accidentally (Figure 5.13).

Most people who may be referred to as 'blind' do have some usable vision. They find it helpful if contrasting paint, fabric or waterproof sticky tape are used to mark handles, entrances, the edges of steps and ramps, or to warn of hazards to avoid.

A safety-rail is recommended on paths where a wrong step could result in a fall, such as next to a pond, or on a steep river bank. If the rail is also used for support, it must be strong enough to bear the users' weight (see pages 126 to 133 on support-rails). It must be high enough (80 – 100cm) so that it does not become a trip hazard.

Rails are helpful to other users in the community, such as children and elderly people. Guide- or safety-rails at the right height for adults, however, will be too high and too thick for children to use safely and comfortably. An additional lower rail (H: ~75cm) with a smaller diameter can be provided, which will also be useful for wheelchair users. A rail that obstructs other users should be avoided.

Entrances – getting in

A level platform is needed immediately outside any door so that users can open the door without their wheelchair rolling backwards, or stand on crutches without losing their balance.

For a wheelchair user, where the door opens outwards, the flat area should provide enough space for a wheelchair user to manoeuvre to open the door. The minimum dimensions will change, depending on the direction of approach (Figure 5.15). A crutch user is likely to need a similar amount of space.
A handrail next to the door is useful for a person who is unsteady on their feet while opening the door. This can be attached to the outside wall if the wall is strong enough, or fixed to the ground (see page 102, Support rails).

Entrance width

The entrance should be wide enough for wheelchair access: 80cm is a recommended minimum width. For most crutch users, a widened door is convenient, but not essential.

Threshold

The transition from outside to inside should be as level as possible for easy access (Figure 5.17). Where a kerb is necessary, such as for flood prevention, this should be as smooth and rounded as possible (Figure 5.16).

If the inside is higher than outside, a ramp is recommended for easy wheelchair entry. If there has to be a step, a handrail is helpful for crutch users, for people crawling, and those with poor balance or co-ordination. For other users, see page 51 on Steps.

Signs

In a communal setting there may be a row of toilets or bathrooms, not all of which are accessible to disabled users. A brightly coloured visual sign on the door, such as the international disability symbol, can show which is the accessible facility. This can be helpful to all users, including those with a visual impairment. It can also have the function of raising awareness of the community about accessibility.

Issues for blind and visually impaired people

For many people with visual impairments, highlighting the edge of a step or entrance is helpful. This can be done with brightly coloured paint or waterproof tape to improve the contrast.

The entrance needs to be signalled in a way that the blind person can see or feel. A common way of doing this is by a change of floor texture, from concrete to brick, or from earth to stones. A blind person can feel the difference with their feet or with a cane.

For further resources about blind and visually impaired people, see Appendix A1.9, on page 265.

Examples of entrances

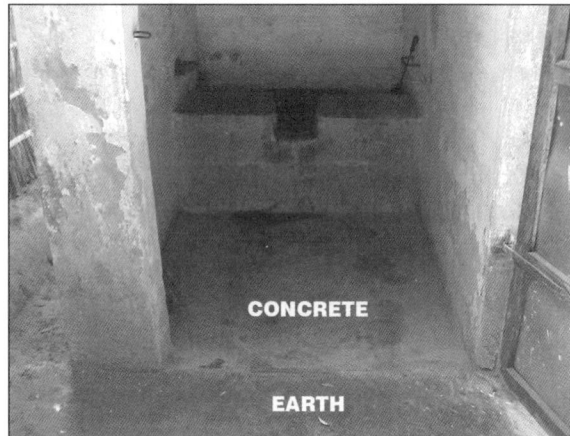

Figure 5.16. Toilet entrance.
(Case-study 9.1, page 154)

Description	Smooth concrete floor and threshold, with toilet floor only 1-2cm above the surrounding yard.
Dimensions	Entrance width: 90cm.
Key features	A level area of packed earth in front of the latrine for wheelchair stability while the user opens the door. The earth in front of the toilet is level with the floor inside, making wheelchair access easy. The user annually replaces the earth washed away by the rain. This takes about 1 hour.

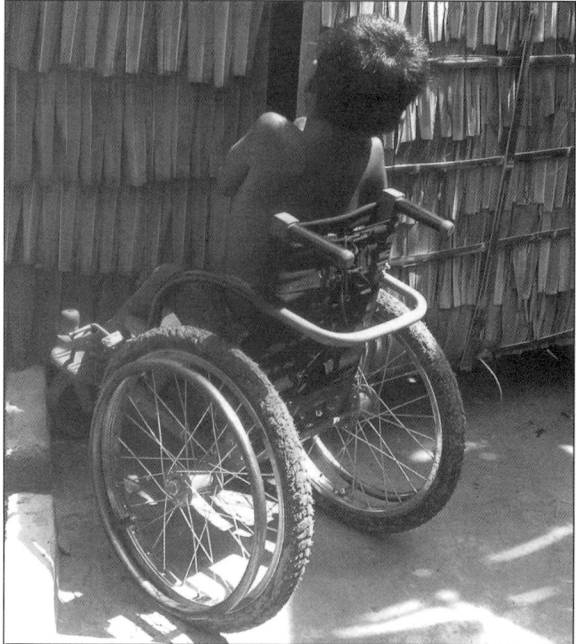

Figure 5.17. Wheelchair user opening a door on a flat area.
(Case-study 9.15, page 201)

Description	Flat platform area at the top of a ramp (see Figure 5.9) for wheelchair stability while opening the door.
Dimensions	100cm x 134cm. Height of kerb around platform: 6cm; width: 6cm.
Key features	Platform is level with the toilet floor, making wheelchair access easy. Platform has space for the wheelchair to move around the door. Kerb around the platform prevents wheelchair falling over the edge.
Drawbacks	High cost. Only a minimum flat area is provided. For a larger wheelchair, the area will need to be widened. It would be cheaper to make it wider at the outset, e.g. 150cm x 150cm.

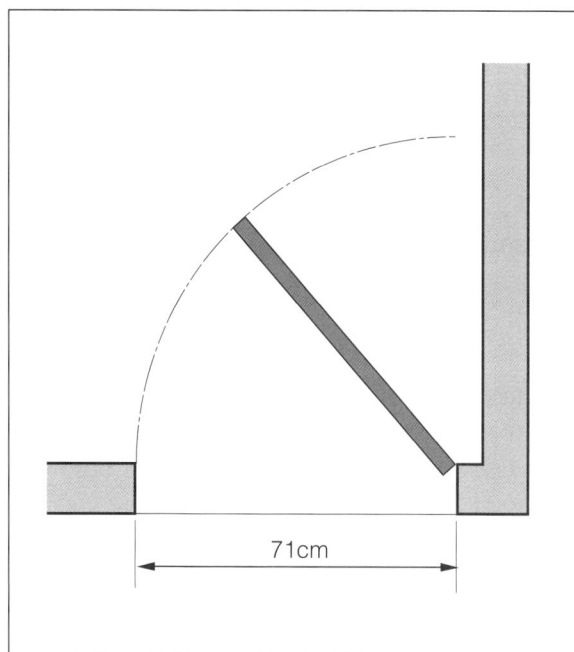

Figure 5.18. Inward opening door that opens flat against a side-wall.

71cm

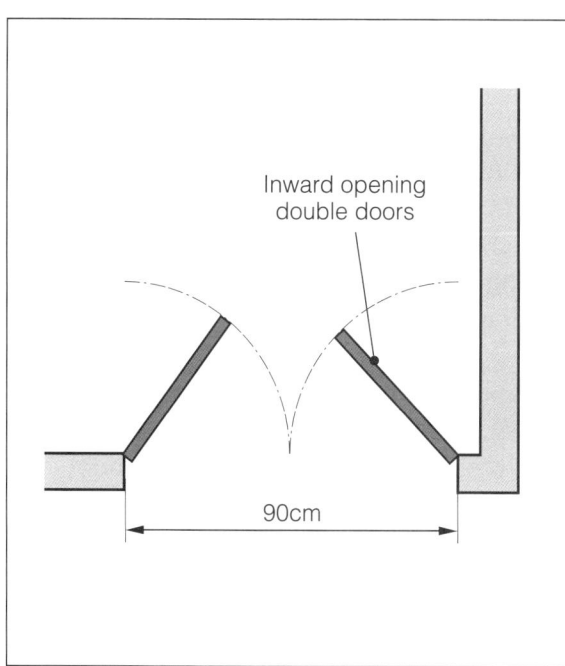

Inward opening double doors

90cm

Figure 5.19. Double doors take up less room when opened.

Doors and their features

A door that opens outwards leaves more space for a wheelchair to move around inside. Outward opening doors may be hazardous if they open onto a footpath, as they may hit another user. They therefore need to be positioned so as not to obstruct footpaths or corridors.

Where the door opens inwards, extra space may need to be provided for a wheelchair to move around – this can be more costly if the floor is concrete. To maximise available space, the door hinge should be placed so that the door opens flat against a side-wall (Figure 5.18).

A two-way hinge has the advantage of allowing the door to be pushed or pulled from either inside or outside (Figure 5.20). It is generally easier to push than to pull a door open.

Double doors, each of which is half the width of the opening, are less obstructive but a more costly option (Figure 5.19). They are difficult for a wheelchair user to open.

A sacking or plastic curtain instead of a solid door allows more flexibility in the space required. For example, the user's legs can stick out under the curtain. However it is not recommended because of concerns about privacy and security for the user (see the section on and privacy and security issues on page 60).

An outward opening door can be more difficult to close from the inside. A rail or rope on the inside of the door is helpful. Large bolts and/or handles on both inside and outside are good for easy grip.

If the rail extends the full width of the door, it allows the user to close the door without having to stretch too far (Figure 5.21).

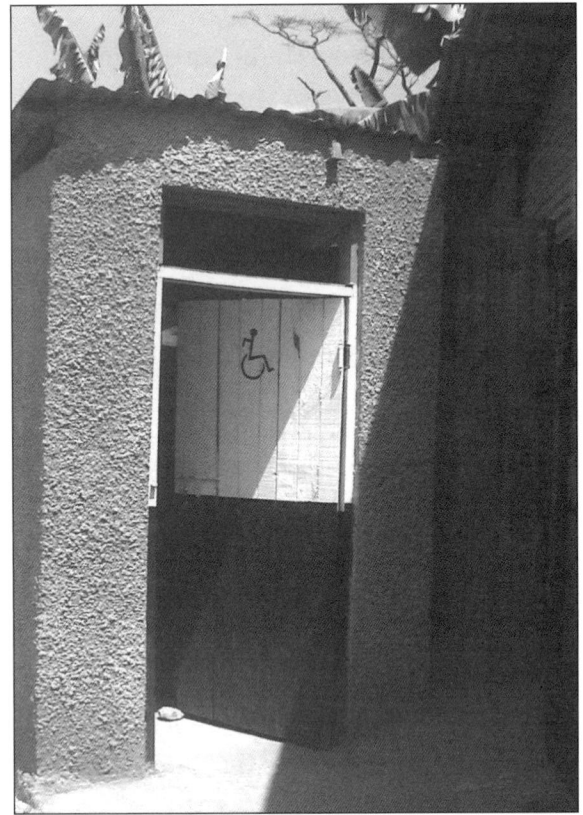

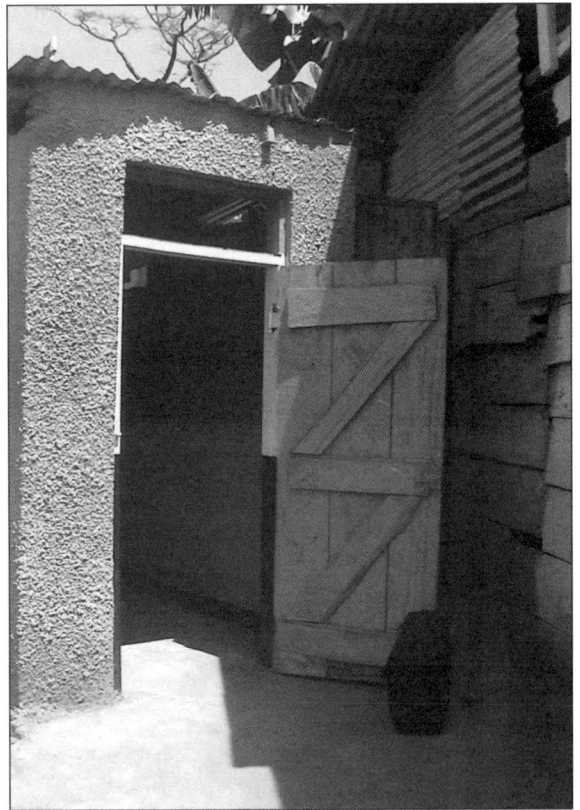

Figure 5.20. Toilet door with a two-way hinge allows this door to open outwards and inwards. Note the international disability symbol on the door.
(Case-study 9.25, page 229)

A self-closing door may be helpful to some people. By installing the door frame slightly inward leaning makes the door swing shut by itself.

A door-stop is recommended to prevent the door opening more than 90 degrees, otherwise it is more difficult to close (Figure 5.15).

Privacy and security
Privacy and security are a high priority for many people when using the toilet or bathing, especially for women. Lack of security can lead to anxiety about latrine use. This may lead to urine retention, and subsequently to medical problems.

Holes for light and ventilation must be high up, so that outsiders cannot see inside. Doors must be high (and low) enough to prevent outsiders looking over or under them. A secure door fastening is needed, which should ideally be a large, easy-to-grasp bolt, but may be as simple as a string or chain that hooks over a nail on the inside of the door.

A curtain is a widely used low-cost replacement for a door, which does not restrict space inside, and does not need closing. It is not an ideal solution, especially if facilities are communal, as it is not as secure.

In some circumstances it may be necessary to enable the door to be opened from outside in an emergency, for example in a school or hospital. One solution is to have a small window near the fastening to allow someone outside to put their hand through to undo the bolt (Figure 5.23). This has the disadvantage that other users could also open the door from the outside, and could look in.

Internal dimensions and layout
Disabled people usually need more space to move around inside a facility than non-disabled people. How much they need will vary. Where a number of disabled people with

See Appendix A 1.1 page 255 for a list of publications on inclusive design.

different needs use a facility, the preferred option is to provide more space, rather than less (see Section 5.3).

In designing toilet and bathing spaces, the following issues need to be considered:

- What functions will it be used for: toileting, bathing, washing clothes, other?

- What kind of mobility aid is used, how much room does it need?

- Does there need to be space for a support person to also move around?

- Wheelchair/trolley manoeuvring: is the need to enter and turn, or enter and reverse out (Figure 5.25), or will it be left outside?

- For sideways wheelchair transfer, which side of the toilet is space needed?

- Space for an internal water source for anal cleansing, handwashing and/or cleaning the toilet.

- Space for a toilet seat to be moved to one side of the toilet.

- Shelf or hook for aids or equipment, or anal cleansing materials.

Placing the toilet in one corner leaves more space for a wheelchair, if the user does not need access from two sides. (Figure 5.24).

Floors
The floor should be even and smooth for easy cleaning, but not so smooth as to make it slippery when wet. Any surface can become slippery if it is frequently wet because of poor drainage, and algae are allowed to grow. Every effort must be made to ensure good water drainage away from the user, to minimise this risk.

Concrete or cement mortar are easier to keep clean than an earth floor, but more costly. A slightly roughened finish is advised where crutches will be used. This should not be so rough, however, that a person crawling hurts

Adapted from Handicap International (8)

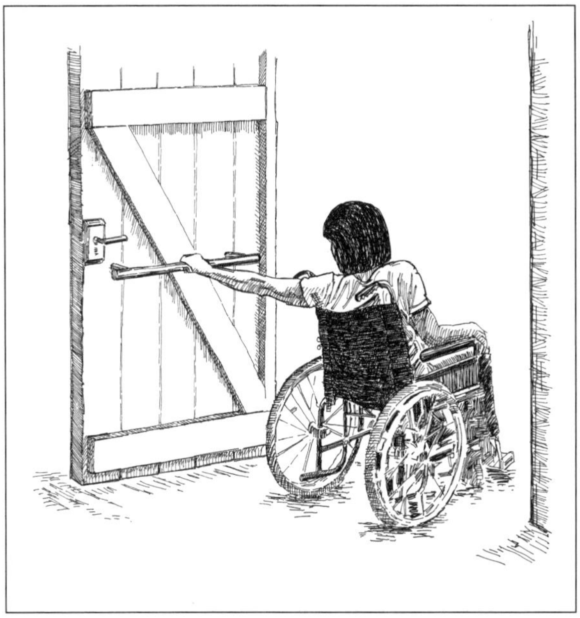

Figure 5.21. Door-rail extending the full width of the door.

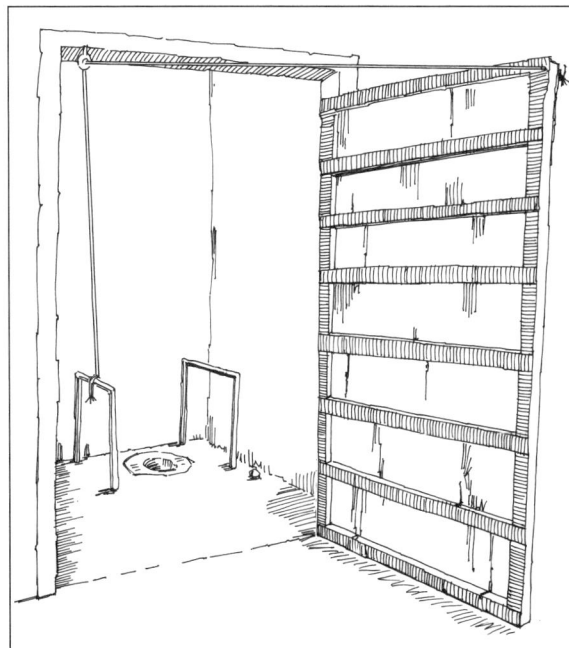

Figure 5.22. String attached to the door threads through a hook. User pulls the string to close the door and ties the end to the handrail.
(Case-study 9.16, page 207)

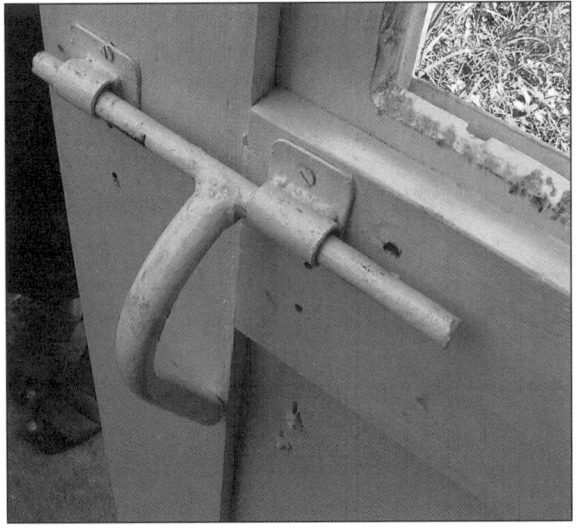

Figure 5.23. Large bolt, easy to grasp.
The small window allows the door to be opened from outside.

their hands or knees. Alternatively, ridges can be created in the concrete to provide a non-slip surface.

The disadvantage of concrete or mortar is that they absorb urine, so painting them makes them moisture resistant and easier to keep clean and hygienic. For more details about surfaces of paths and steps, see Section 5.4, page 51.

The starting point for deciding what features to include is to talk to the users, to find out their needs and preferences (see the sections in Chapter 8 on working with families, on pages 137 and 147).

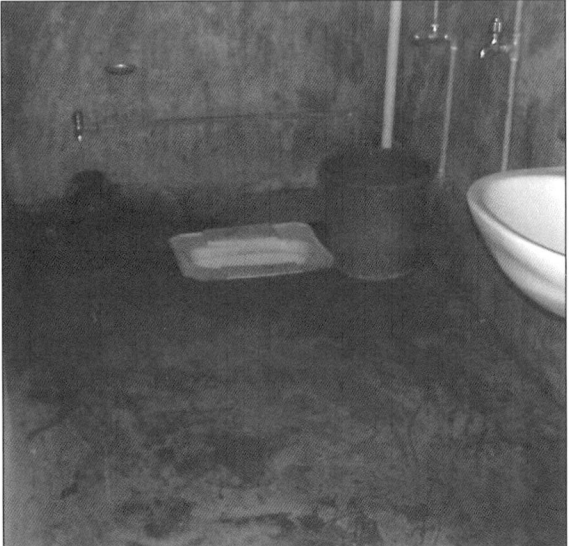

Figure 5.24. Combined bathroom and toilet.
Note toilet in the corner to maximise space.

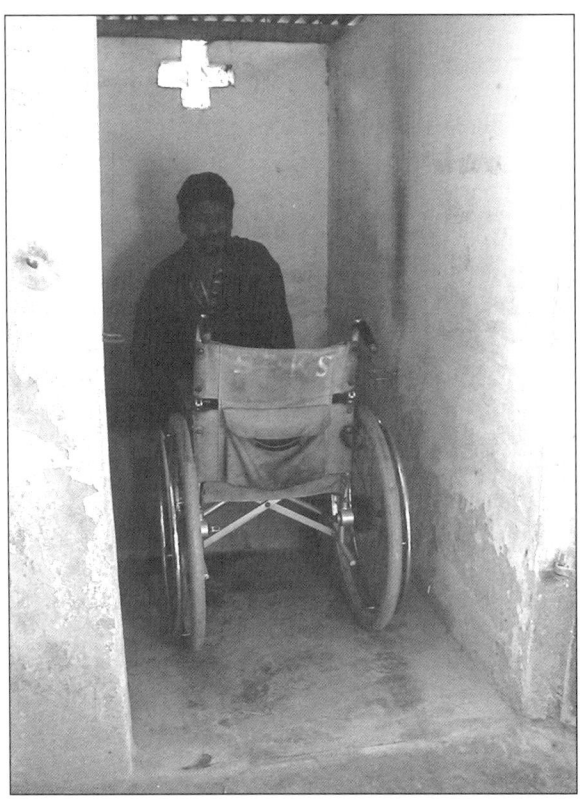

Figure 5.25. Toilet with space for wheelchair user to enter, but not to turn. User must reverse out. *(Case-study 9.1, page 154)*

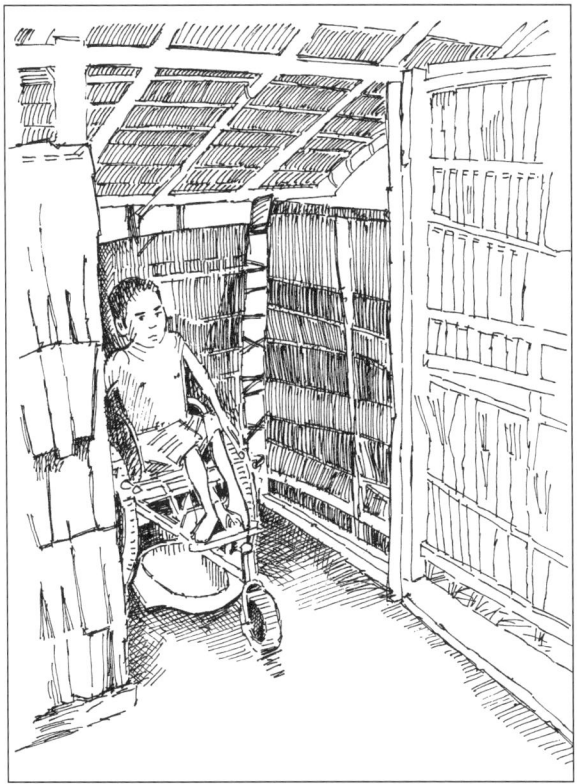

Figure 5.26. Toilet with space to position wheelchair over toilet, but not beside it. The user must reverse in. *(Case-study 9.15, page 201)*

Accessibility

References

1. Disability Rights Commission (2003) *Creating an Inclusive Environment - a report on improving the Built Environment*. http://www.drc-gb.org/publicationsandreports/ publicationdetails.asp?id=157&section=access

2. UNESCAP (1995) *Promotion of Non-handicapping physical environments for Disabled Persons: Guidelines*. United Nations Economic and Social Commission for Asia and the Pacific: UN: New York. http://www.unescap.org/esid/psis/disability/decade/publications/ z15009gl/z1500901.htm

3. Venter, C.J. et al (2004) *Overseas Road Note 21: Enhancing the mobility of disabled people: Guidelines for Practitioners*. Transport Research Laboratory & DFID, UK. http://www.transport-links.org/transport_links/filearea/publications/1_831_ORN%2021.pdf

4. Jones, H.E. and Reed, R.A. (2003) *Water Supply and Sanitation Access and Use by Physically Disabled People*. Report of field-work in Uganda. WEDC, Loughborough University and DFID: UK.

5. Jones, H.E. and Reed, R.A. (2003) *Water supply and sanitation access and use by physically disabled people: report of field-work in Bangladesh*. WEDC, Loughborough University and DFID: UK.

6. Centre for Accessible Environments (2002) *Designing for Accessibility*. CAE and RIBA Enterprises: London.

7. Barker, P. Barrick, J. and Wilson, R. (1995) *Building Sight. A Handbook of building and interior design solutions to include the needs of visually impaired people*. HMSO & Royal National Institute for the Blind: London.

8. Handicap International Belgium. *Booklet on household adaptations for daily living*. PRC, Siem Reap: Cambodia. (drawings and text in Khmer)

Chapter 6

Water supply – access and use

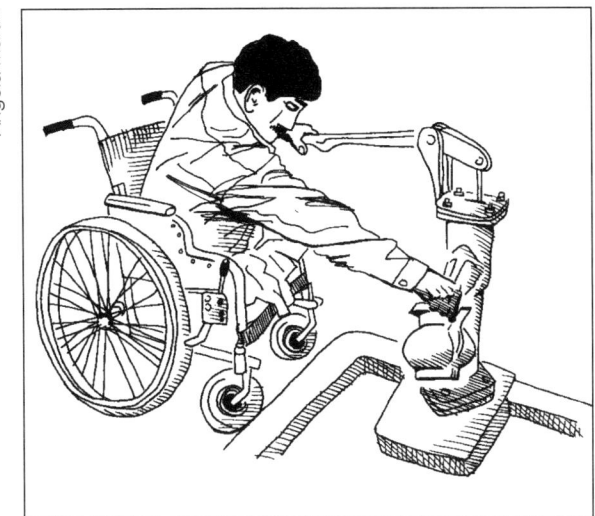

Figure 6.1. Handpump sited close to edge of apron.

A range of water sources are dealt with in this section, including taps, handpumps, wells, rainwater storage facilities, and natural water sources.

6.1 Benefits of access to water

Improved access to water and activities related to water bring far-reaching benefits, including:

- Increased self-reliance and dignity for disabled people: being able to carry out an activity unaided, whereas before they relied on the family for support.

- Improved health and well-being of disabled people.

- Savings in time and effort for the whole family, which frees up more time for other household activities.

- Increased productivity and income generation opportunities: increased quantities of water means the surplus is available for domestic production of vegetables, fruit or for animal raising.

Benefits of accessible facilities are felt not only by the disabled person, but by the whole family, and often neighbours too.

- Improved health and well-being of the whole family.

- Other family members and neighbours, who previously spent a lot of time fetching water, now have time to spend on other activities. Children have time to play, or go to school.

Note:
Technical details of water supply facilities can be found in a range of other publications (See Appendix A1.2, page 256, for a list of resources).

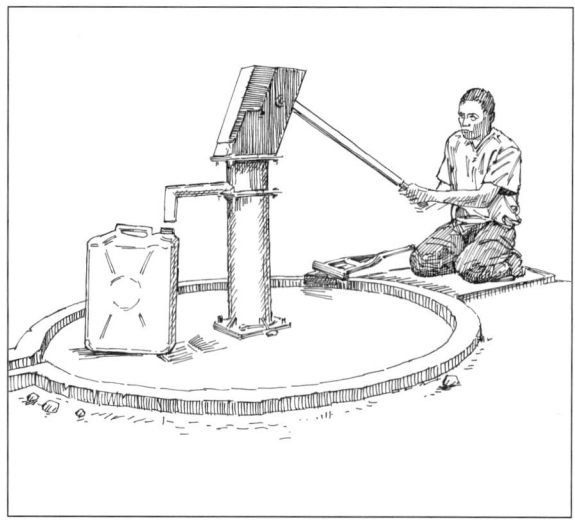

Figure 6.2. Crutch user operating handpump from a platform on the outside edge of the apron.

6.2 Principles of inclusive design

In making a water facility easy to access and use, the principles of inclusive design should be aimed for, i.e. ease of use, freedom of choice and access to mainstream activities, diversity and difference, safety and predictability.

6.3 Drawing water

Accessibility

At the water source, the user needs to be able to get into a position to reach the water drawing mechanism, to be able to operate it, and to reach the water produced.

Handpump aprons

Where a handpump has a concrete apron, this is liable to be slippery when wet, and treacherous for a user with poor balance. For many users, it may be better to avoid the risks of a slippery surface by designing the handpump to be used from outside the apron. This can be done by:

- Installing the pump near the edge of the apron, so that it can be operated from outside the apron (Figure 6.1),

- Lengthening the pump handle so that it is long enough to operate from the edge of the apron (Figure 6.2). Help may still be needed to collect the water.

- Constructing the apron so that it is level with the surrounding ground, or so that any kerb or threshold has a rounded edge, to enable wheelchairs to wheel onto them if necessary.

Some pumps have a concrete platform outside the edge of the apron for the pump operator to stand on. This should be level with the surrounding ground, so it is accessible to wheelchair or crutch users (Figure 6.2). The concrete should have a roughened finish so that it is not slippery when wet, and kerbs should have smooth edges.

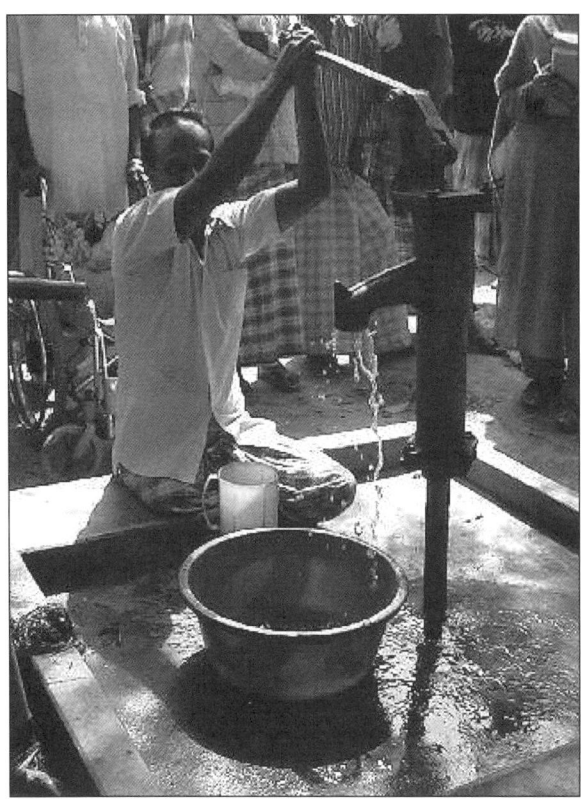

Figure 6.3. Low concrete sitting platform built into pump apron.
(Case-study 9.2, page 161)

Figure 6.4. Handpump with apron showing direction of water drainage away from pump. Note lengthened handle for extra leverage.
(Case-study 9.3, page 164)

An alternative is to build a concrete platform so that it is inset into the pump apron. This brings the user nearer to the pump handle, which can be used either sitting or standing (Figure 6.3). This also helps other family members, children, and women washing clothes or bathing children, to operate it more easily. A basic design of platform can be adapted in terms of height, width, and distance from the pump, to suit individual households or users.

As rain washes away the earth, the ground around the apron will get lower, so regular maintenance is needed to replace the earth to keep it at the required level.

Accessing the concrete apron
If a wheelchair or crutch user needs to go onto the apron to reach the handle or lifting device, a ramp, preferably of concrete, can make this possible (Figures 6.5 and 6.6).

There should be a level area at least 1 metre wide on the platform or surrounding ground to stand, sit or position a wheelchair next to the handle. Where possible, especially if the pump is used by several disabled people, this level area should be on three sides of the handle, allowing *all* users the option of accessing it from the side most suitable for them. This would allow them to use either hand, depending on whether they are left or right-handed.

A slippery floor can cause difficulties for a range of users. Slipperiness can be minimised by:

- Constructing the drainage slope so that water drains away from the ramp and user platform, to minimise water on the platform (Figures 6.4 and 6.6).

- Using a slightly rough finish to the apron where the user sits or stands.

Handpump equipment
Factors that make the equipment or facility easier to operate include:

6

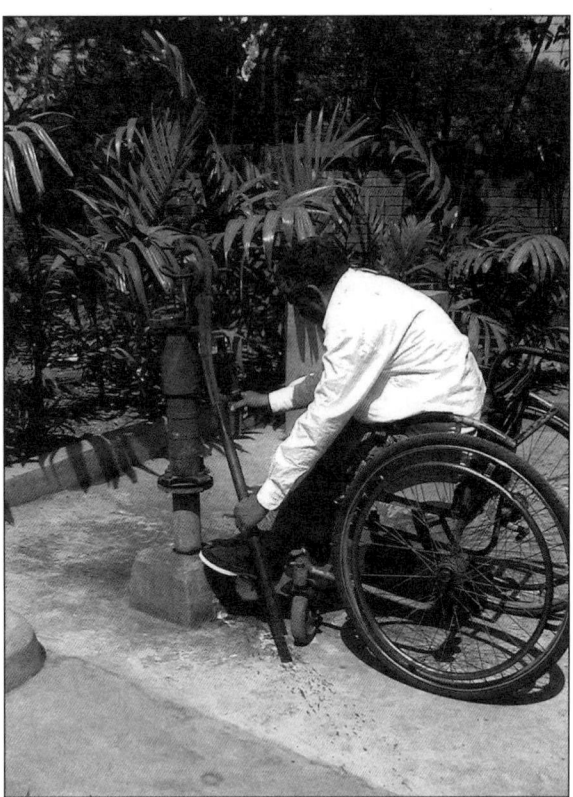

Figure 6.5. The same handpump operated by a wheelchair user on a level apron.
(Case-study 9.3, page164)

- Installing the pump at a height from which the handle can be reached, either from sitting in a chair or from sitting nearer ground level.

- Lengthening the pump handle to provide more leverage, so less strength is needed to operate it (Figures 6.4 and 6.5). It also allows the handle to be reached from outside the apron, or from lower down by a person sitting. The drawback is that a greater range of movement is needed to pump the same amount of water, which is a disadvantage for a person with limited arm movement.

- Installing the spout and pump handle at 90 degrees to each other. This allows the user to pump water and hold the container to collect water at the same time (although this is only possible from one side of the pump – see Figure 6.5). This is an advantage for someone with limited mobility, as it reduces the amount of walking between the handle and the container. Even if the container is placed on the ground to be filled, it is still less distance to move from the pump handle to the container. Also, it is possible to hold the container steady while it is being filled.

Open wells
Lifting devices benefit everyone, especially those with weak arms or grip, such as children and the elderly. Various types of lifting device are widely used, including the following devices used by disabled people:

Simple pulley arrangement on a wooden frame over a shallow well (Figure 6.8 and Case-study 9.12 on page 191). This has the following advantages:

- The user pulls down on the rope to lift water, which is easier than pulling upwards;

- A pulley can be operated from either a standing or sitting position;

![Figure 6.6 illustration]

Figure 6.6. Well apron with access ramp. NB the ramp is on the opposite side to the direction of drainage to ensure it stays as dry as possible.

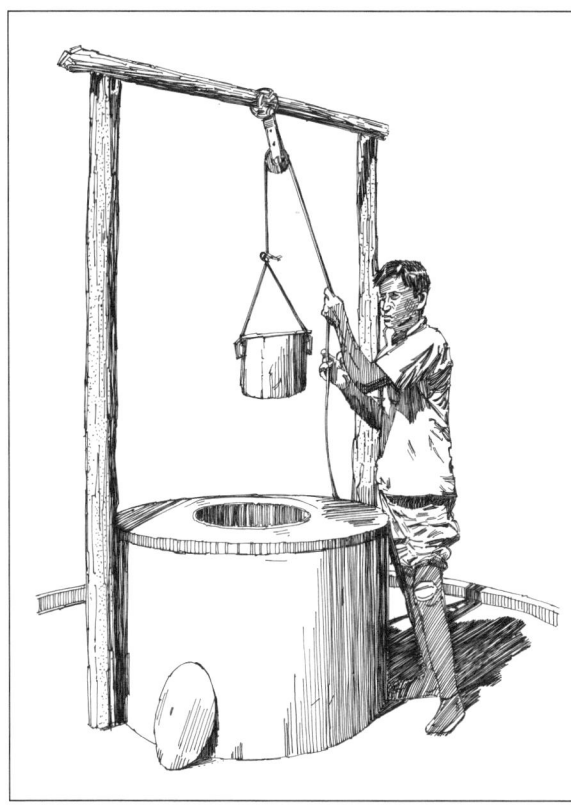

Figure 6.7. Rope and pulley over a shallow well.
(Case-study 9.12, page 191)

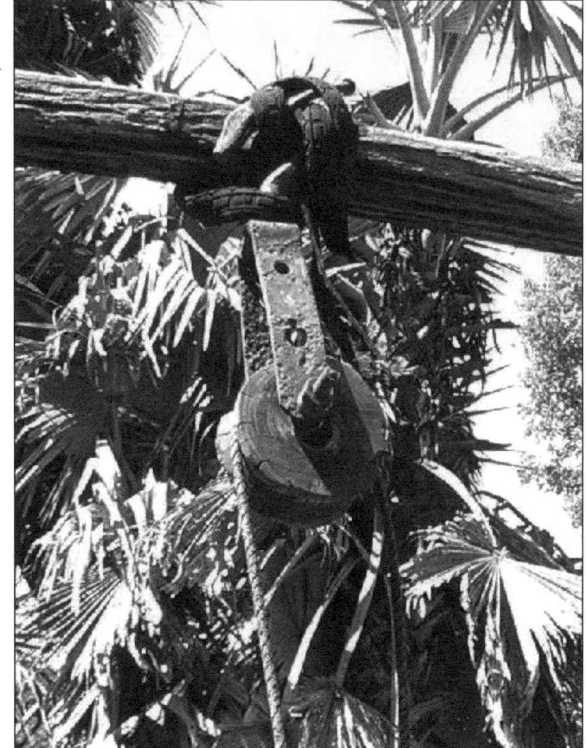

Figure 6.8. Detail of pulley lifting mechanism.
(Case-study 9.12, page 191)

- There is no need to lean over the edge of the well to lift water, so a person sitting beside the well, such as an elderly person or wheelchair/trolley user, can operate it.

The user does however need to lean across to reach the water container once it is raised. People with limited reach could use a long-handled hook to do this. Once the container is raised, it is also useful to be able to tie off the rope, round a pole or cleat for example, so that both arms are free to handle the container.

A cantilever lifting mechanism with a pulley over the well can be made easier to use by the addition of a **ratchet and pawl** winding and locking mechanism for the rope (Figure 6.9). The ratchet and pawl can be made out of wood, which is cheaper than metal, but easily damaged. Metal is more expensive but more durable. Its advantages are that:

- Less strength is needed to raise water, and it prevents the rope burning hands or stumps of arms.

- This is useful for a disabled person with only one arm, or a user with limited strength, as it gives additional control. For this reason it could also be of wider benefit to all users of deep wells.

Treadle pump designed to be operated using the feet (Figure 6.10). The user pushes down alternately on the ends of two lengths of wood, which are pivoted around a metal bar. The wooden beams are connected to a simple twin cylinder suction pump that draws water through a pipe from a nearby shallow well or borehole. Its advantage is that:

- It can be operated using either hands or feet and is easy to use by people with a range of impairments.

However, it is only useful for water tables less than 7m below the surface.

Maintenance
All the above types of lifting devices can be repaired and maintained by the disabled

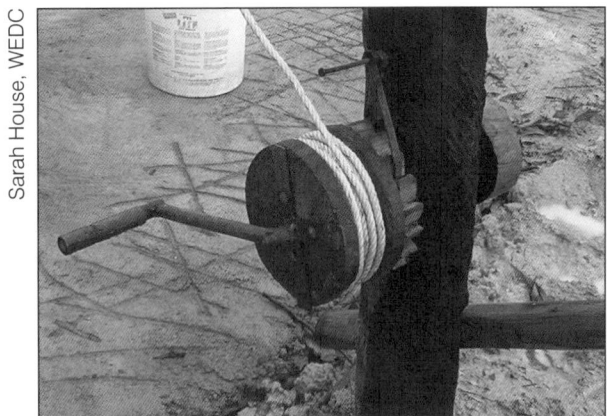

Figure 6.9. Detail of ratchet and pawl winding mechanism.
(Case-study 9.11, page 187)

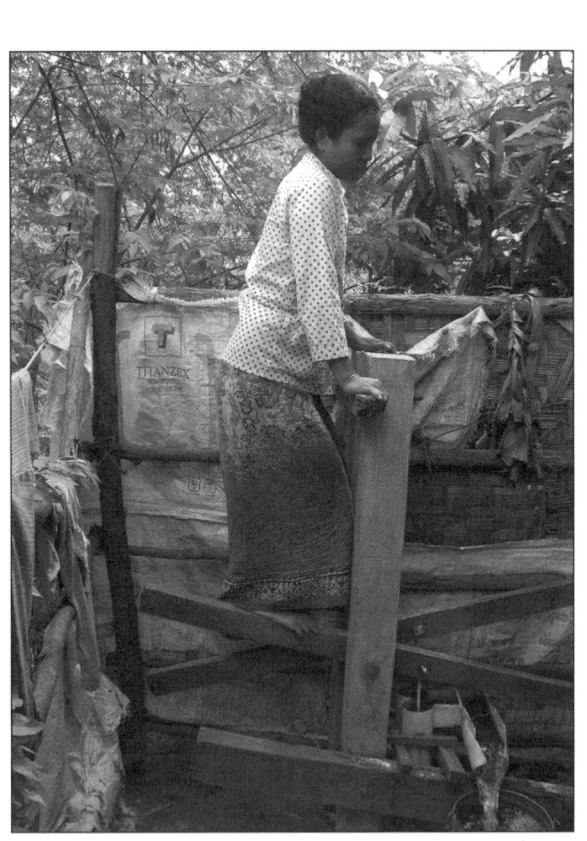

Figure 6.10. Treadle pump in operation.
(Case-study 9.13, page 193)

owners themselves. The spare parts of the pulley mechanism (Figure 6.8) and the treadle pump (Figure 6.10) could be purchased locally and replaced by the user. The ratchet and pawl winding mechanism (Figure 6.9) was designed and constructed by the disabled user.

The benefit of equipment that can be maintained by the user is that it can lead to greater self-reliance and sustainability (Box 6.1).

Handpump
Installing a handpump directly over a well makes water lifting easier and also generally improves the quality of water provided (see pages 66 to 68 for more on handpumps).

Open well without lifting mechanism
If the well is open with no lifting mechanism, there should be somewhere safe for the user to stand or sit (see pages 56, 66 and 67 for suggestions on flat platform areas).

A raised well wall, while reducing the risk of water contamination, is helpful for a person who is standing to draw water, to lean against for balance. The height of the wall should be between an adult's hip and waist, or approximately 80cm high. The wall should be strong enough to support the weight of a person leaning on it while lifting water.

For a wheelchair user, or any person sitting, the wall should not be above the height of their waist or chair arm (approximately 50cm high). This will allow them to reach over the side of the wall to lift water.
Wells used by a range of disabled and non-disabled people should have a wall at various heights to suit different users (Figure 6.11). The minimum height of an open well wall should be 50cm, to reduce the risk of small children falling in.

A flat cover over the well, of concrete or wood, with an access hatch, provides an additional surface to lean on, and to rest the container before and after filling (Figures 6.12 and

Mr Lann watched carefully as the treadle pump was being installed, as he knew that when the agency had gone he would have to repair the pump himself – which he does,. replacing valves and pipes as needed. Mr Lann's skills in repairing the pumps have also led to him being asked to repair his neighbours pumps and he is paid for this service in cash or in rice. Mr Lann and his family hold spares at their home and purchase them from local suppliers. Mr Lann has thus become a community resource person and his family have gained increased respect. *(Case-study 9.13, page 193)*

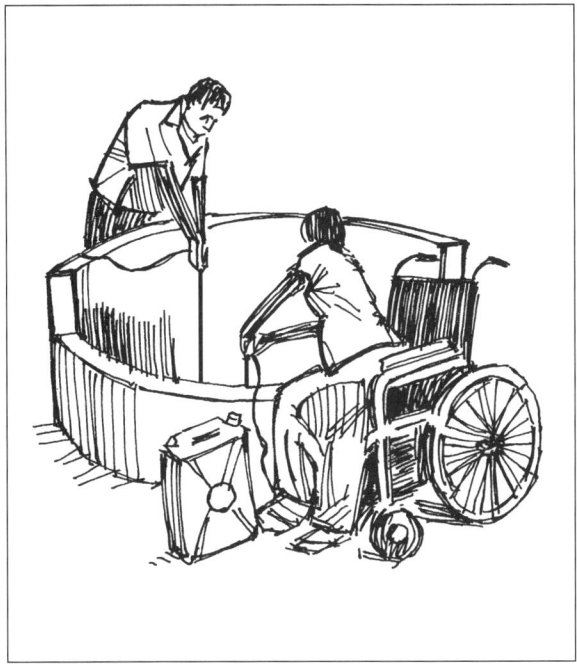

Figure 6.11. Well wall of different heights.

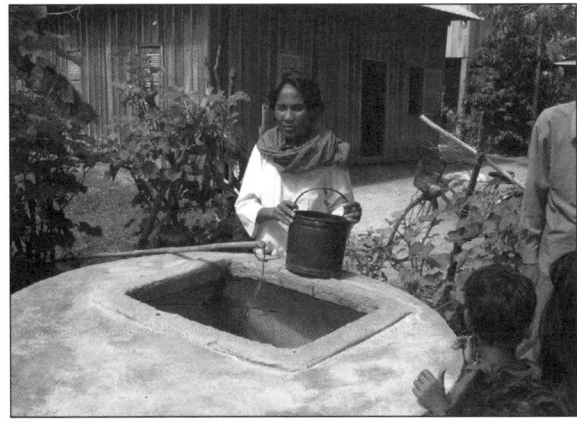

Figure 6.12. A concrete slab cover over the well provides a surface to rest a container.

6.13). This avoids the need for the user to bend down, reduces the risk of accidents and reduces contamination of the water in the well. The hatch must be at the edge of the cover so that it is within reach of all users.

Taps and tapstands

The advantage of a tap is that it requires little strength to operate, compared with water lifting devices. It can be installed at any convenient height, to suit a variety of users, and to allow the filling of any size of container. The rate of flow can be controlled easily, so there should be less wastage.

Height of tap

A communal tapstand needs to have taps at different levels to suit different users.

80 – 100cm is suitable for someone sitting on a seat or wheelchair and for many crutch users (Figures 6.14 and 6.16). A higher tap may be more suitable for people who have difficulty bending (Figures 6.13, 6.17 and 6.18).

A low tap is useful for a person crawling, and can result in less water being lost between spout and opening. If the height of the tap from the floor or shelf is too low, however, larger sizes of container cannot be used (Figure 6.15).

If the tap is over a basin or shelf, it needs to be positioned so that it can be reached from a sitting or standing position. In addition, there should be enough space for the wheelchair user to get their knees under the basin and

6

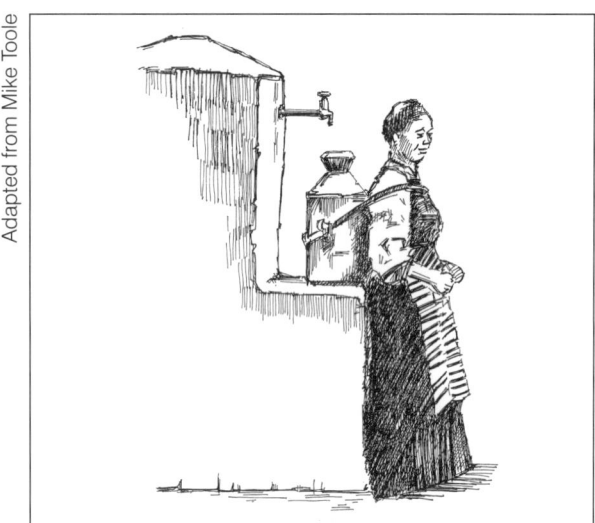

Figure 6.13. Tapstand in Tibet with higher tap and shelf that does not require the user to bend.
(Case-study 9.32, page 252)

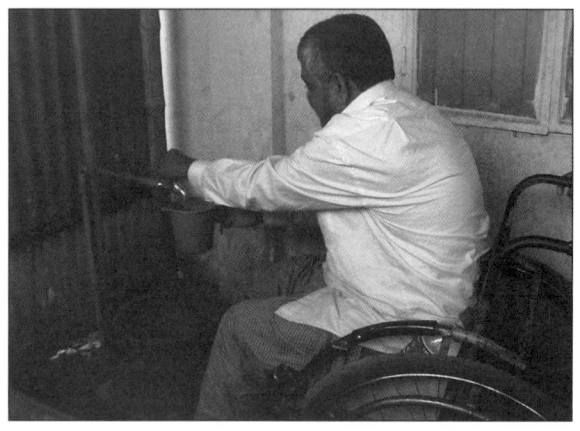

Figure 6.14. A wheelchair user collects water from a tap ~90cm high.
(Case-study 9.3, page 164)

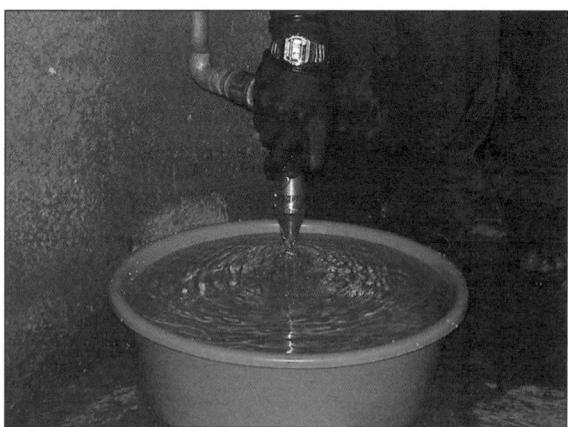

Figure 6.15. A low tap (25cm high) is useful for a person crawling or using a trolley.
(Case-study 9.20, page 217)

close enough to reach the tap (Figures 6.17 and 6.18).

Place to rest the container
A shelf or platform should be provided to rest a container while filling (Figures 6.13, 6.17, 6.18 and 6.19). This is beneficial for all users, especially those with weak arms, weak backs, women and girls carrying babies and elderly people.

The shelf should bear the weight of a full container of water.

Types of tap
Taps are an efficient way of accessing piped or stored water. Standard twist action taps are generally easy to use and control the flow of water easily. Large size taps (22mm diameter) are better than small ones (12mm diameter) because they are more robust and easier to operate.

A 'hospital tap' with a long lever is recommended (Figure 6.20), as it is easy to operate with almost any body part although it may be difficult to find in many areas. Instead, a tap turner can be made with nails or notches that fit over the twist tap (Figure 6.21). A lever which can be padlocked enables the owner to control who has access to their water (Figure 6.22).

Twist action taps may be difficult to use for some people because of the twisting wrist movement required. A press action tap may be more suitable for users with stiff wrists. However, the spring mechanism makes it more difficult to control the flow, and continuous pressure is needed to keep the tap open, which is difficult for those who lack strength, so press action taps are not generally recommended.

A flexible hose attached to a tap allows water to be directed into a container without lifting it off the floor. This can be done with one hand only (Figure 6.23). It can be cut to a length that allows a disabled person to direct

Adapted from Mike Toole

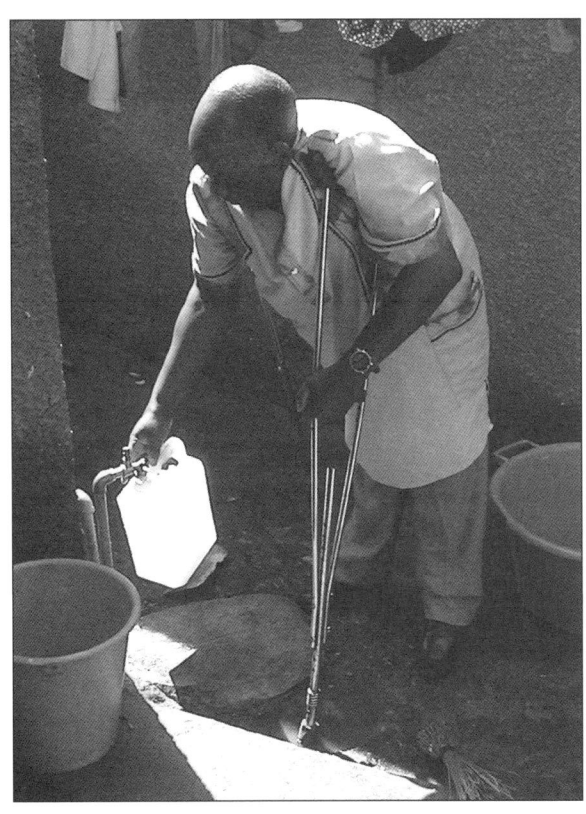

Figure 6.16. A man using crutches collects water from a 40cm high tap.
(Case-study 9.24, page 224)

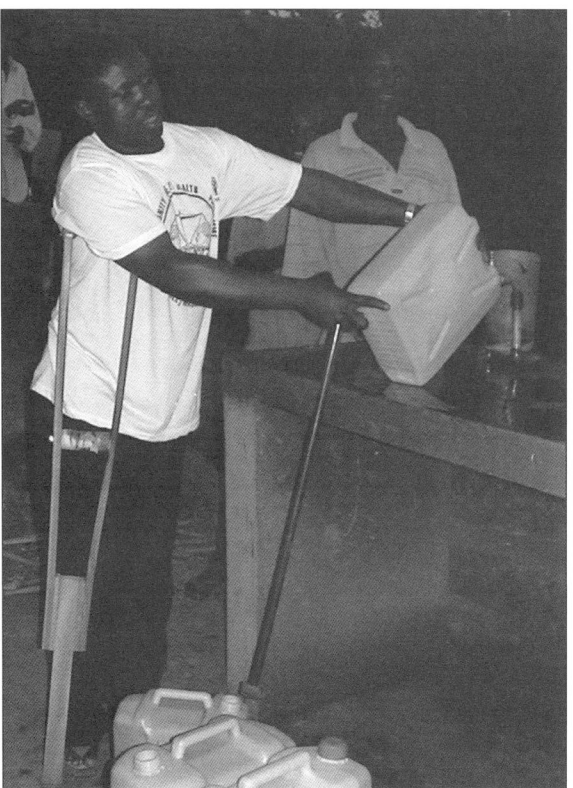

Figure 6.17. Taps ~25cm above a concrete shelf (H: ~1m) do not require the user to bend.
(Case-study 9.20, page 217)

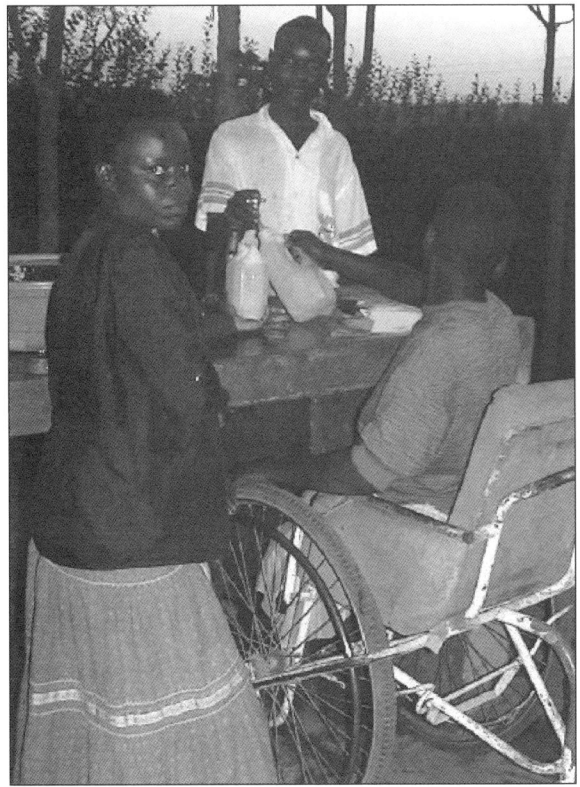

Figure 6.18. A user parks his wheelchair with his knees under the concrete shelf of a tapstand.
(Case-study 9.20, page 217)

6

Brian Reed, WEDC

Source: Internet (1)

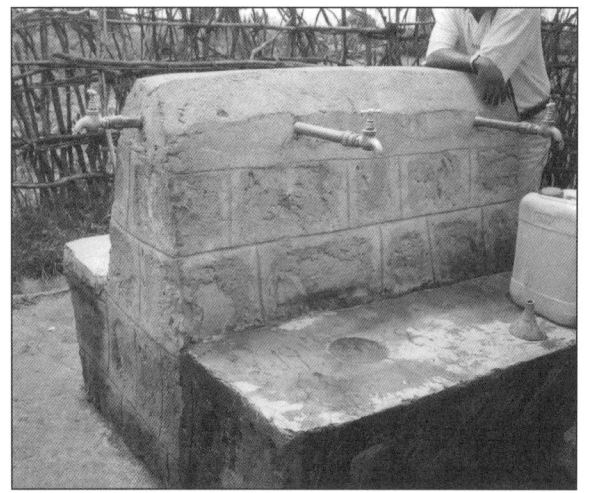

Figure 6.19. Tapstand in Ethiopia.
Note the indentation in the shelf to sit round-bottomed containers in while they are filled.

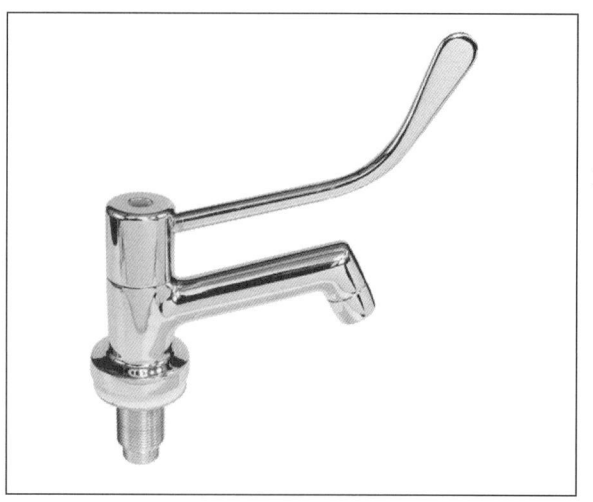

Figure 6.20. Lever operated tap.

Source: Van der Hulst et al (2)

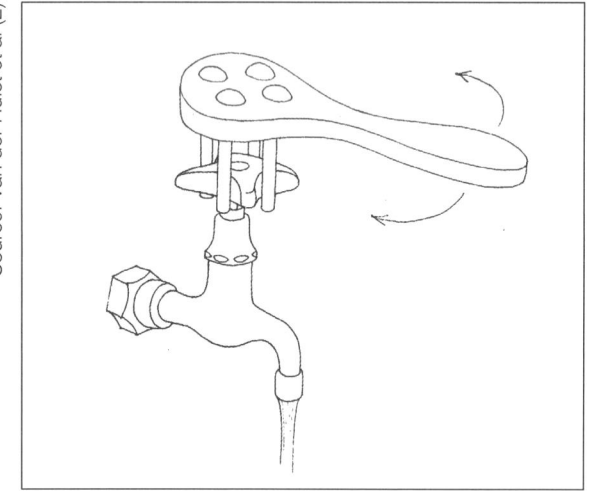

Figure 6.21. Tap turner made by driving nails through a piece of wood.

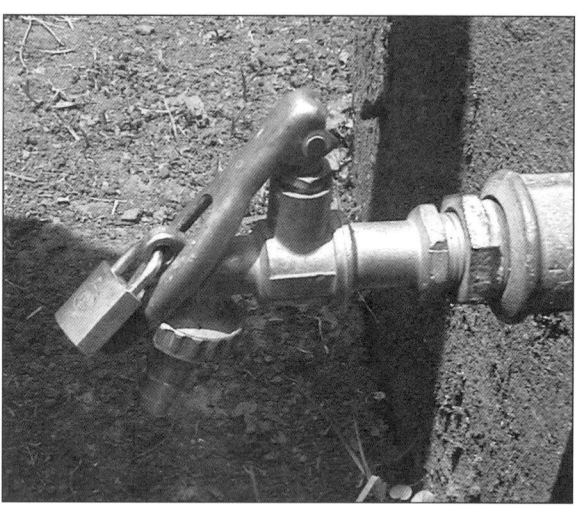

Figure 6.22. Lever operated tap with padlock. Unsuitable for a person with limited grip or stiff fingers.
(Case-study 9.21, page 219)

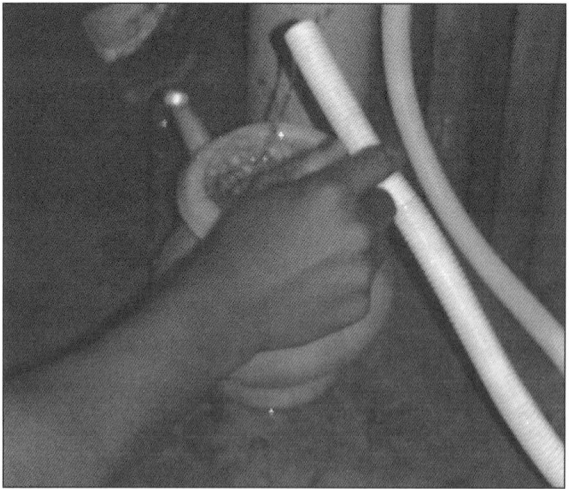

Figure 6.23. A flexible hose attached to a tap allows water to be poured into a container with one hand. *(Case-study 9.6, page 177)*

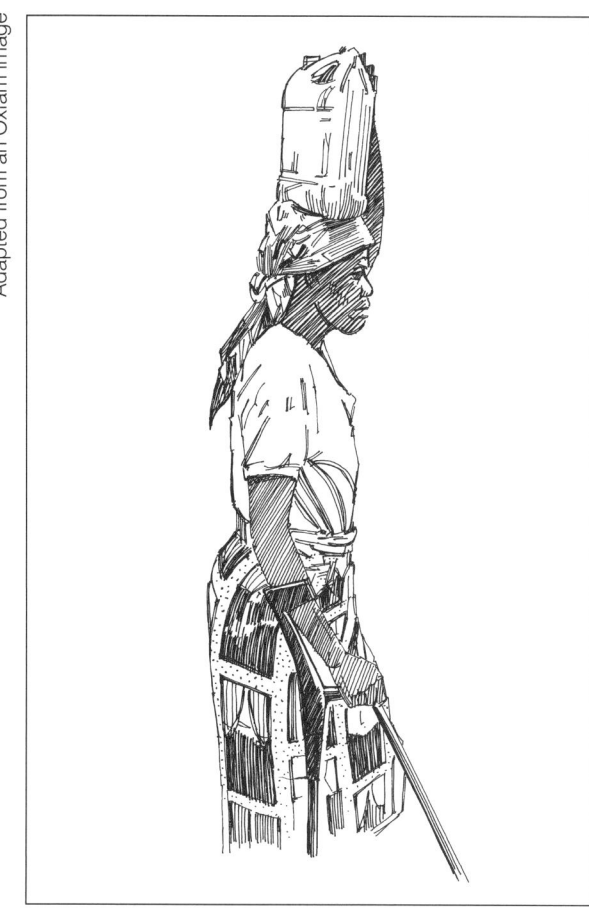

Figure 6.24. Carrying a jerry-can on the head.

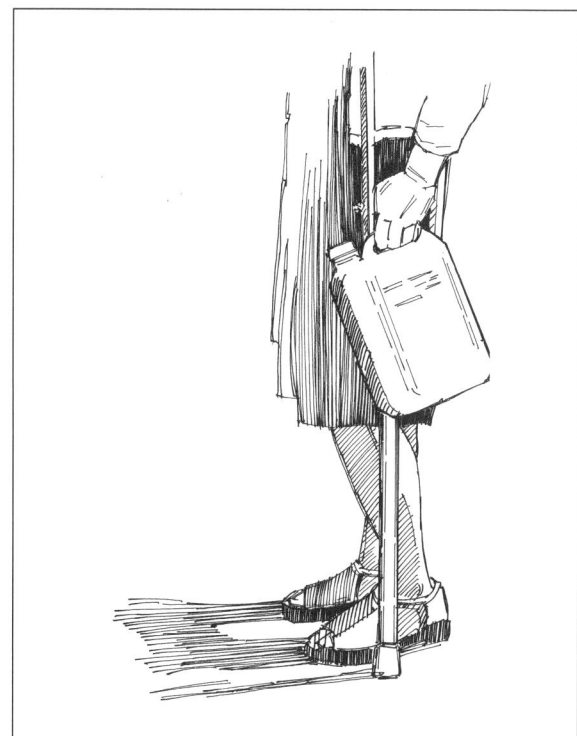

Figure 6.25. Crutch user carrying a jerry-can with three fingers.

Adapted from an Oxfam image

the flow of water more easily, for washing and other uses. The hose should be stored off the ground when not in use, to stop it resting on the ground and getting dirty, and contaminating the water and container.

The tap needs to be positioned high enough from the ground or shelf to allow a range of sizes of container to be filled. If it is very low, or over a hand-basin, it may be difficult to fill large water containers.

6.4   Transporting water

The need to transport water can be reduced by (a) bringing the water point nearer to the user (see Section 5.4 under Proximity on page 45), and (b) taking water-related tasks to the water source, such as bathing and washing clothes.

It is the norm in many countries to see children and women fetching water in pairs or groups. Often, one person pumps water while the other holds the container. In this context, the contribution of a disabled person to the group activity is often valued, even if they can only do one aspect of the task, such as carrying, but not drawing water.

Few devices or containers are specifically designed for use by disabled people, but the advantages and disadvantages of equipment and containers in general use are discussed here.

Ways of carrying water
Direct carrying
Water can be carried by disabled people in a number of ways: on the head (Figure 6.24), on the back (Figure 6.13), on crutches – either in the hand (Figure 6.25), or in an adapted container (Figure 6.26).

Wooden yoke
A wooden or bamboo pole rests on one or both shoulders with a container on each end. This method allows more weight to be carried

6

Water supply – access and use

75

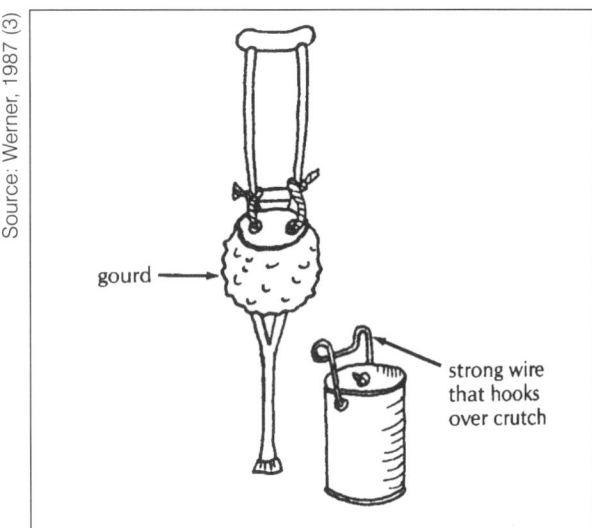

Source: Werner, 1987 (3)

gourd →

strong wire that hooks over crutch →

Figure 6.26. Adaptations for carrying things with crutches.

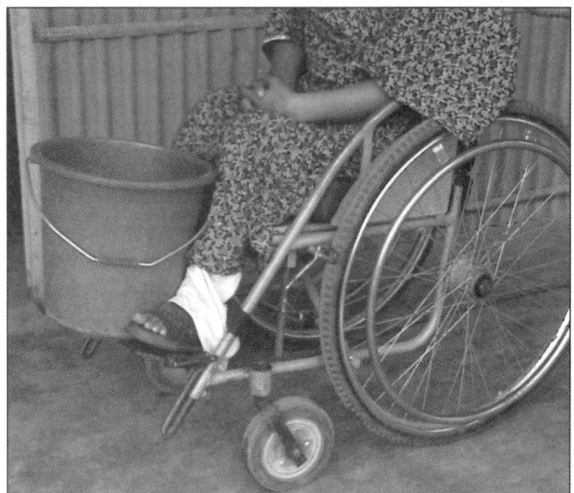

Figure 6.27. Plastic bucket carried on the footrest of a wheelchair. A rubber strap would help keep it in place. *(Case-study 9.4, page 169)*

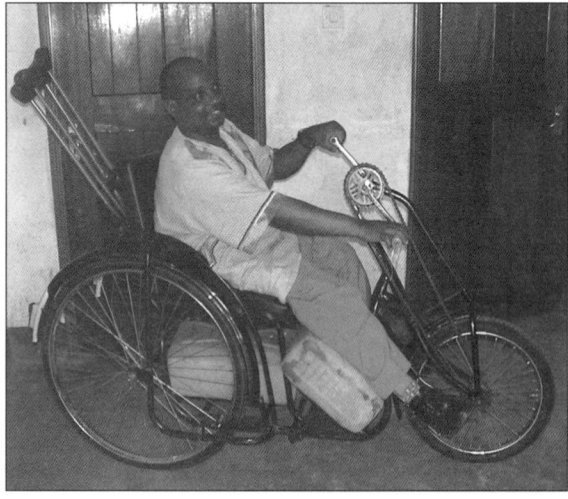

Figure 6.28. Two jerry-cans carried under the seat of this wheelchair. *(Case-study 9.24, page 224)*

than in a hand-held container, and is widely used by the general population in East and South-east Asia (see Case-study 9.11 on page 187). The yoke is suitable for users who may have damaged arms or hands, or limited grip, but who can walk.

Weight can be shared by carrying a pole on the shoulders of two people, with a container of water suspended from the pole between them. In this way a person with limited strength can contribute to carrying water.

Indirect carrying – using equipment

Wheelchair
Water containers can be carried on a wheelchair in various ways:

- On the footrest: Jerry-cans (see page 77) are most suitable for this, because their square shape can be wedged between the user's legs. Round containers such as buckets or jars are more difficult to carry on a footrest (Figure 6.27). They may need to be kept in place with a strap, hooked onto the frame on each side of the chair and round the container. Straps can be made from recycled inner tube (Figure 6.39).

- Under the seat: this is possible with some designs of wheelchair (Figure 6.28).

- On the knee or beside the user – suitable for small containers up to 5 litres.

- Hooked onto the handles on the back of the chair. A bag with a long strap, or a sling made from a local cloth, sarong or wrapper can be used. Care must be taken not to carry too much weight, otherwise the wheelchair could tip up.

Wheelchair trailer
A trailer can be attached behind a wheelchair, and carry more weight than could be carried directly on a wheelchair or on the head. It can also be used to carry goods to market, or even young children! A wooden two-wheeled trailer hooks onto the back of a wheelchair, which can easily be detached when not in use (Figures 6.29 and 6.30). This could also be

6

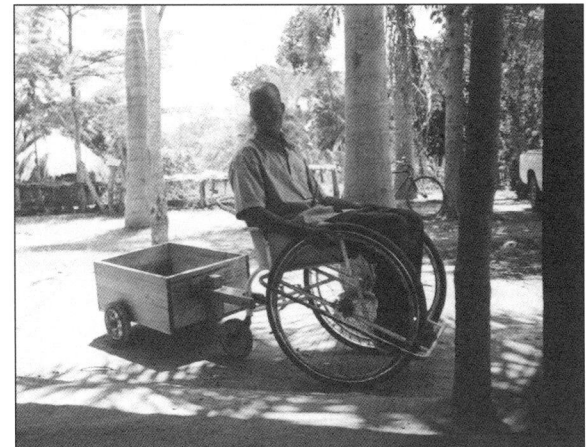

Figure 6.29. Two-wheeled wooden wheelchair trailer.

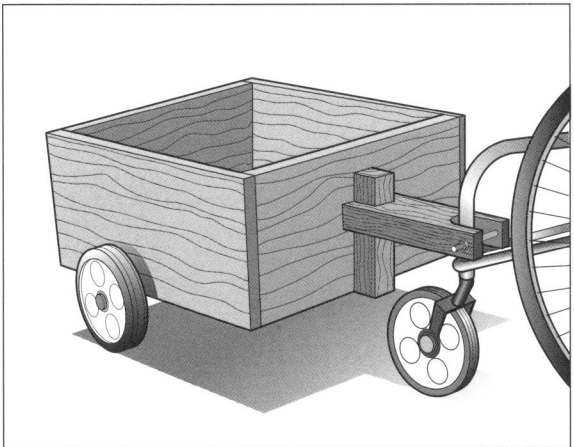

Figure 6.30. Detail of how the trailer attaches to the wheelchair frame.

used as a hand-drawn trailer, with a different pulling arrangement, such as a rope.

A trailer may not be suitable for rough, narrow paths.

Types of water container
Jerry-cans

A **jerry-can** is a plastic or metal container with a handle and screw lid. They are widely used in Africa to transport and store water in various ways. They have a number of features that make them convenient for disabled people:

- They are cheap, durable and widely available in Africa.

- They are available in different sizes, from 1 to 25 litres. The smallest – 1 litre – is small and light enough for a disabled child to carry when filled (Figure 6.32).

- Wheelchair users can select the size of jerry-can that suits them. It needs to fit the space available, such as the footrest of the chair, and be light enough to be lifted on and off without unbalancing the wheelchair.

- The handle makes it possible to carry using two or three fingers, which means it can be carried while walking with crutches (Figure 6.25). Threading the rope through a short piece of pipe, bamboo or used bicycle inner tube can make the handle wider and more comfortable to carry.

- Using rope or string, the handle can be made any length for the convenience of the user when either filling or carrying water. This can be useful for someone with a lack of reach or who has trouble bending.

- The square shape makes it easy to carry on its side, and the screw-on lid prevents spilling, even when the container is carried on its side, or moved erratically.

6

Source: Werner, 1987 (3)

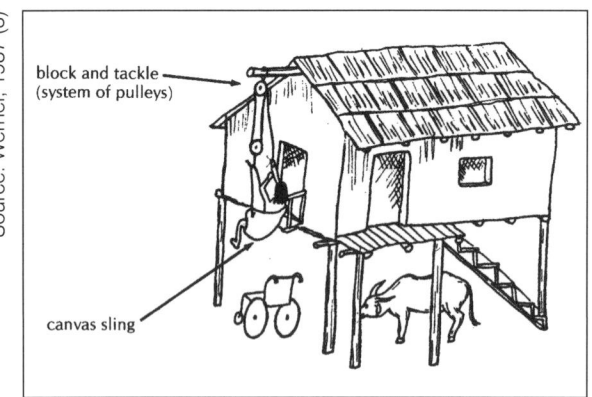

Figure 6.31. Rope and pulley system could be used to lift water, or even people.

- The square shape allows jerry-cans to be packed closely together, which makes good use of available space under a wheelchair (Figure 6.28) or on the footrest. They can also be carried on the head.

- The plastic is strong but flexible enough to be adapted by cutting and piercing (Figure 6.33).

Drawbacks of jerry-cans
- Less widely available outside Africa.

- The lid is easily lost, so bananas, leaves or other unhygienic objects are often used to close the opening to prevent spilling, which can cause contamination.

- They are difficult to clean inside, so contamination and unsightly algal growth (green slime) can be a problem.

- A lot of spillage occurs when filling because of the narrow opening.

Buckets and bowls
Buckets and bowls have an advantage for disabled people in being easy to fill because of their wide opening. They can be placed on the floor, and even if there is a long distance between the water spout and the bucket, little water is wasted in collection.

Box 6.2. Houses built on stilts

In many parts of the world, entry to the house is up a steep wooden ladder. Carrying a bucket of water upstairs to the house is possible for a person with only one leg, or weak legs, who cannot walk up the steps. This can be done by sitting on one step at a time and pulling the container up to balance on each subsequent step. This task can be made easier if the ladder, rather than having round rungs, has steps, which provide a flat surface to rest the bucket on. (4)

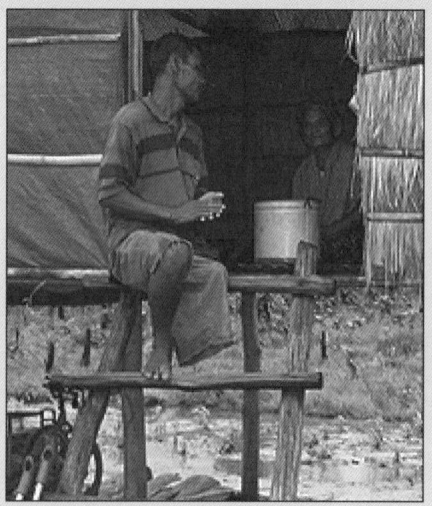

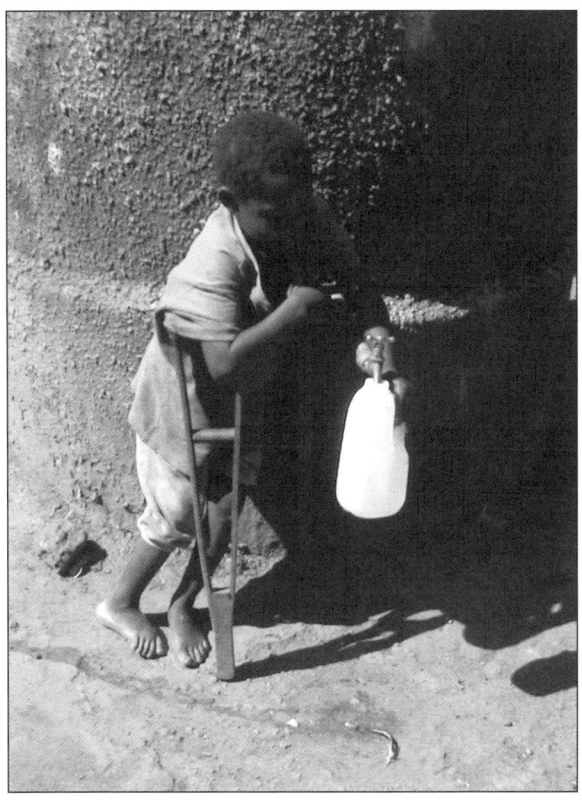

Figure 6.32. A full 1 litre jerry-can is light enough for a child to hold in one hand.
(Case-study 9.30, page 245)

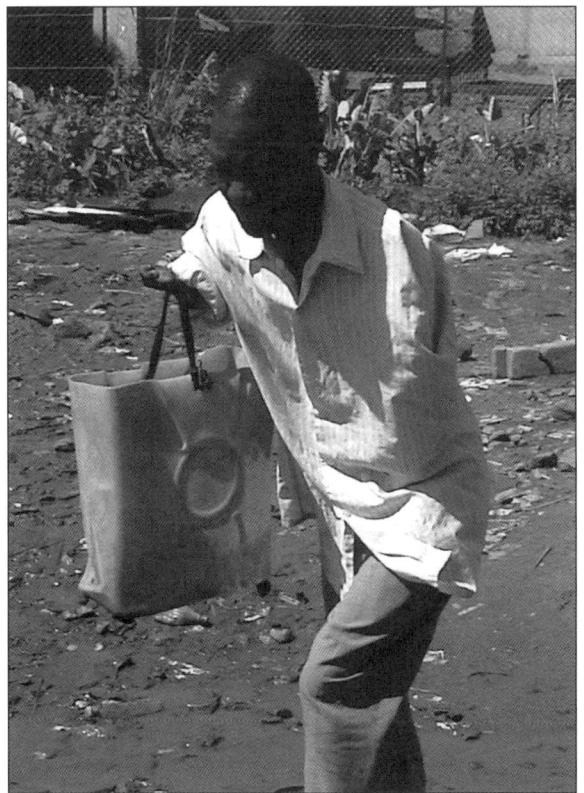

Figure 6.33. A man with one very short arm carries an adapted jerry-can one third full.
(Case-study 9.22, page 221)

Buckets are suitable for large quantities of water. Both bowls and buckets are easy to empty and clean. A tight fitting lid can reduce spillage during transport, and contamination during transport and storage.

Used food cans and other containers can be adapted for collection and storage of water.

For lifting water from a well, the size of container can be adjusted to suit the strength of the user. In this way, the weight of water and any risk of rope burn are reduced, which is of particular benefit to people with limited strength or poor grip, such as elderly people and children. Water can then be emptied into a larger container for transporting if required.

Drawbacks: Bowls are very difficult to carry without spilling water. Buckets are easier to carry than bowls, but are still inconvenient to carry because of their width, and the wide opening, which makes it easy to spill water.

Tight fitting lids are hard to make and not always widely available.

Traditional water jars
Traditional aluminium and clay water jars are widely available in a range of sizes. Their wide opening makes them easy to fill and to clean. However, they have no handle, which makes them difficult for disabled people to carry, as they must be carried by holding the rim of the jar. They have no lid, which means there is the risk of spilling water, and of contamination.

A handle could be made with string or rope tied round the neck of the jar.

Soda bottles
Soda bottles (1 litre), with a screw-top to prevent spilling and contamination, can be carried easily by a wheelchair user, as they do not need to be carried upright, and can be carried on the knee, or tucked between the chair arm and the user's side.

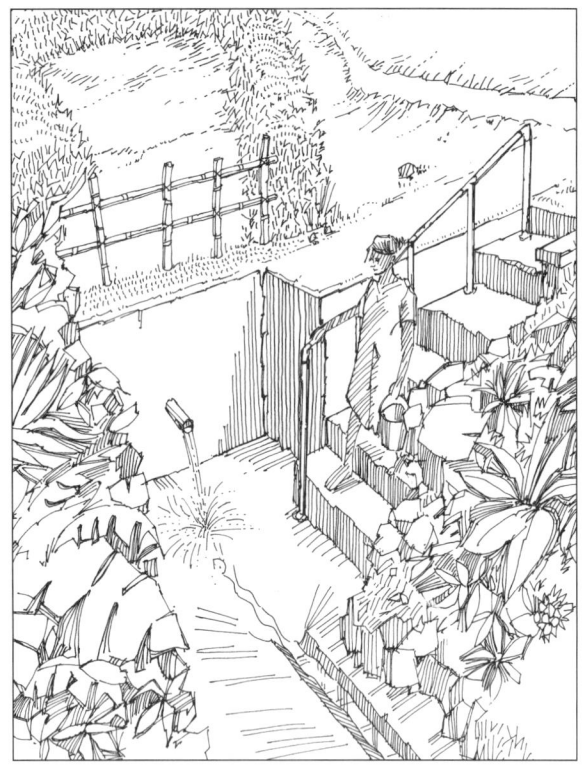

Figure 6.34. Protected spring with a rail for guidance and safety.

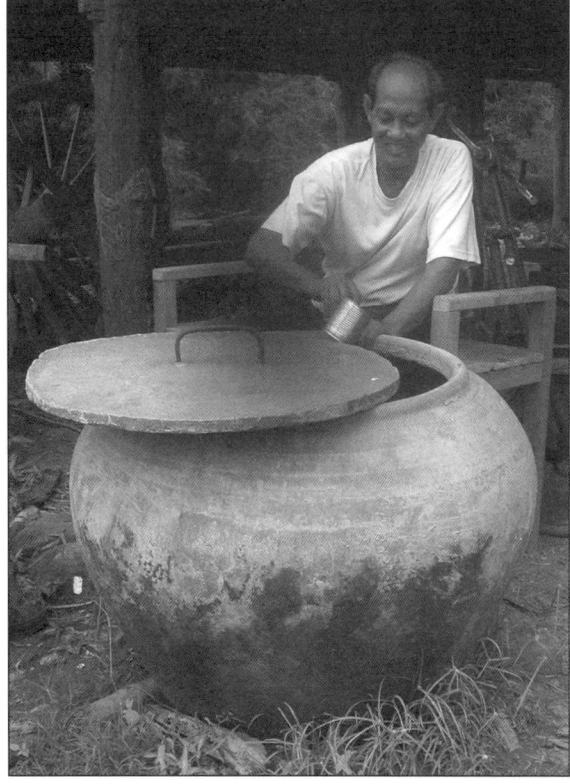

Figure 6.35. Ferrocement water storage jar. Water is scooped from the top using a mug.
(Case-study 9.17, page 209)

Drawbacks: The narrow neck makes them slow to fill at a tap, and almost impossible to fill at a handpump without using some type of funnel. They have no handle, which makes them difficult to carry for a crutch user or someone with poor grip. Some bottles can be fitted with a carrying handle made of string or rope.

Issues for blind and visually impaired people

Getting to and from a water source can be particularly hazardous for people with visual impairment, especially if they are carrying a container of water and have only one hand to feel their way and to steady themselves.

A safety rail or rope is recommended for paths that lead to or past an open water source (Figure 6.34). This is useful for everyone, especially young children, and others with unstable balance, such as pregnant women, elderly people and people with epilepsy. This must be installed at a height of 100cm (adult waist height), otherwise it can become a trip hazard for many users. A lower rail of 75cm high can be added for children.

See also page 57 in Section 5.4 on issues of mobility for blind people.

6.5 Storing water and accessing stored water

Water can be stored in the home in a variety of containers, varying in size from 1 to 500 litres and beyond.

Accessing the water

In general, containers with a wide open top, such as buckets and wide-mouthed jars, are easier for disabled people to use, as they can scoop water from the top with a small container (Figures 6.35 and 6.36). This is possible for most people with a reasonable range of arm movement, and no heavy lifting or pouring is needed. A wide opening also makes the container easy to clean. A lid reduces the risk of contamination.

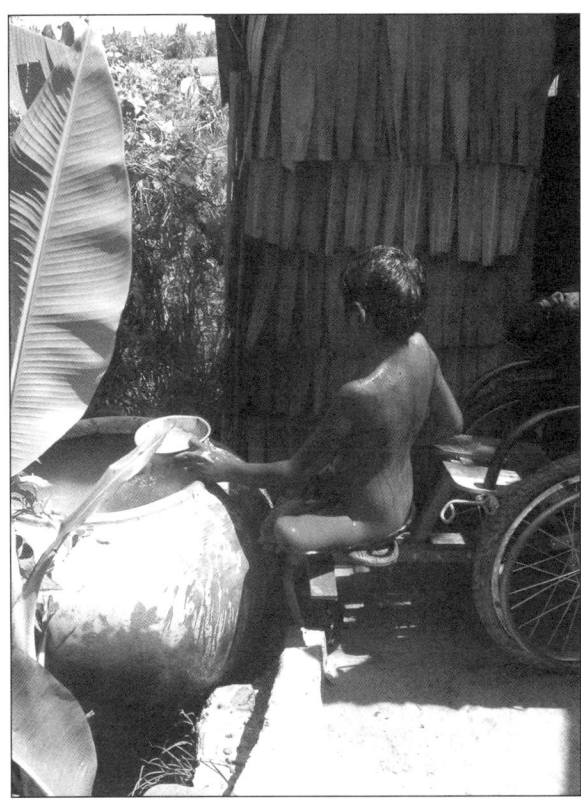

Figure 6.36. Water jar placed below the user, to make it easy to reach in.*
(Case-study 9.15, page 201)

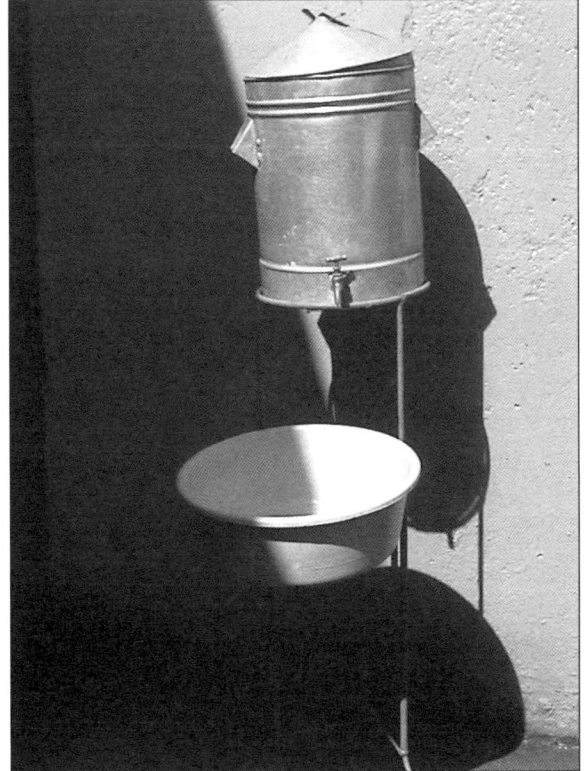

Figure 6.37. Water for handwashing.
(Case-study 9.24, page 224)

The drawback is that the water in a wide-mouthed container is easily contaminated, as any cover must be removed for access, and a scoop repeatedly dipped in the water. This is not a problem if the water is used for bathing or washing clothes, but it is not recommended for storing drinking water.

For people with limited arm movement, a tap fitted near the bottom of a container makes it easier to draw water (Figure 6.37 and 6.38). The container needs to be raised off the ground so that the tap is at a convenient height. However, raising the container can also make it more difficult for the disabled user to fill and clean.

A flexible hose attached to a storage container, or to a tap, can be useful for bathing and anal cleansing (Figures 6.70 and 7.55). This can either be attached to a tap, or have a tap on the end of the hose to control the flow. The end of the hose must be hooked off the floor when not in use to avoid getting it dirty.

For handwashing a 'tippy tap' can be used. This consists of a can which releases a small amount of water – just enough for a clean handwash – each time it is tipped. It can be used with one hand.

Drinking water is best stored in a container with a close-fitting lid to reduce contamination. Ideally the water should be delivered through a tap as described above (Figure 6.38). If the water has to be scooped from the top, a two-cup system should be used. This means that the scoop is used only for scooping into other containers, and never for drinking from.

Plastic jugs with handles and a lid are widely available in different sizes, from 2 to 3.5 litres. These are suitable for storing and pouring smaller quantities of water, particularly for drinking. The handle makes it usable by a person with poor grip. The lid prevents contamination.

6

* Note: the footrest of this wheelchair is designed for sitting on. Many wheelchairs will tip over if the user sits on the footrest (see pages 92-93), Wheelchairs for bathing).

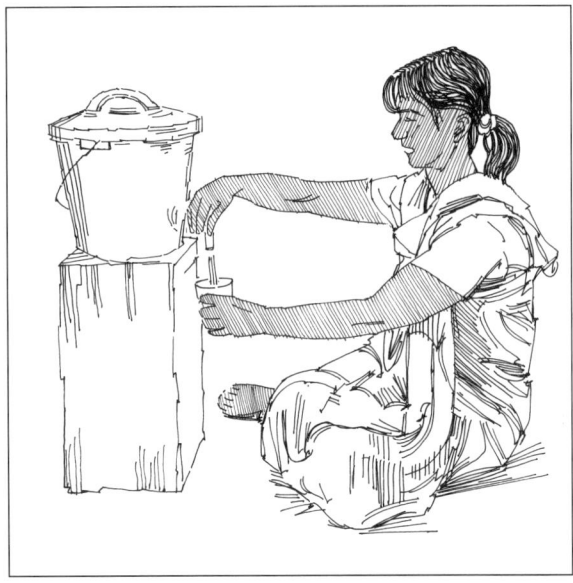

Figure 6.38. Disabled woman pouring a drink of water.

Location

Water is most useful when provided at the point of use, such as next to the bathing/laundry area, or inside a latrine. The container needs to be positioned so that the disabled user can easily access the water. In some cases this means raising the container (Figure 6.37), and in other cases lowering it in relation to the user, so that it is easier to reach in and scoop water (Figure 6.36).

If the container is raised off the floor, it needs to be held in place so that it is not knocked over. A wooden or metal stand (Figure 6.37) or a rubber strap made of recycled tyre inner tube (Figure 6.39) are two ways of doing this.

The container can be suspended, as in the case of a tippy tap used for handwashing (Figure 6.40).

Filling the storage container

Water which is stored at the point of use enables disabled people to be more self-reliant, as they can access water when they need it (Figures 6.39 and 6.41). Even if the water container has to be filled by family members, the disabled person does not have to request and wait for water each time he or she needs it. Family members can fill the container at their own convenience, on a daily or weekly basis, rather than each time the disabled person needs it, which may be several times a day.

Water stored at the point of use can be fed by a gravity system from a primary source. A flexible hose leads from the main storage container to the smaller secondary container, which must be positioned lower than the main container (Figure 9.66). The hose has a tap on the end, which allows the user to stop and start the water flow at the point of use, and to fill the secondary jar as required.

Figure 6.39. Water storage jar in bathing area, raised on a wooden stand and held in place with a rubber strap.
(Case-study 9.14, page 197)

Sarah House, WEDC

6

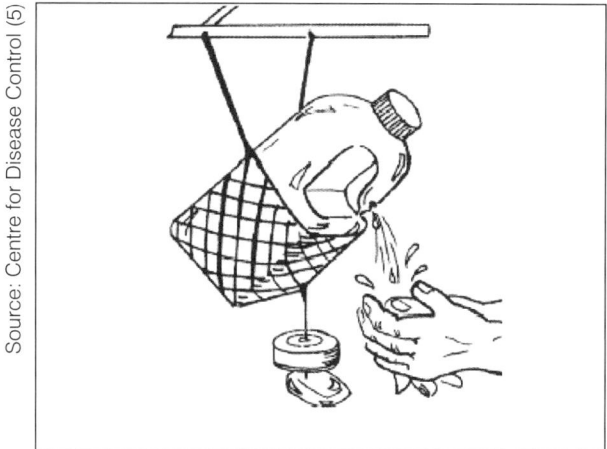

Figure 6.40. Tippy tap for handwashing.

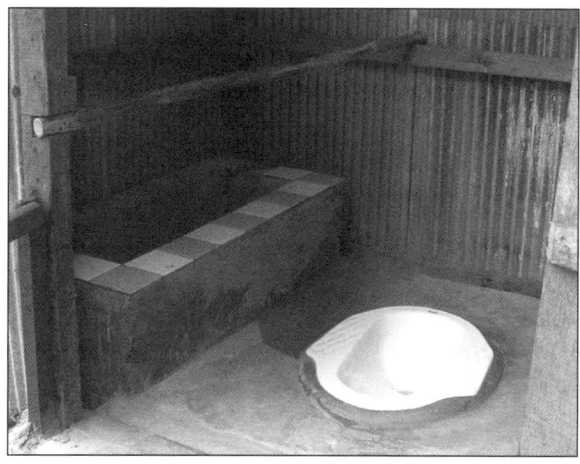

Figure 6.41. Water trough next to the toilet.
(Case-study 9.19, page 215)

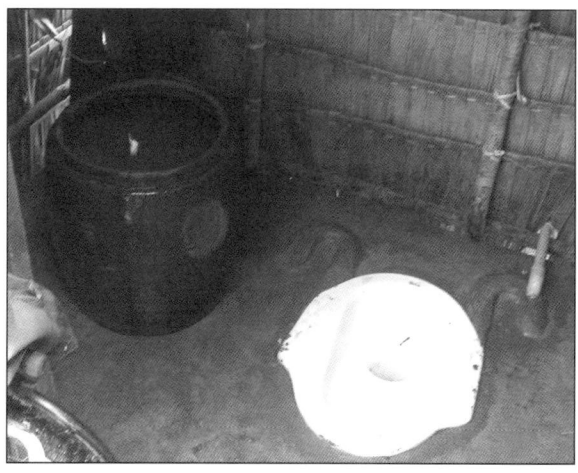

Figure 6.42. Water jar next to the toilet.
(Case-study 9.15, page 201)

6.6　Bathing

Bathing facilities can take a range of forms, levels of sophistication and cost, from specially designed brick built rooms with internal piped water to bathing in a pond.

Benefits of inclusive facilities

Wherever possible, the aim should be for the disabled person to use the same facilities as the rest of the family. None of the features described here excludes non-disabled people from using the same facilities. Accessible facilities can promote inclusiveness, but also bring positive benefits to other family members, especially frail elderly people, women and children.

At the same time, some individual equipment can provide more flexibility for disabled users. For example, they may wish to move a bathing seat to a different location, depending on the time of year, or use it for a different purpose, such as washing clothes. Such equipment can be moved out of the way when not in use, to prevent it getting dirty or damaged, and to prevent it obstructing other users.

Accessible bathing facilities have a number of features in common.

Getting there and getting in

See pages 45 to 60 for issues related to getting to and into facilities.

Privacy

In many countries and communities, it is traditional for both men and women to bathe in the open, usually in separate areas, or at separate times. A piece of cloth such as a wrapper or sarong is often used for personal privacy. Many people with movement or co-ordination problems may have difficulty manipulating a wrapper in this way. This can be made easier by adding elastic to the top of the wrapper to keep it in place at the waist, below the arms or around the neck.

6

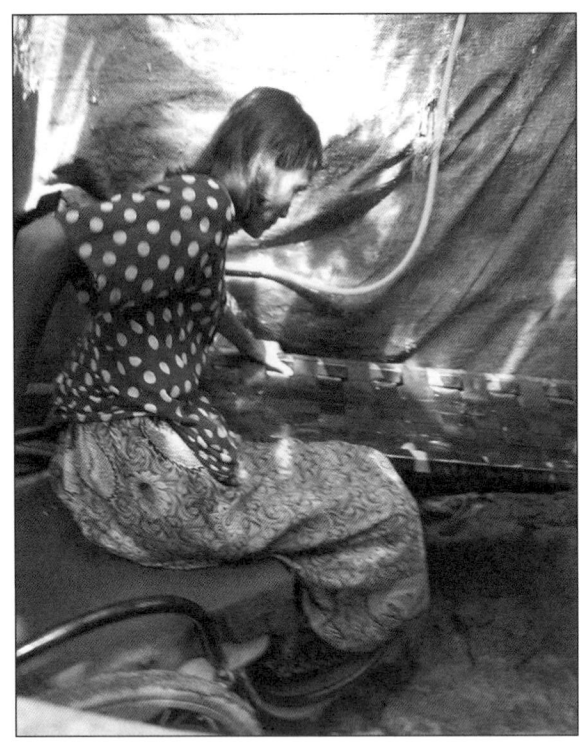

Figure 6.43. Space for the wheelchair beside the bathing seat for easy transfer.

Figure 6.44. Sitting on a low stool to bathe.

Additional privacy may be needed while bathing, especially for women. A private bathing area can be created at low cost, using screens of locally available materials, such as leaves (Figure 6.45), wood, or plastic sheets (Figure 6.47).

See page 60 in Section 5.4 for further discussion of privacy and security.

Internal space and layout
See Section 5.4 on page 60 for issues related to internal dimensions and extra space to suit the needs of different users.

If the bather needs to transfer from a wheelchair to a bathing seat, space should be provided so that a wheelchair can be positioned beside the seat for easy transfer (Figure 6.43).

Floor
The floor should be level with a slight fall for drainage, and it needs to be even, to allow a wheelchair to stand firm while the user transfers, and so that bathers who are blind, or unsteady on their feet do not risk falling. The floor should not be too smooth, to prevent it from becoming slippery when wet. Good drainage also helps to reduce slipperiness. The drainage outlet should encourage water to flow away from the bathing area.

See pages 51, Surface of paths and step, and page 61, Floors, for detailed discussion of materials for floor surfaces.

Internal water source
A water source at or inside the bathing area is a great advantage, as it saves the disabled person carrying water or having to ask a family member to fetch water.

See Section 6.5, pages 80 - 82, for discussion of water storage options and pages 92 and 94 for ideas for simple showers.

6

Examples of screening materials for bathing areas

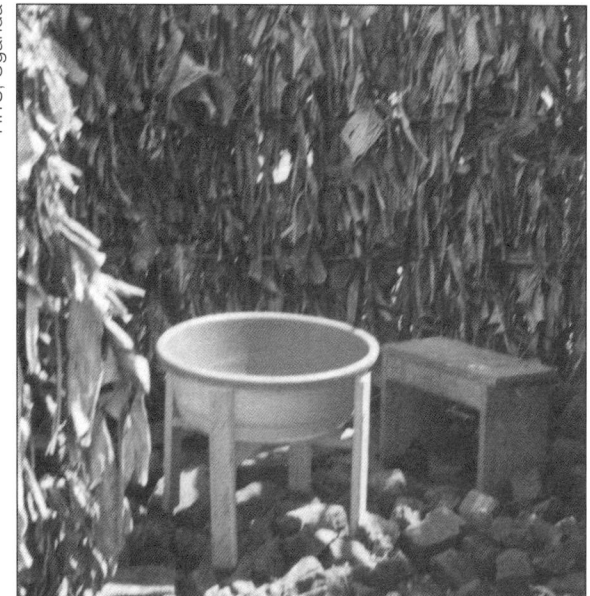

Figure 6.45. Demonstration bathing area (the floor surface is not recommended). *(Case-study 9.31 on page 247)*

Wall	Leaves on a wood frame
Cost	Low
Longevity	6 – 12 months

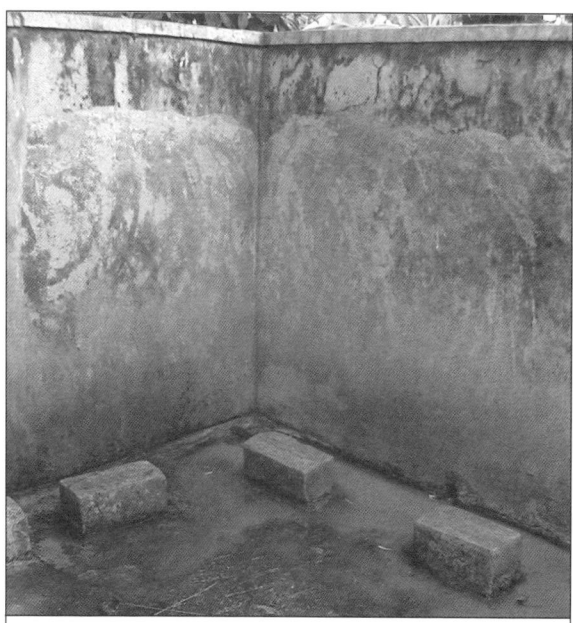

Figure 6.46. Communal bathing area in residential school. *(Case-study 9.25 on page 229)*

Wall	Cement-plastered brick
Cost	High
Longevity	5 years +

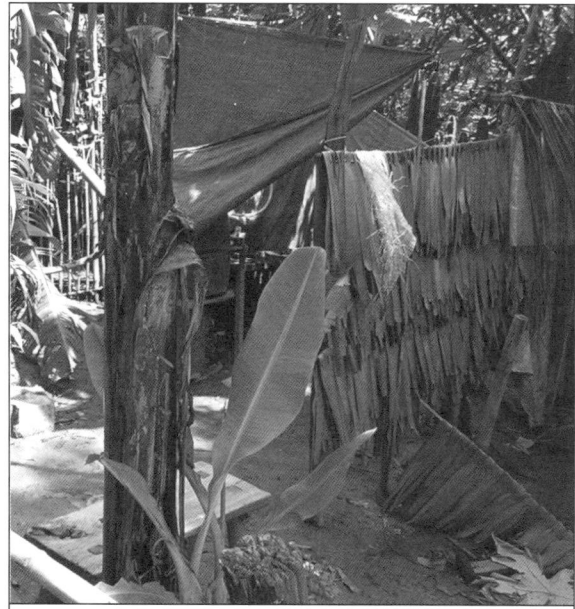

Figure 6.47. Household bathing area. *(Case-study 9.14 on page 197)*

Wall	Palm leaves on bamboo frame
Cost	Low
Longevity	6 – 12 months

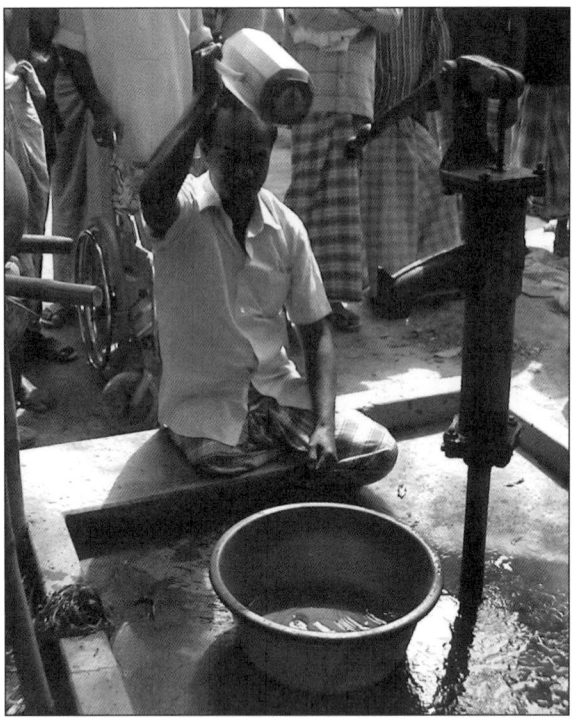

Figure 6.48. Low concrete sitting platform.
(Case-study 9.2, page 161)

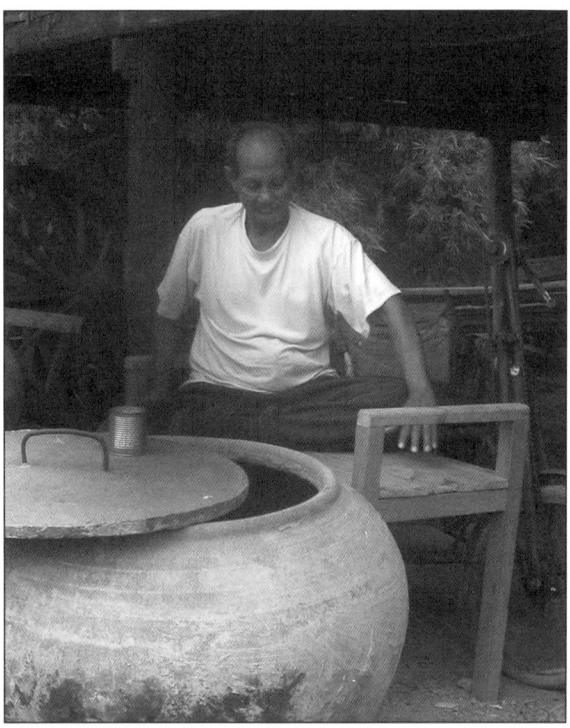

Figure 6.49. Wooden bathing bench next to water source.
(Case-study 9.17, page 209)

Bathing at the water source

In many communities, it is usual to bathe at the water source rather than to carry water to a separate bathing area. There are a number of design and equipment options to enable disabled people to bathe at a water source comfortably.

A water point may be designed and constructed to enable bathing and other water-related activities to take place there. A sitting area next to the water is comfortable not only for disabled people but also for women and elderly people. For example, a flat concrete platform built on the edge of a handpump apron allows a disabled bather to sit at the pump to bathe (Figure 6.48). It also allows the women in the family to sit comfortably to do their laundry and bathe their children, it reduces back-ache and injury from too much bending, and reduces accidents from slipping on the wet apron.

A seat or bench placed next to a water source can allow a disabled person to bathe with less help (Figures 6.49, 6.62 and 6.69).

Bathing in natural water sources

Where a pond or river is used for bathing, the bank around the edge is often muddy and slippery, which can cause problems for many people, especially people who are unsteady on their feet. For a person who can walk, but may need support, a rail of rope or bamboo or similar local materials may be useful to reach the water safely. The rail should also extend into the water, to provide support to hold onto whilst bathing (Figure 6.50).

An alternative is to place a bathing seat beside the pond, so that the person can sit on it to bathe.

Bathing seats

A seat is needed for the bather to avoid sitting or lying on a wet or dirty floor, in his own wastewater. It may be a fixed feature of the facility, such as the concrete platform in Figure 6.48. Or it may be a piece of furniture, such as a stool or bench, chosen or designed for the individual disabled user as in Figure 6.49.

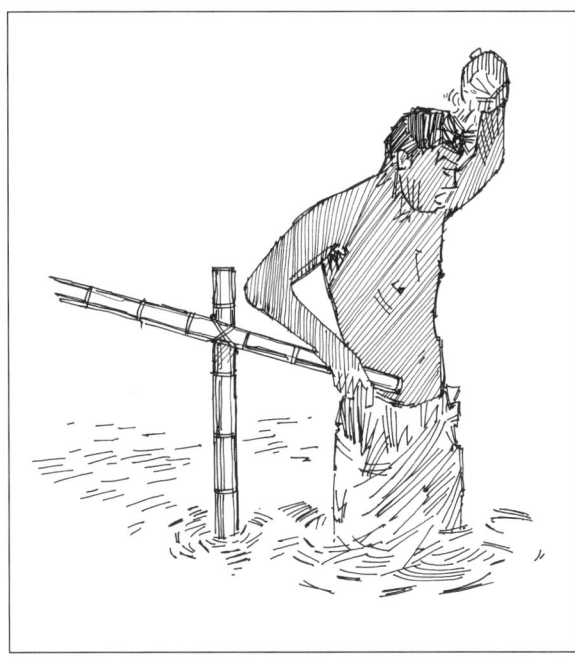

Figure 6.50. Bamboo rail leading into the bathing pond.

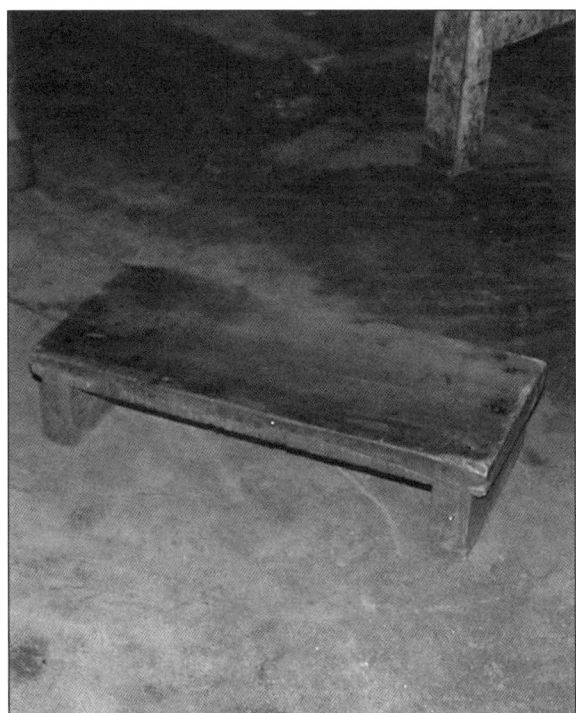

Figure 6.51. Low wooden stool, widely used throughout South Asia to carry out floor level tasks.
(Case-study 9.4, page 169)

---

* People who lie or sit in one position for long periods risk developing pressure sores. These can take a long time to heal, and can cause permanent damage if left untreated (3).

A bathing seat needs the following features: Appropriate height and support, good drainage, and to be hygienic.

Height
The height of the seat needs to be suitable for transferring easily, whether from standing, crawling or from a wheelchair. This should be decided in consultation with the user as far as possible.

A **low seat** (height: 10 – 25 cm) makes it easy to use a washbowl placed on the floor, and reduces the risk of injury if the bather falls, but makes independent transfer to and from a wheelchair more difficult for some (Figures 6.44, 6.45, 6.51 and 6.52).

A **seat at similar height to a wheelchair seat**, or **at knee height** or above, is convenient for transfer to and from a wheelchair, and is easy for a bather with poor balance or difficulty bending to sit down and get up again (Figures 6.61 and 6.62).

Support
People with poor sitting balance need a back support to lean against. Side-rails on one or both sides of the seat are good for the person to hold onto for balance while moving on and off the seat, and whilst bathing (Figure 6.49). These can also provide a handle for picking up and moving the seat without having to bend too low (Figure 6.52). However, side-rails can be an obstacle to sideways transfer from a wheelchair. See page 108, Support and safety, and Figures 7.20 and 7.21 for flexible options for side-rails.

Good support needs to be balanced against comfort. Seating materials that provide a high level of support may be the least comfortable. Concrete is firm, but could feel cold and harsh. Concrete edges need to be smoothed and rounded, to avoid injury if the user falls, and to avoid rubbing the skin or making pressure sores worse*. A wooden or bamboo seat can be firm and supportive, but again the edges must be smooth to avoid splinters. Softer, flexible materials, such as

6

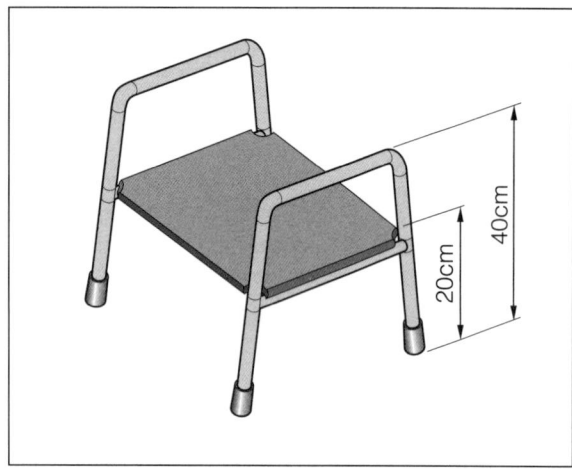

Figure 6.52. Low stool with side-rails.
(Case-study 9.4, page 169)

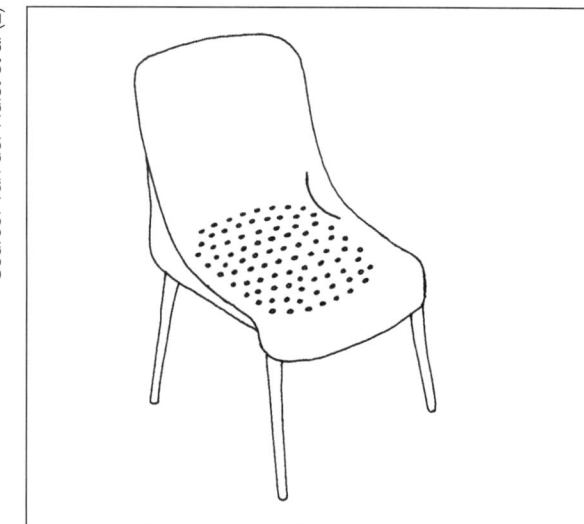

Figure 6.53. Moulded plastic bathing chair
with holes in seat.

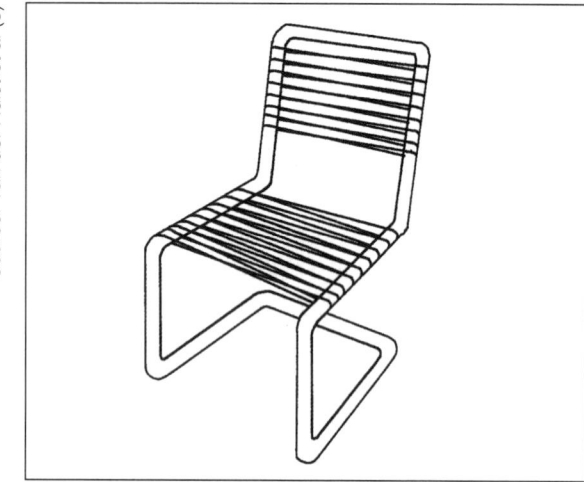

Figure 6.54. Steel tube frame bathing chair with
seat and back of woven plastic strips.

rubber or plastic, are more comfortable to
sit on but may provide less support, so that
a person with poor balance may need extra
support from a raised back and/ or side-rails.
A good compromise can be a supportive
wood or metal frame, but with a softer surface
for sitting or lying, such as woven rubber or
plastic strips (Figures 6.53, 6.54 and 6.61).

Drainage and hygiene

Water needs to drain easily away from the
surface of the seat, so that the bather is not
sitting in his or her own bathwater, which
can be uncomfortable and unhygienic.
Good drainage will also enable the surface
of the seat to dry more quickly, so it does
not deteriorate rapidly. Drainage can be
encouraged in the following ways:

- A narrow seat that lets water run off easily
  (Figures 6.45, 6.51, 6.52 and 6.68);

- Holes or gaps in the seat to let water flow
  through, such as wood or bamboo slats,
  or woven rubber or plastic strips (Figures
  6.53, 6.54 and 6.61).

Materials such as rubber and plastic are easy
to clean and therefore hygienic. If wood,
bamboo, metal or concrete are used, they
should be painted or varnished to make them
moisture resistant, easy to clean and therefore
more hygienic (Figure 6.55).

Bathing while sitting down can make it
difficult for the bather to wash their buttocks.
Solutions to this include using a bathing seat
with a large hole in the middle (Figures 6.55
and 6.56), or with a cut-away section at the
front (Figures 6.57 and 6.58), or raising the
buttocks off the seat, with a cushioned ring
such as a tyre inner tube (Figures 6.59 and
6.67).

Materials

A range of materials can be used to construct
bathing seats, such as concrete, metal,
plastic, rubber, wood, bamboo and even
paper*. In general, the higher the cost of
materials, the greater their durability. Table 6.1
summarises the strengths and weaknesses of
different materials.

Table 6.1 Summary of strengths of different materials

Material	Durability	Cost	Hygiene	Comfort	Support
Concrete	High	High	Good if painted Poor if unpainted	Low	Good
Metal	High	High	Good if painted	Low	Good
Plastic	Good	High	Good at first, but cracks and peels in sun and heat.	Good	Good
Rubber	Good	Medium	Good	Good	Low
Wood	Good	Medium	Good if painted/ varnished	Fair	Good
Bamboo	Low	Low/none	Good if painted/ varnished	Fair	Good
Paper	Low (especially if it gets wet)	Low	Good if painted/ varnished	Good	Good

For information on making furniture from paper, see Appropriate Paper-based Technology (APT) Appendix A2.6, page 273.

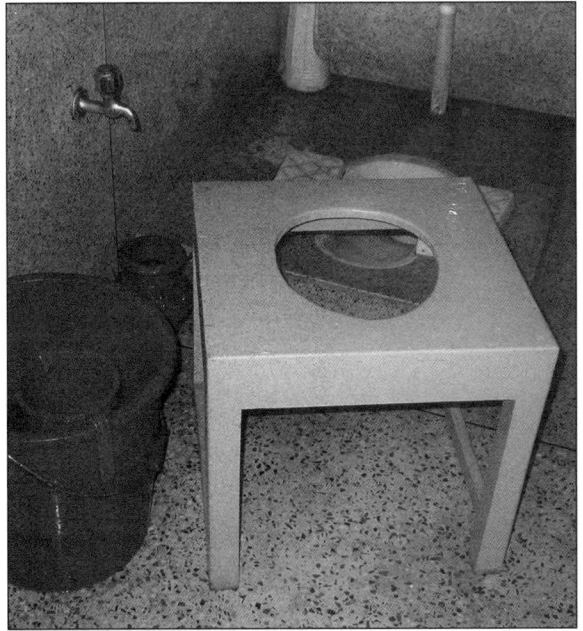

Figure 6.55. Painted wood bathing/toilet seat is moisture resistant and easy to clean.

Bathing benches

If resources and space are available, a bathing bench can provide enough space for the user to put a water container, soap, and clothes beside them when they sit to bathe (Figures 6.61 and 6.62). In this way the bather does not have to bend or reach too far for these items.

The drawback is that a bench takes up more space than a chair or stool. If the bench has more than one function, however, the use of space can be justified. For example, a bathing bench can also be used for eating or sleeping or by other family members.

Advantages

- Saving space – one piece of equipment generally takes up less space than several.

- Reduced cost – only one piece of equipment to pay for.

- Less need for the user to transfer from one seat to another.

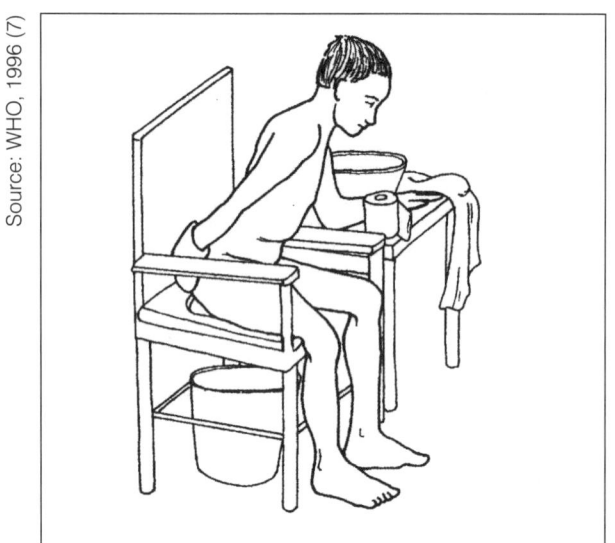

Figure 6.56. Using a bathing chair. Bather washing anal and genital area from behind. To do this, the bather must be able to lift his weight off the seat.

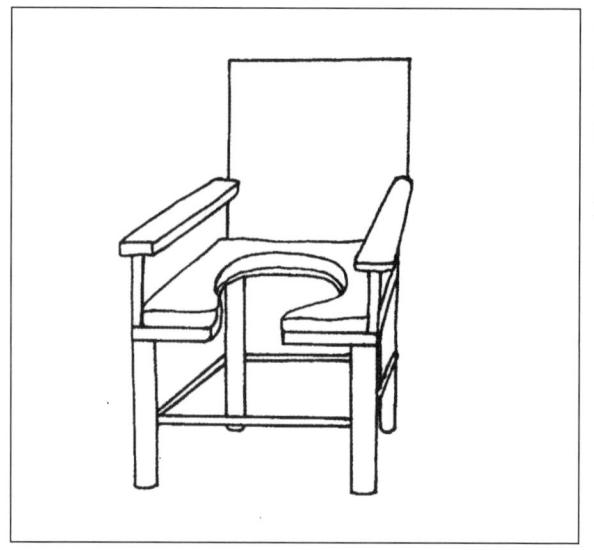

Figure 6.57. Wooden bathing/ toilet chair. The gap in the seat allows access for anal cleansing from the front, but may be uncomfortable for some people to use.

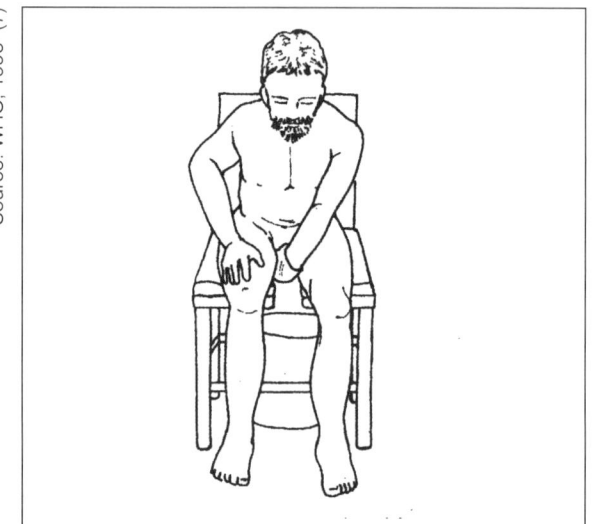

Figure 6.58. Anal cleansing from the front, without the bather lifting his weight off the seat.

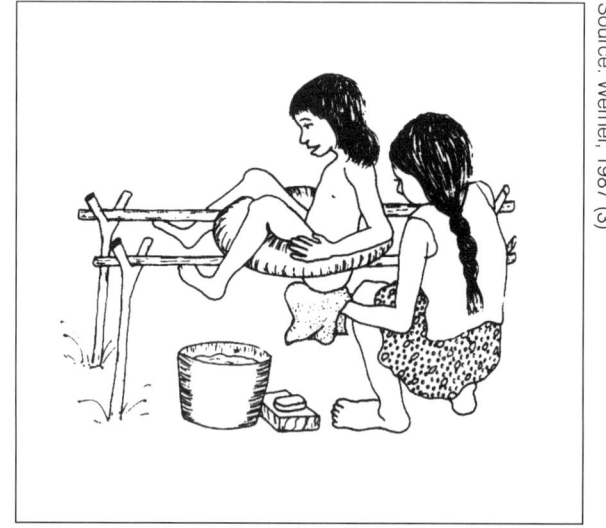

Figure 6.59. An inner tube on poles used as a bathing seat.

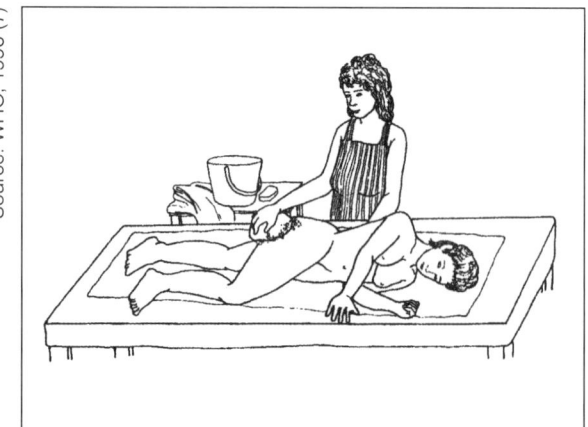

Figure 6.60. Lying on one side to bathe.

6

Water supply – access and use

Examples of multiple use bathing benches

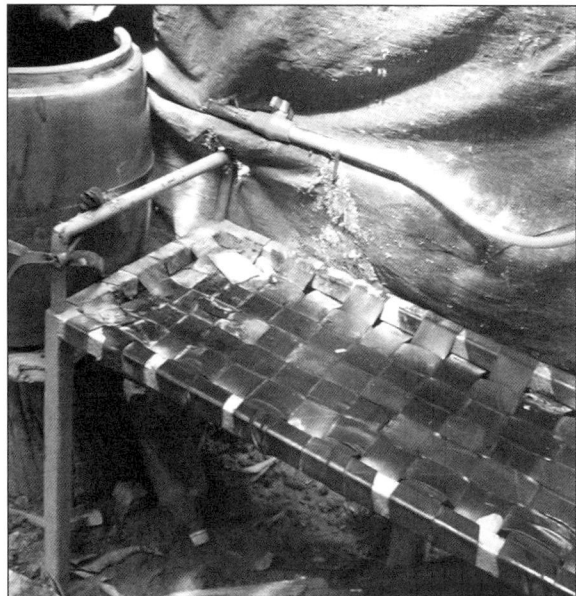

Figure 6.61. Metal framed bathing bench.
(Case-study 9.14, page 197)

Description	Metal framed bathing bench with seat of rubber webbing (woven strips of recycled rubber)
Uses	Bathing, washing clothes
Key features	Rubber webbing is low cost, locally available, durable, easy to clean and comfortable. Good drainage, the bather is not sitting in her own bath water. A rail at each end of the bench for the bather to hold on to for balance.
Drawbacks	Rubber webbing is not very supportive. No back support, so suitable only for users with good balance.

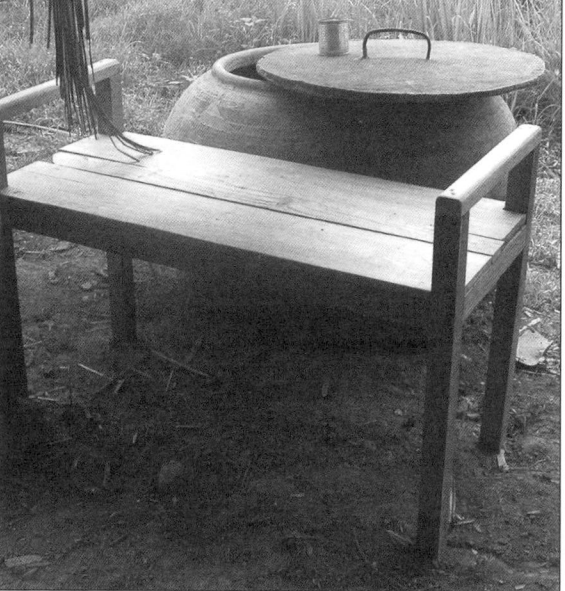

Figure 6.62. Wooden bathing bench.
(Case-study 9.17, page 209)

Description	Wooden bathing bench
Uses	Bathing, washing clothes
Key features	Locally made, reasonable cost. Wood is fairly durable, and easy to clean. A rail at each end for user to hold onto for balance.
Drawbacks	The wide solid surface makes drainage poor, so the wood may deteriorate if it is always wet. No back support – unsuitable for people with poor balance.

6

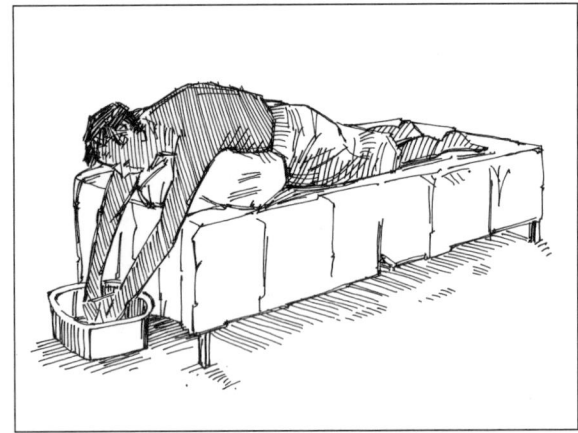

Figure 6.63. Bather lies on his front to bathe. *(Case-study 9.23 on page 223)*

Source: Werner, 1987 (3)

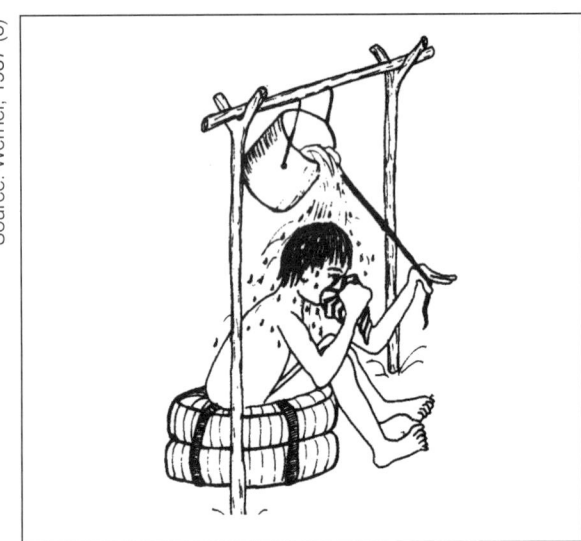

Figure 6.64. Simple shower arrangement.

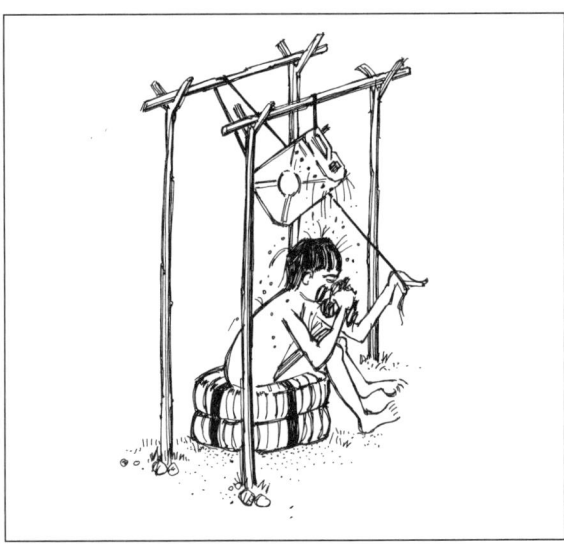

Figure 6.65. Adapted jerry-can with holes pierced around top. *(Case-study 9.27, page 237)*

Drawbacks
Poor drainage – water drains less easily off a wide bench with a solid surface, so the bather sits in a pool of water while bathing. This can result in discomfort and pressure sores. After bathing the seat remains wet, which is a problem if the bench is also used for eating or sleeping.

A woven seat can reduce this problem (Figure 6.61) (see also previous section under Drainage and hygiene, page 188). Rigid wooden slats would also improve drainage, and have the advantage of providing something to hold on to for support.

Wheelchairs for bathing

If a wheelchair is used for bathing, it is important that it is designed for this use. If not, always check for stability, especially when putting weight onto the footrest, which may tip the chair over and cause injury.

Bathing lying down

For disabled people who have difficulty supporting themselves in a sitting position, it may be suitable to bathe lying down, with or without help.

Bathing may be done lying on one side (Figure 6.60), with equipment next to the bather, or lying face down, with the wash-basin on the floor (Figure 6.63).

For comfort, and to prevent the bedclothes getting wet, a towel or plastic sheet may be spread under the bather.

Equipment used for bathing

A variety of equipment can be used by disabled people and their family members to enable them to bathe more easily and independently.

Water supply – access and use

Examples of wheelchairs used for bathing

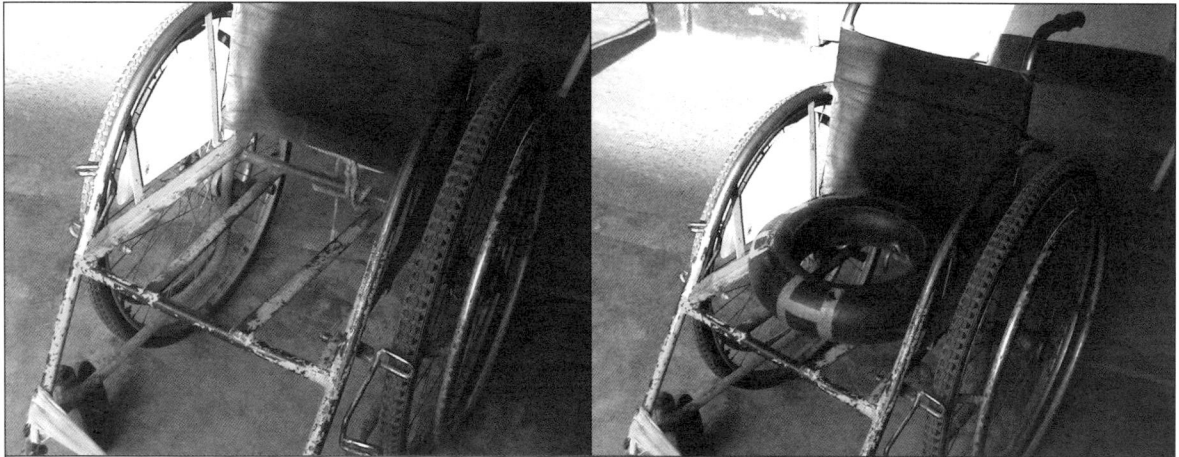

Figures 6.66 and 6.67. Wheelchair convertible to a bathing seat. Wheelchair with cushion and seat board removed and tyre inner tube in place.
(Case-study 9.3, page 164)

Description	The wheelchair has a removable seat board and cushion. These are replaced by a small tyre inner tube, which is supported on two metal struts, but with a wide enough gap for drainage.
Use	The bather enters the bathroom in the wheelchair, replaces the seat with the inner tube, which he or she sits on while bathing.

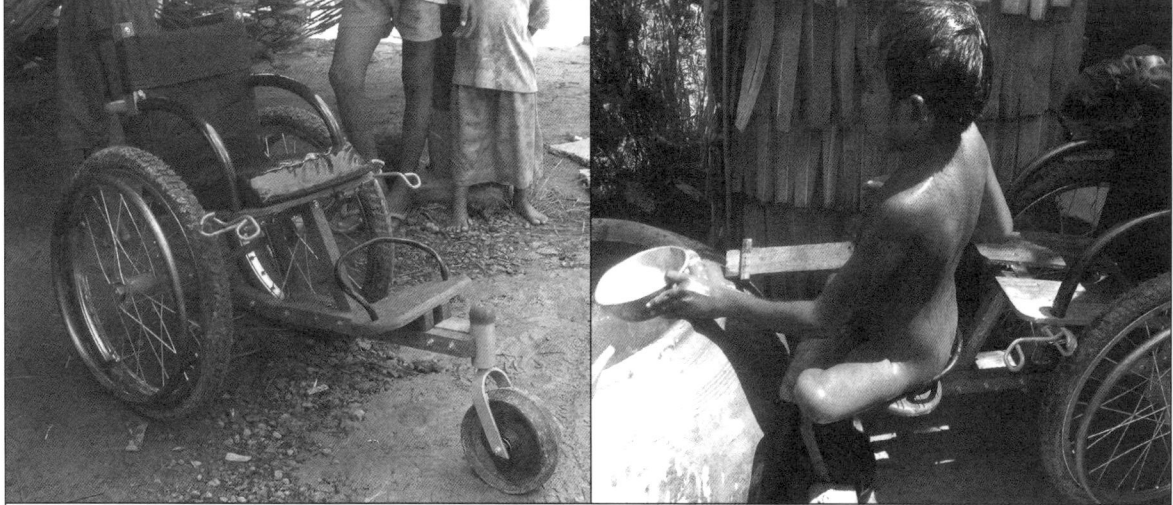

Figures 6.68 and 6.69. Wheelchair with wooden footrest and child sitting on footrest to bathe.
(Case-study 9.15, page 201)

Description	Wheelchair with wooden footrest located behind the single front wheel. It also serves as a 'transfer' seat between the seat and the ground. A metal rail holds the feet in place, and also acts as seat back.
Use	Bather parks the wheelchair next to the water source and lowers himself to sit on the footrest. He bathes sitting on the footrest. When he has finished, he lifts himself back onto the chair seat.

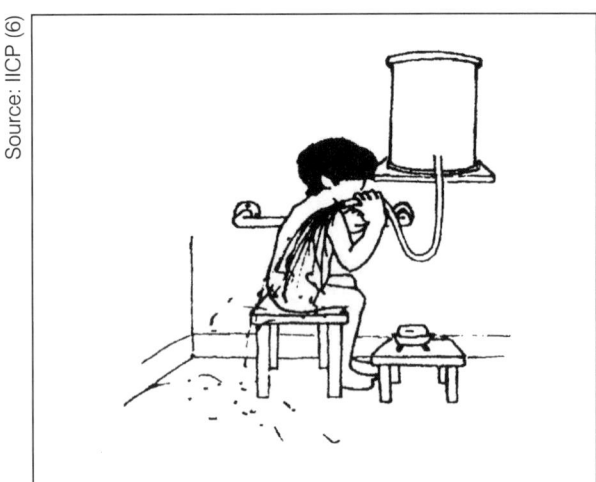

Figure 6.70. Bathing with a flexible hose connected to a water container.

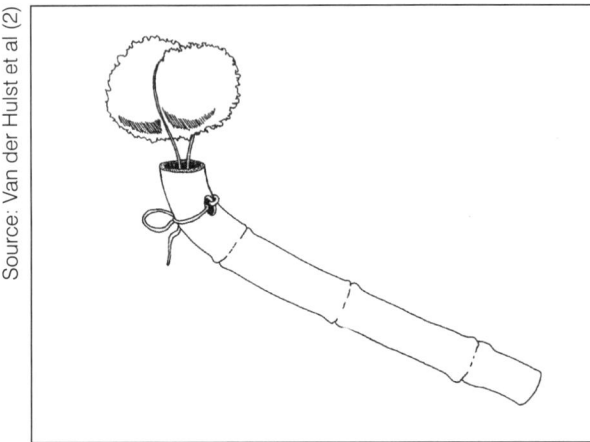

Figure 6.71. Bathing sponge on a bamboo stick.

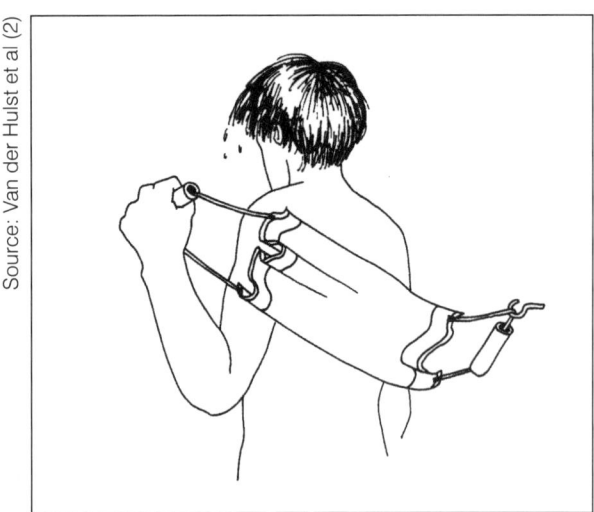

Figure 6.72. Towel with a loop at each end. One end is attached to a hook in the wall, so it can be used with one hand.

Simple showers

Many disabled people find it difficult to move their arms enough to scoop water over themselves, because of poor co-ordination or stiff or weak arms. Simple shower arrangements can make it easier for many people to bathe more independently (Figures 6.64 and 6.65 and 6.70).

Family members may still need to fill the container, but this is probably less time consuming than helping the person bathe.

Cloths and brushes

People with stiffness or limited movement of one or both arms can use a long-handled bath brush or long loofah to wash all parts of the body, so long as they have a good grip (Figure 6.71).

For people with weak grip, loops may be sewn on each end of an ordinary wash-cloth, which the bather can hold one in each hand. The cloth can be made of any length, to suit the bather. If the person only uses one hand, they could hold one loop with a foot, or attach it to a fixed object (Figure 6.72).

A person with the use of only one arm may have difficulty washing that arm. Some kind of sponge or brush can be fixed to a wall for the bather to rub their arm against (Figure 6.73).

Implement holders

An implement holder can be useful for people with limited use of their hands (Figure 6.74). This can be made to any height, to stand on the floor or table, or be fixed to a table or other furniture as needed. A holder that can be used to hold any implement – toothbrush, spoon, comb, etc. – is the most useful (Figure 6.75).

Artificial arm attachment

Some types of artificial arm for amputees are designed with attachments that can be interchanged. A bowl or scoop for pouring water over the body when bathing is one possible option (Figures 6.76, 6.77 and 6.78). A double amputee would need help to attach

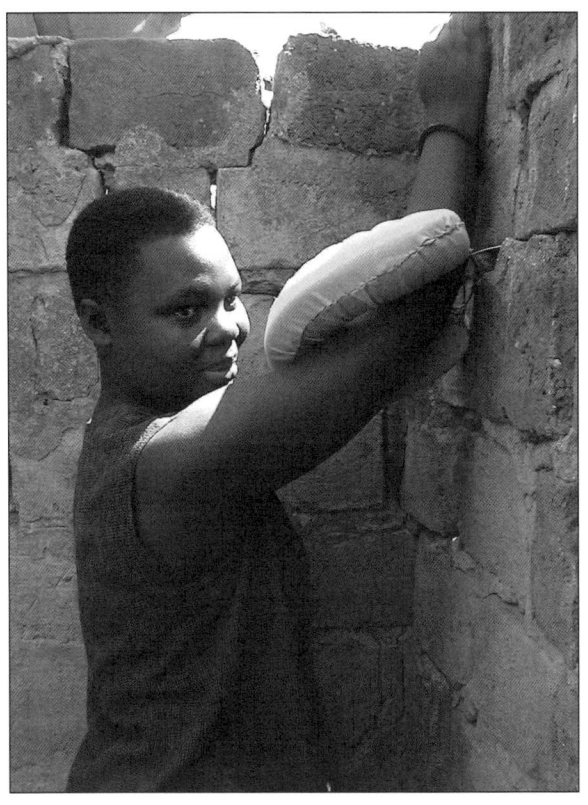

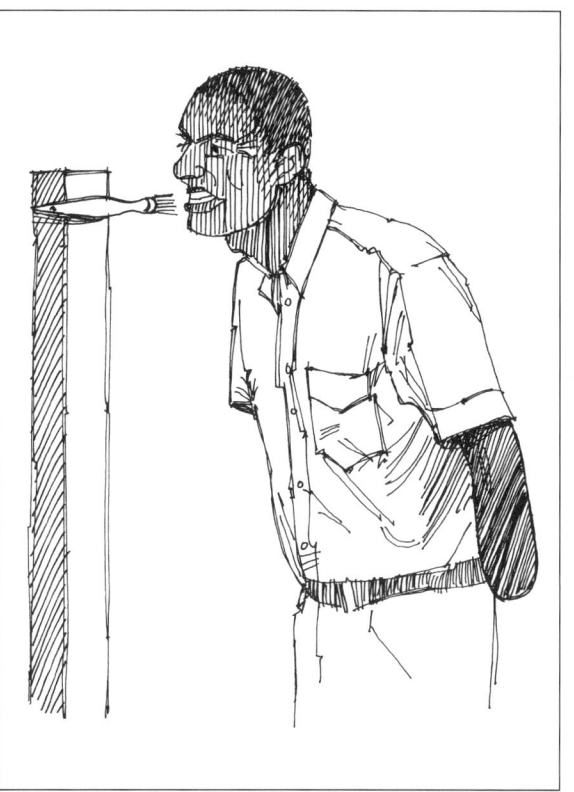

Adapted from information from HITS, Uganda

Figure 6.73. Bather using a padded bathing ring to wash her one arm.
(Case-study 9.28, page 241)

Figure 6.74. Floor-standing wooden toothbrush stand, with toothbrush nailed to post at the required height.

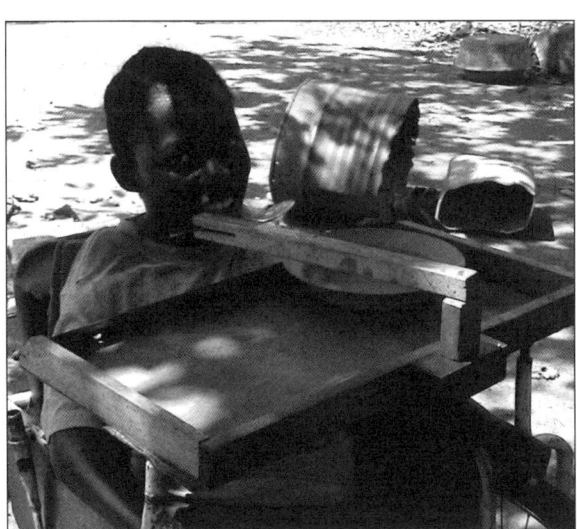

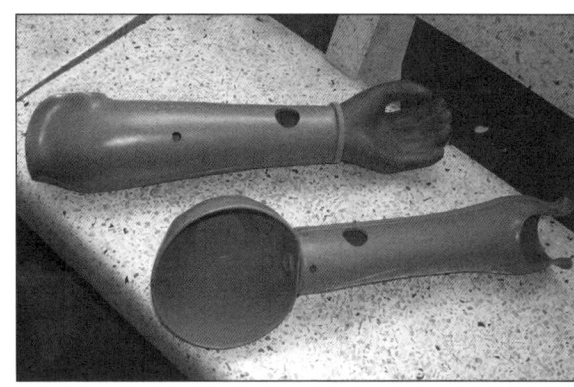

Figure 6.76. Interchangeable bowl and hand attachments on an artificial arm.

Figure 6.75. Implement holder attached to wheelchair tray, used with spoon, toothbrush or other tool.
(Case-study 9.27, page 237)

6

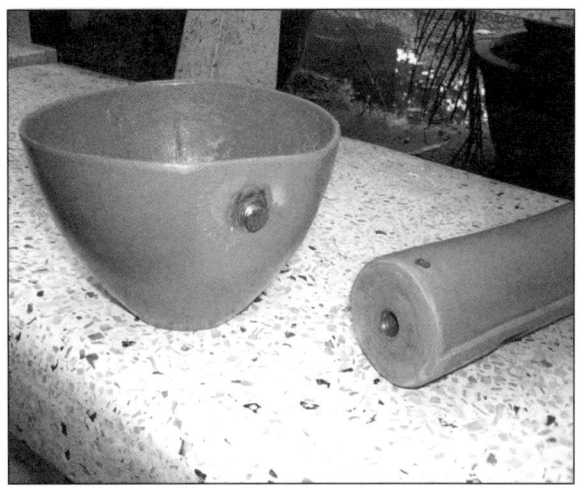

Figure 6.77. Screw attachment on a bowl for an artificial arm.

Figure 6.78. Bather uses bowl attachment to scoop water over himself.

it, but could then bathe independently. There are other functions for which it could be used, such as scooping rice, or bathing one's children.

Drawbacks
This is a high cost option. Most wearers prefer to remove their artificial arm or leg for bathing. A single arm amputee is unlikely to need it, as he could use his one hand to hold a scoop to bathe.

Issues for blind people
Blind people need a well ordered bathing area, as storing objects consistently in the same place makes them easier to find. They should preferably be on open shelves, or on hooks, rather than on the floor where they can trip up a blind person. The advantage of this approach is that it costs nothing, but it does depend on a co-operative and tidy family!

Containers of different shapes, which can be identified by touch, can be used for different purposes.

This orderly approach is also helpful for elderly people who are becoming confused, and for people who have difficulty learning and remembering everyday tasks.

Further ideas for people with limited use of their arms and hands

Werner, 1987 (3)

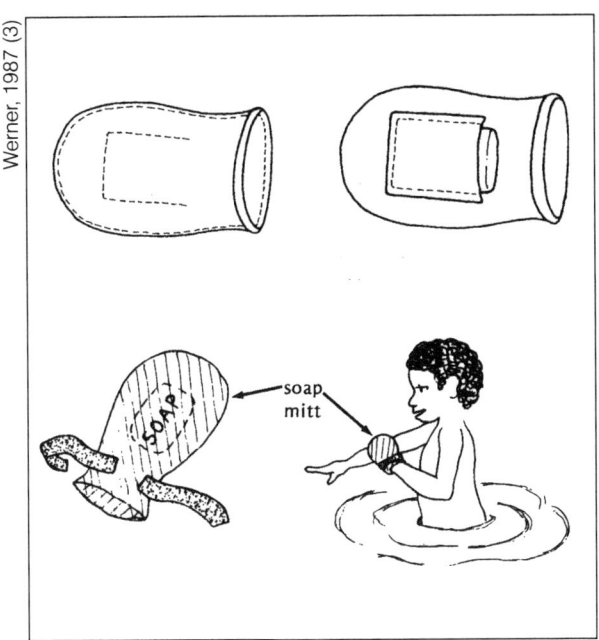

WHO, 1996 (7)

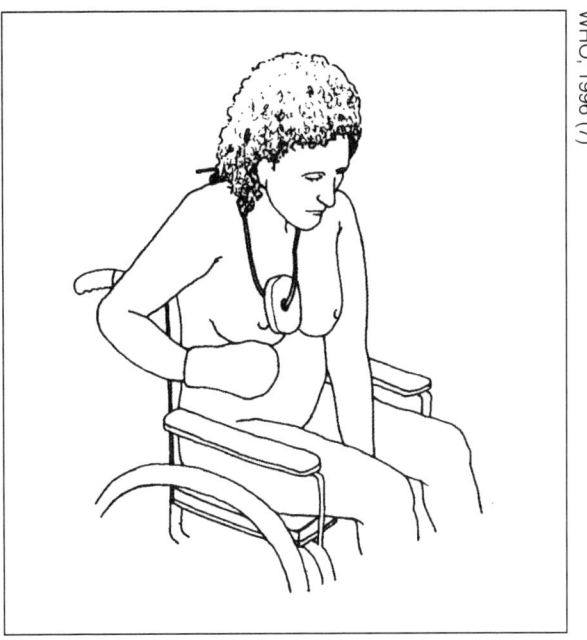

Figure 6.78. Soap mitt made from two pieces of towel with pocket for soap, fits over bather's hand.

Figure 6.79. Soap on a rope – string threaded through hole drilled in soap, hung round bather's neck while washing.

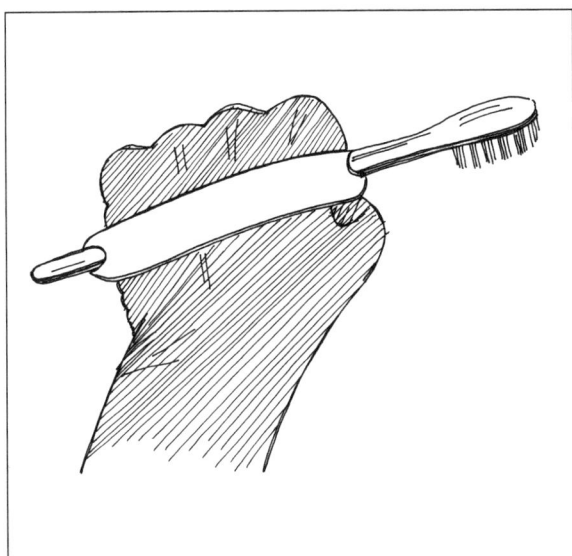

Figure 6.80. A cuff or strap used to hold a toothbrush. Can be made from a strip of recycled rubber inner tube.

6

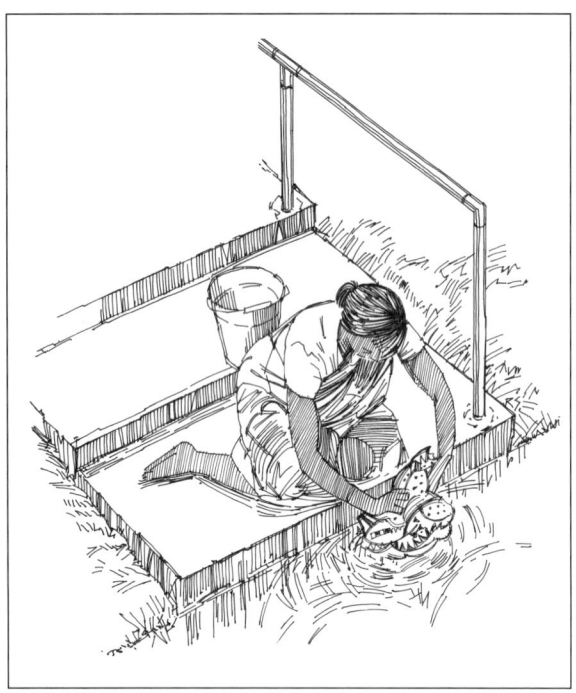

Figure 6.81. Disabled woman washing clothes at a natural water source.

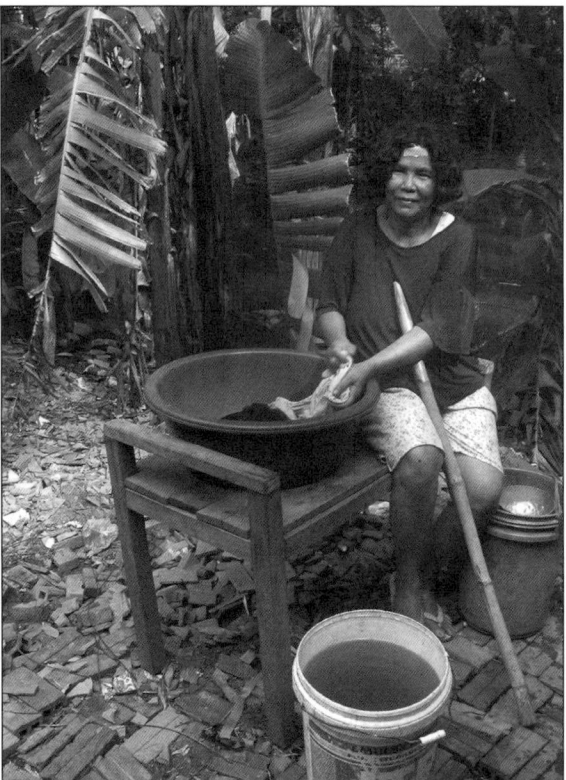

Figure 6.82. Wooden bench for bathing and washing clothes.
(Case-study 9.18, page 214)

6.7 Washing clothes and dishes

Household tasks such as washing clothes and dishes are often carried out at facilities, including washrooms and water points, where a range of water-related activities take place.

Where it is usual to wash clothes and dishes at floor level, whether at a handpump or a tap, providing a place to sit can improve accessibility for many users, including disabled people. This may be designed and constructed as part of the facility, such as the low level concrete platform described on page 86 (Figure 6.48). Low stools (10-25cm) are also suitable for a number of floor level tasks, such as preparing vegetables and cooking, and are widely used throughout the world. A metal-framed seat is durable, but costly (Figure 6.52), whilst wood or bamboo is less durable, but usually cheaper (Figure 6.51).

Washing clothes

Clothes washing is often carried out next to the same water source as bathing. It is therefore helpful if bathing equipment, such as benches, can be designed for more than one function, including bathing, washing clothes and dishes. This can be done by providing enough space on the seat next to the user for objects such as washing bowl, clothes and soap (Figure 6.82). (See also the section on Bathing benches, page 89).

A height of 30 – 60cm is convenient for wheelchair transfer, and for those who have difficulty lowering themselves onto a low seat (check the best height with the person concerned). The user needs to have good sitting balance.

For wheelchair users who prefer to stay in their chair, a concrete laundry slab at waist height is a useful option, with enough space beneath for the user's knees to fit under (Figures 6.83 and 6.84). It can also be used

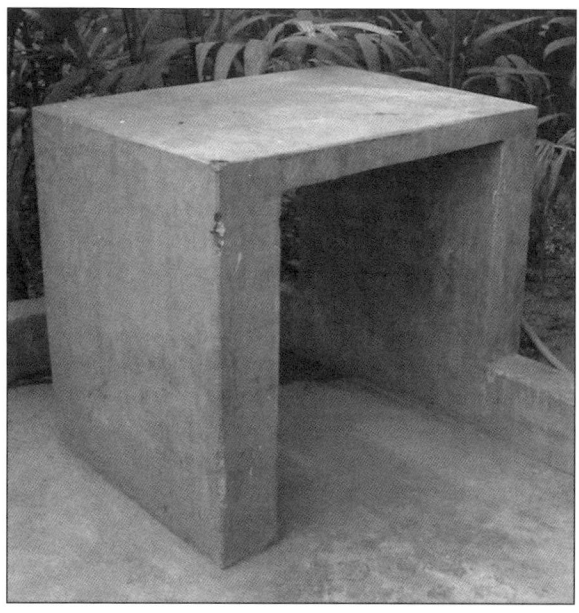

Figure 6.83. Concrete slab for washing clothes. *(Case-study 9.3, page 166)*

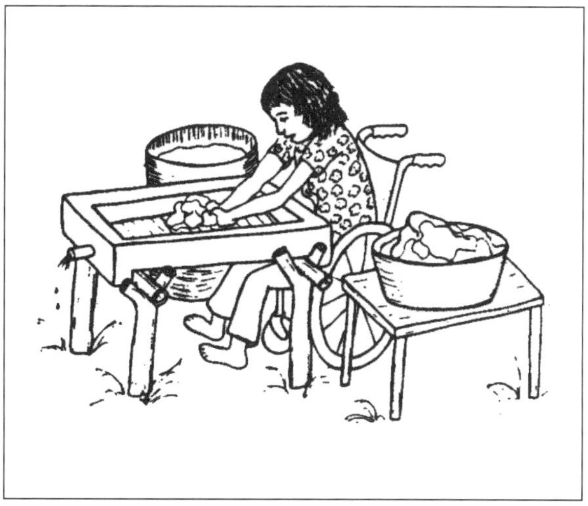

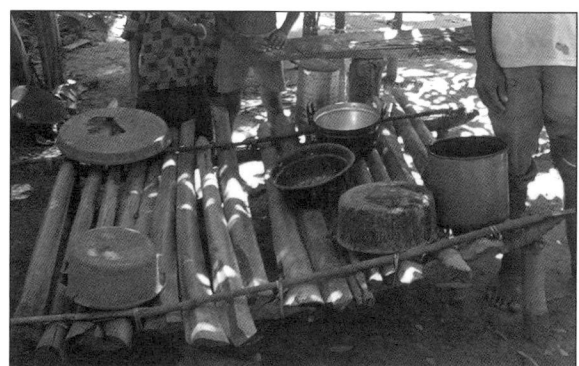

Figure 6.84. Concrete or wooden washstand with ridged bottom for washing clothes.

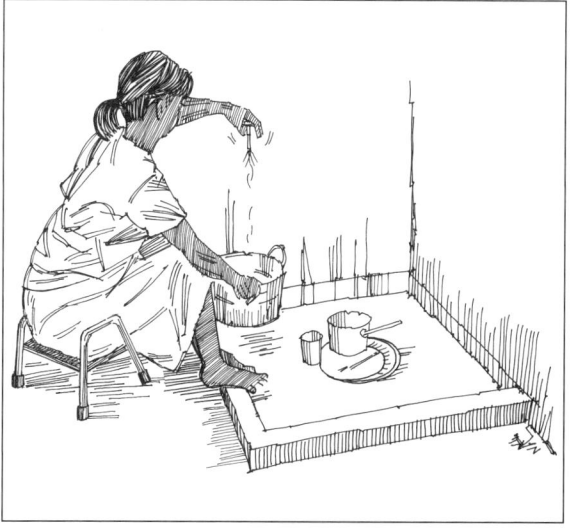

Figure 6.85. A dish draining rack made of split bamboo.
(Case-study 9.12, page 191)

by people standing up. Both these options need to be located as near as possible to a water point for convenience.

Containers used for washing may be commercially available plastic or enamel bowls or, more cheaply, adapted from used food cans or large jerry-cans with the top cut off.

Washing dishes

Washing dishes can be carried out at floor level using a low-level stool, as described above (Figure 6.86).

A dish draining rack can be made at little or no cost out of wood or split bamboo attached to a frame (Figure 6.85). This promotes general good hygiene and can be constructed at a height suitable for the user, either high enough for a wheelchair user to get their knees under, or low enough for a person to use while sitting at ground level.

Issues for blind people

As with bathing, an orderly environment is helpful for blind people, and for people who have difficulty learning or remembering everyday tasks, such as confused elderly people (see page 96 for suggestions).

Figure 6.86. A floor level dish-washing facility in the corner of the kitchen.
(Case-study 9.4, page 169)

References

1. From results of a search on keywords 'lever' and tap' on Google image search http://www.google.co.uk/imghp?hl=en&tab=wi&q=

2. Van der Hulst, G., Velthuys, M. and de Haan, G. (1993) *More with Less: Aids for disabled people in daily life*. TOOL: Amsterdam.

3. Werner, D. (1987) Disabled Village Children. *A guide for community health workers, rehabilitation workers, and families*. Hesperian Foundation: USA.

4. Jones, H., Reed, R.A. and House, S.J. (2003) *Water supply and sanitation access and use by physically disabled people. Report of field-work in Cambodia*. WEDC, Loughborough University and DFID: UK.

5. Centre for Disease Control Centre for Disease Control Tippy Taps http://www.cdc.gov/safewater/tippy-tap.pdf

6. IICP (1999) Series of booklets: *Cleanliness for the Child with Cerebral Palsy, Special Furniture, Toileting for the Child with Cerebral Palsy*. Indian Institute of Cerebral Palsy: Kolkata, India.

7. WHO (1996) *Promoting Independence following a Spinal Cord Injury*. A manual for mid-level rehabilitation workers. World Health Organization: Geneva.

6

Chapter 7

Toilets – access and use

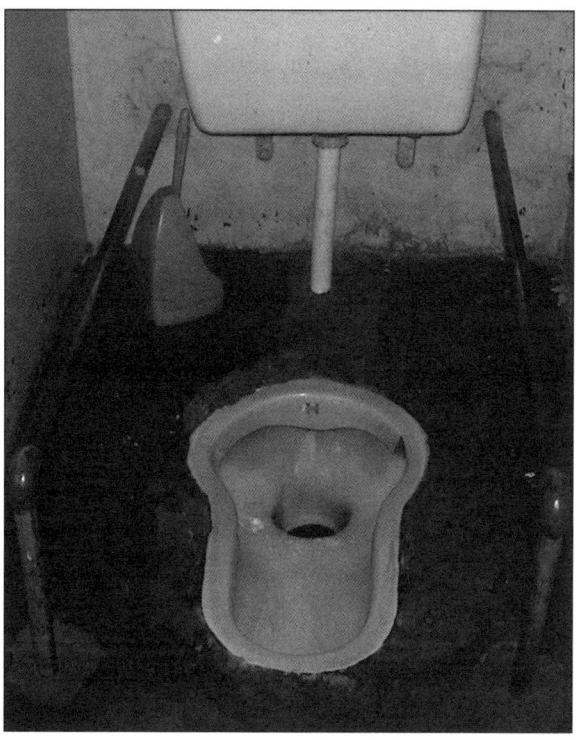

Figure 7.1. Handrail attached to floor on both sides of a squat toilet. H: ~30cm. (The wide toilet pan is not recommended.)

This section considers a wide range of toilet facilities and their alternatives, from sanitary water-flush systems to open defecation, because these are the current living conditions of many people in the world, including many disabled people.

7.1 Benefits of more accessible toilets

Benefits reported to be felt by disabled people themselves:

- Greater self-reliance, dignity and privacy – those who previously relied on a family member to stay with them, to provide support, can now be left to use the toilet in private. This includes elderly people who are enabled to use the toilet independently until later in life.

- Disabled people are able to use the toilet more promptly and hygienically, which helps them avoid soiling their clothes and the toilet, resulting in health benefits, and also greater comfort, dignity and self-esteem.

- Improvements in health – a user who may previously have had to place their hands on the floor to balance, can now avoid getting them wet and dirty.

- The disabled user's clothes stay dry and clean because they are not dragging on the dirty floor. This reduces the risk of contamination.

Benefits are felt by the whole family:
- Less soiling of clothes and toilet creates easier, more pleasant work for the clothes washer and toilet cleaner (usually women in the family).

For a list of resources providing inclusive design recommendations for toilets, see Appendix A1.1, page 255.

For resources on types of latrines, see under Technical Information, Appendix A1.2, page 256.

7

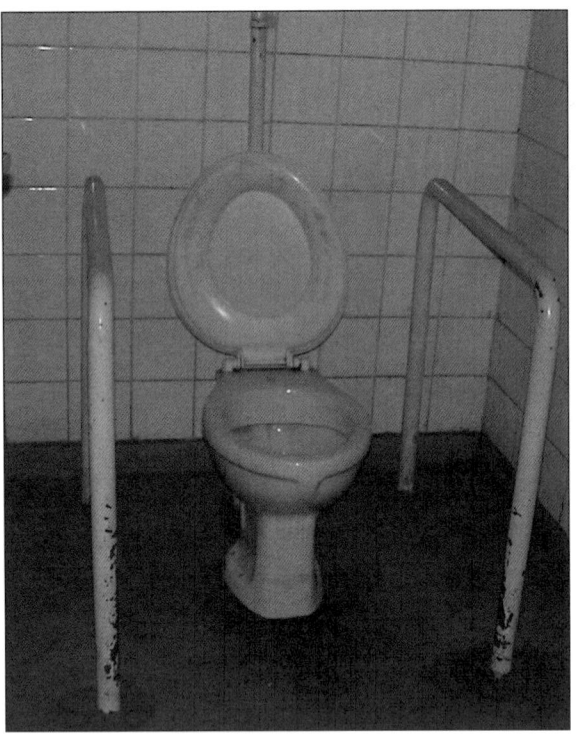

Figure 7.2. Painted handrails cemented to floor on both sides of pedestal toilet. 50mm Ø g.i. pipe; H: ~80cm.

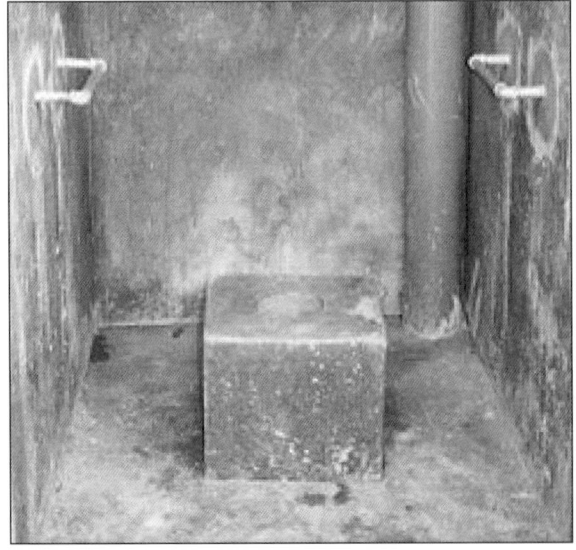

Figure 7.3. Handrails cemented to each side wall of toilet cubicle. H: ~ 80cm – likely to be too high and too far apart for some child users. *(Case-study 9.29, page 242)*

- Savings in time and effort for family members, which frees up more time for other activities, such as income generation opportunities, or time for children to play or go to school.

- Helps avoid injury from falling while using the toilet (an environment which is often slippery, dark and with inadequate space to manoeuvre).

- Greater accessibility for disabled people usually means facilities that are also more child-friendly, and more accessible for pregnant women.

- Overall family health benefits.

7.2   Getting there and getting in

Many of the difficulties of getting to the toilet can be reduced by bringing the toilet as near to the house as possible, allowing for technical considerations. See section 5.4 on 'Getting there' on page 45 for discussion of ways to make it easier to reach a facility. Where technology and the household allow, there are many benefits to installing a toilet inside the house. This is most likely to be acceptable if a water-seal toilet is an available option.

See Section 5.4 on pages 56-62 for details of ways to make it easy for a disabled person to enter a facility.

7.3   Support rails

The most common need is to provide support for a person unable to squat or sit independently. This can be with handles or support rails, or somewhere to sit while urinating or defecating. (The information in this section can also be applied in other situations, such as bathing and clothes washing.)

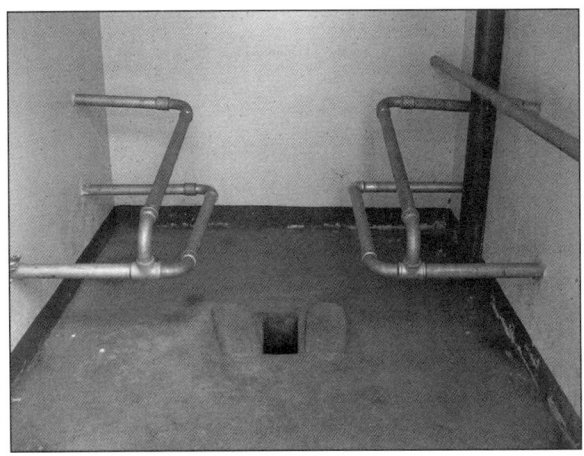

Figure 7.4. Diagonal and horizontal rails fixed to side walls at different heights. Note additional horizontal rail from front to back of wall on the right.
(Case-study 9.26, page 232)

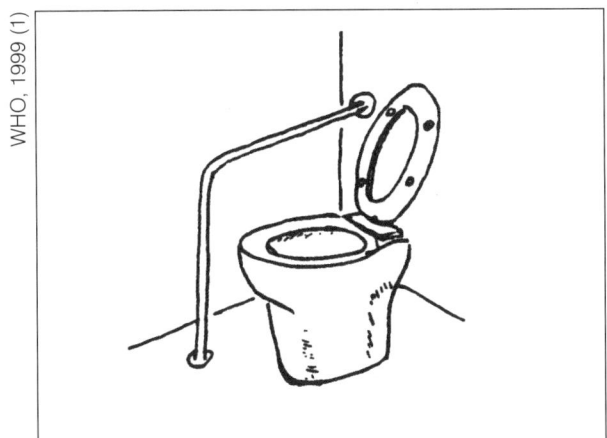

Figure 7.5. Rail on one side only allows wheelchair to be positioned beside toilet for easy sideways transfer.

Rails provide support for people to:

- Enter and leave the toilet cubicle or area;

- Stand while undressing and dressing;

- Balance while lowering themselves onto or getting up from the toilet;

- Balance while transferring to and from a wheelchair, crutches or other mobility device;

- Balance while squatting or sitting on the toilet;

- Guide blind and visually impaired toilet users.

These can be provided as:

- An integral part of the latrine structure;

- An adaptation or addition to an existing facility to make it more accessible;

- A piece of equipment which is movable; or

- A combination of any of these.

Types of support rails

Rails can be provided in different locations, depending on the latrine structure, available space and users' needs (see page 107 on consultation with users):

- Two horizontal rails cemented to the floor on each side of a squat toilet (Figure 7.1). Suitable for use by a person with weak legs who has difficulty squatting without support.

- Horizontal rails cemented to the floor on each side of a toilet with a raised seat (Figure 7.2).

- Two horizontal rails, one attached to each wall on either side of the toilet (Figure 7.3). This is only possible if the toilet wall is strong enough. Rails may be too wide apart for many users.

- Two diagonal rails, attached to the wall on each side of the toilet (Figure 7.4). Rails at different heights suit different sized

7

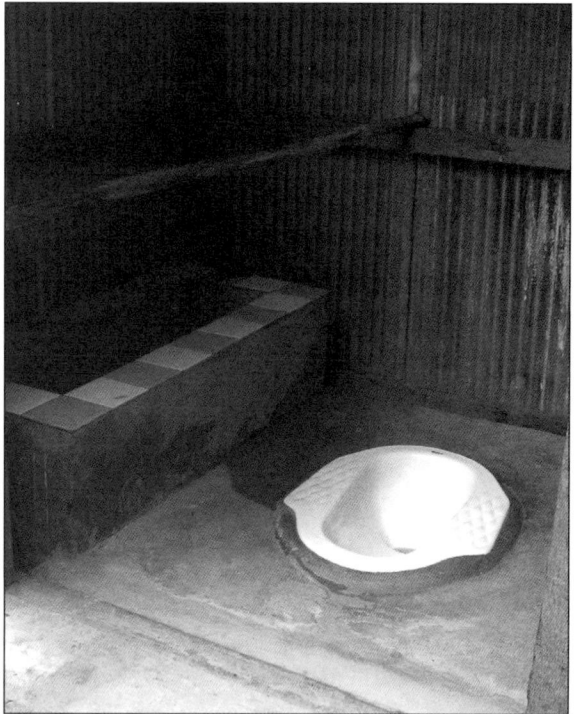

Figure 7.6. Single horizontal wooden rail (H: ~50cm) from door to back wall, for support to enter toilet. Too high for child to hold while squatting.
(Case-study 9.19, page 215)

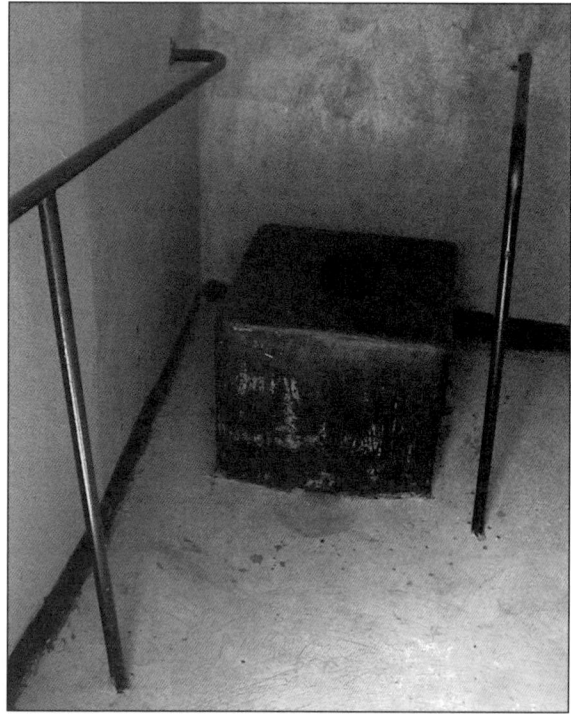

Figure 7.7. Painted rail fixed to floor and walls.
(Case-study 9.25, page 229)

users. The same user can hold a higher rail when standing, and a lower rail when sitting.

- Single horizontal rail beside the toilet, fixed to the wall or floor (Figure 7.5) allows a wheelchair to be positioned on one side of the toilet for easy sideways transfer.

- Single horizontal rail extending from the door to the toilet (Figures 7.6 and 7.7). For use by a person to support themselves while walking from the door to the toilet, and for lowering to sit or squat, and standing up again.

- Horizontal rail in front of the toilet, fixed either to the wall (Figure 7.8) or to vertical support poles (Figure 7.9). A 'ladder' of several rails at different heights can be helpful for a person with limited arm movement, or different sized users (Figure 7.10).

- Two bamboo poles stuck vertically into the ground, one on each side of the latrine slab (Figure 7.11).

- A frame around the toilet, made of wood (Figure 7.12) or metal pipe (Figure 7.13). This is useful if toilet walls and floor are not strong enough to attach rails, or a rail attached to a wall would be too far away, or accommodation is rented or shared, so adaptations to the fabric of the facility are not an option.

- Available furniture, such as a chair or table. This must be stable enough not to fall over when the user leans on it (Figure 7.14).

- Support rails on the toilet seat itself (Figure 7.15).

- A rope suspended from a roof beam for the user to hold on to (Figure 7.16). This is also suitable for use in communal or rented facilities. The rope does not alter the structure of the facility, takes up no extra space, does not inconvenience other users, and is not likely to be stolen.

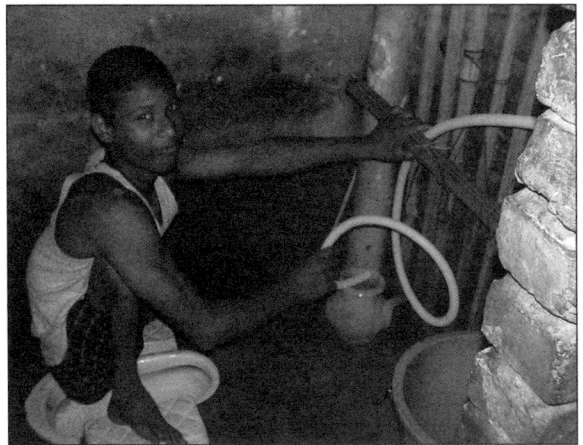

Figure 7.8. Horizontal wooden bar tied to existing pipes in front of toilet. H of bar (~70cm) was decided by user. No choice of distance for bar – nearer would be more comfortable.
(Case-study 9.6, page 177)

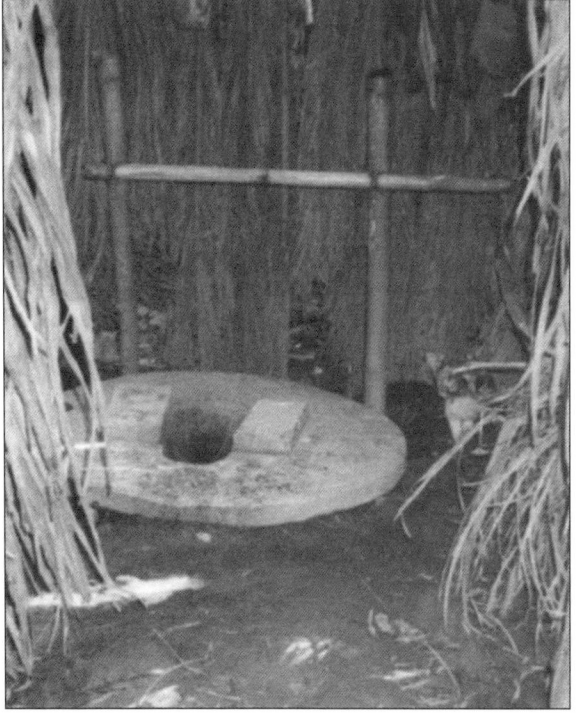

Figure 7.9. Single horizontal bamboo rail in front of toilet.
(Case-study 9.10, page 185)

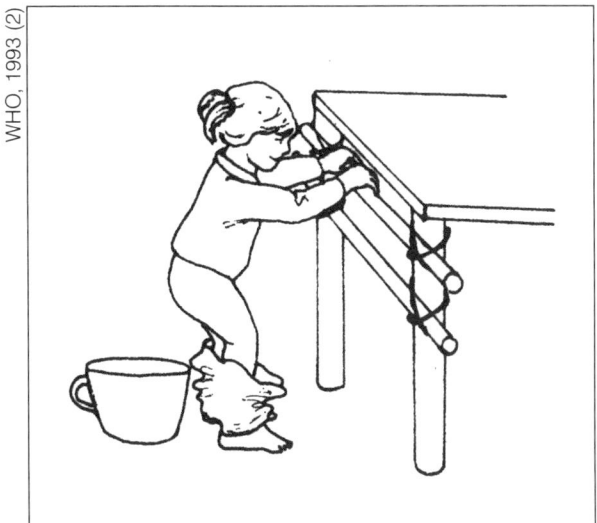

Figure 7.10. 'Ladder' of rails to help a child pull herself up and lower herself down.

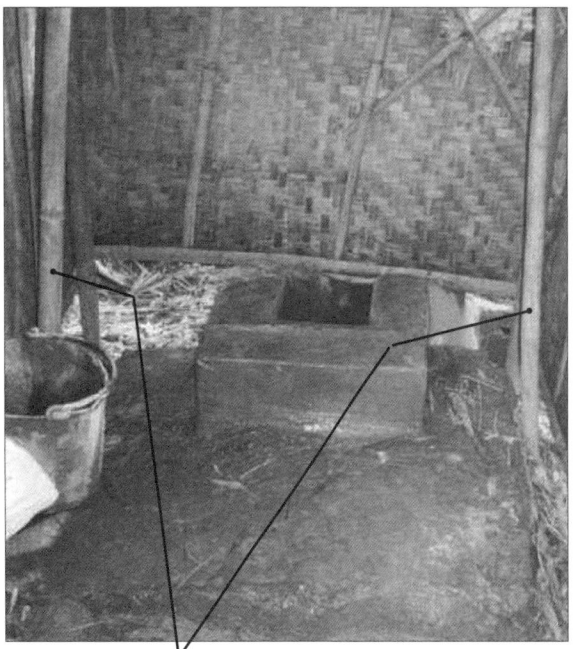

Figure 7.11. Two vertical bamboo support poles one on each side of latrine.
(Case-study 9.9, page 183)

Toilets – access and use

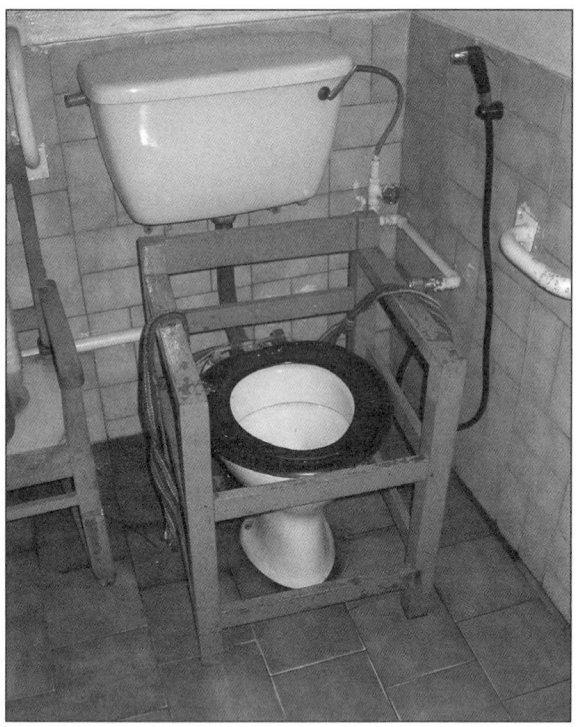

Figure 7.12. Painted wooden frame around pedestal toilet seat.

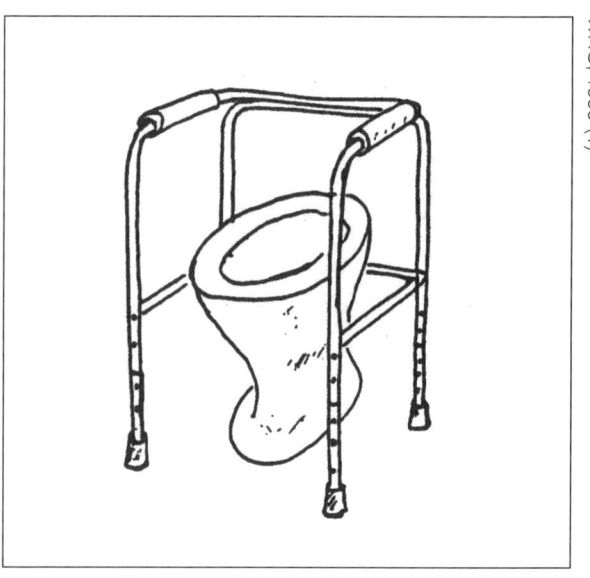

Figure 7.13. Four legged tubular steel frame, with cushioned handles and rubber 'feet'. Adjustable height.

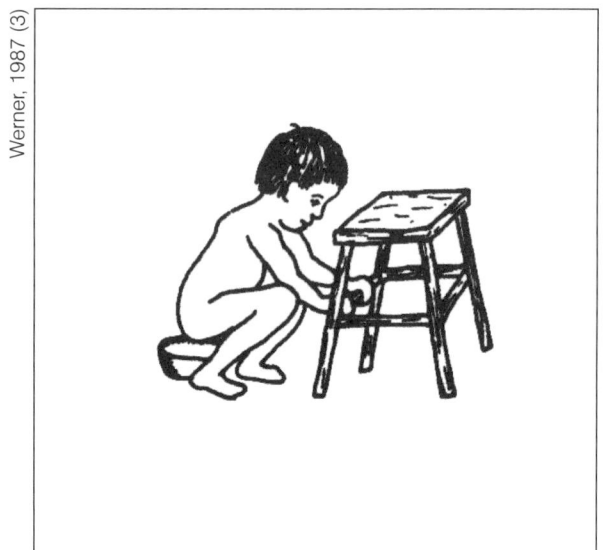

Figure 7.14. Child using available furniture for support.

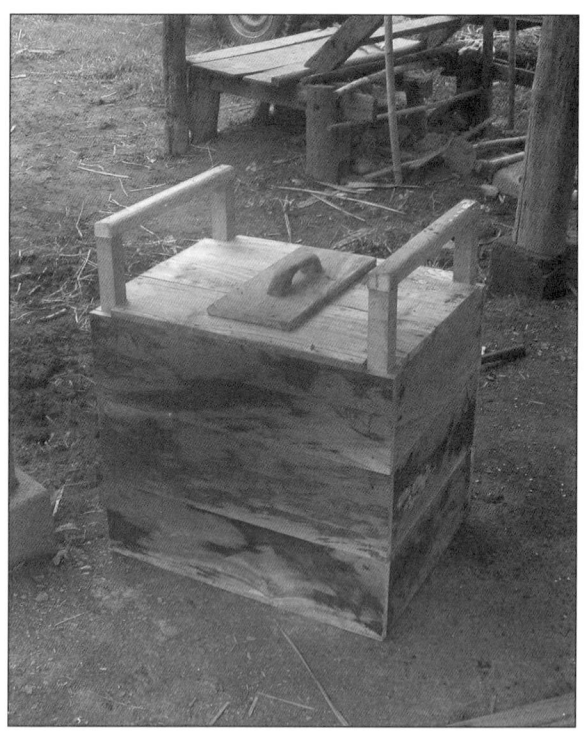

Figure 7.15. Wooden toilet seat with handrails. *(Case-study 9.17, page 209)*

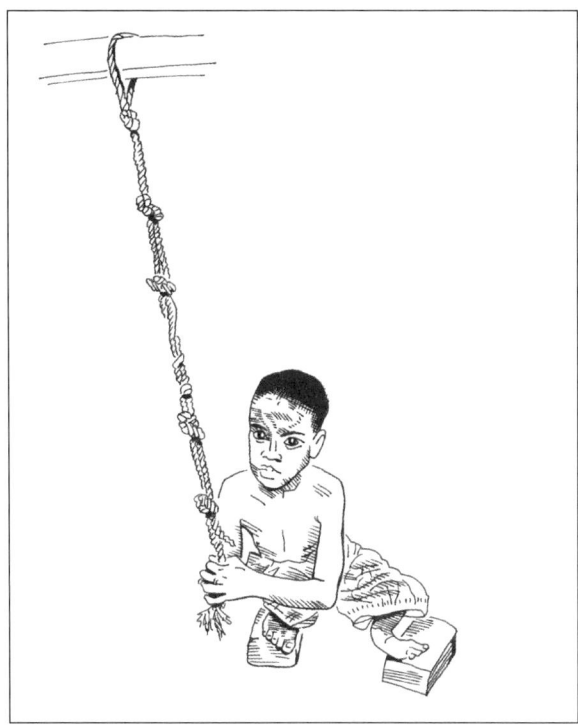

Figure 7.16. Rope suspended from roof beam for support while squatting.
(Case-study 9.7, page 179)

An alternative to rope is knotted recycled bicycle tyre inner tubes. The structure must be strong enough to support the user's full weight.

Characteristics of support rails

Rails may be of galvanised iron (g.i.) pipe (25 – 50mm diameter), bamboo or wood.

50mm g.i. pipe is very robust, and suitable for heavy use by many users, such as in an institutional setting (Figures 7.2 and 7.4). For small children, it is too wide to hold onto comfortably. Narrower pipe (25mm) is suitable for most users at household level (Figure 7.7).

Materials such as bamboo and wood are less durable than iron pipe, but can often be replaced at little or no cost (Figures 7.9 and 7.11).

If rails are made of pipe, the height can also be made adjustable (Figures 7.17 and 7.18). This is useful in the case of a child, as the rails can be raised as the child grows.

Support rails - Issues

Consultation with users: wherever possible, the type, location and dimensions of rails should be chosen to suit the needs of individual users. This needs to be done through a process of consultation, where users participate with the engineer to decide the best place to fit the rails.

Safety: support rails must be strong enough and firmly fixed enough to bear the weight of the user, if this is the function. **A rail that breaks is more dangerous than no rail at all!** Rails intended for help with balance only, or as guidance for blind users may need to be less sturdy. The user/s must be clear about this distinction.

Steel rails should be painted to resist corrosion.

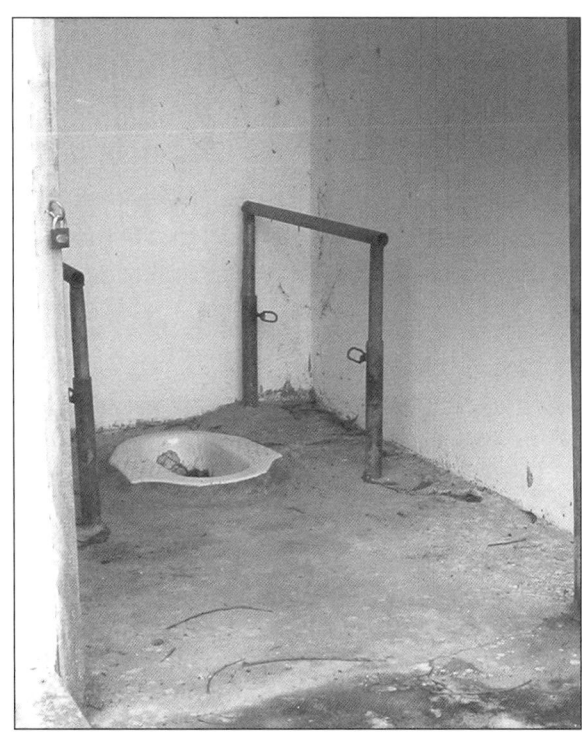

Figure 7.17. Handrails of adjustable height, suitable for a growing child.
(Case-study 9.16, page 207)

If a wheelchair has removable sides, the easiest way to transfer from wheelchair to

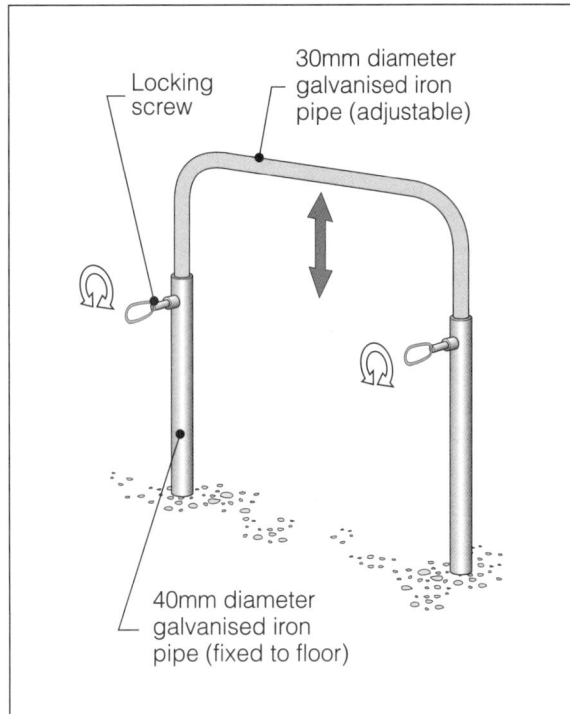

Figure 7.18. Detail of adjustable joint.

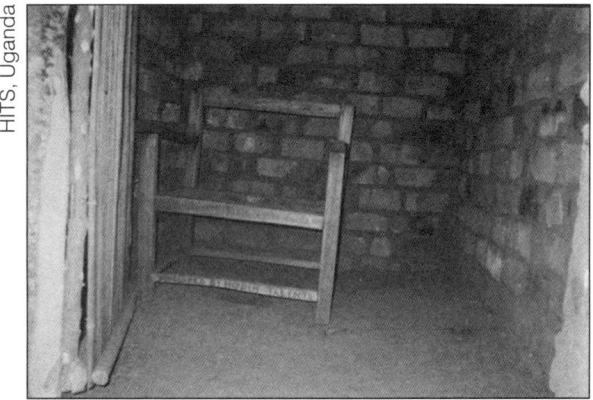

HITS, Uganda

Figure 7.19. Wooden toilet chair with back and side-rails.

toilet is to park the chair beside the toilet, and move sideways. In this case, avoid fixing a rail on the side of the toilet which may obstruct this movement.

7.4 Raised toilet seats

Raised toilet seats are another way of providing support for users. Their advantages are:

*   Convenience for transfer from and to a wheelchair.

*   Convenience for people who have difficulty lowering themselves into a squatting position, and even more difficulty standing up again!

*   Increased comfort - reduced risk of the user getting their clothes dirty and wet.

*   They may help children overcome their fear of using a toilet (they may be afraid of falling into the hole of a squat toilet).

Drawbacks of raised seats

*   A seat may be uncomfortable for people who are used to squatting, or may be perceived as 'Western' and culturally less acceptable.

*   Anal cleansing using water is more difficult when using a seat than when squatting. However, a long gap in the seat from front to back makes this easier.

*   There is the risk that non-disabled users, who prefer to continue squatting, either make the seat dirty by squatting on it, or may need a separate toilet, which increases costs.

Support and safety

Users with poor balance may need support to prevent them falling off the seat. They may be happy to accept support from a family member while they use the toilet. However, if they prefer to be left alone to use the toilet, there are ways to reduce the risk of falling.

7

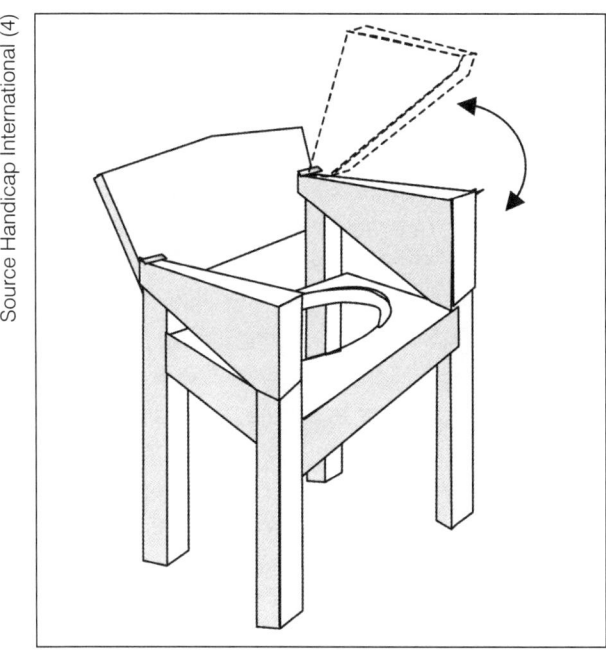

Source Handicap International (4)

Figure 7.20. Chair with hinged side-rails that can be raised out of the way.

Source Handicap International (4)

Figure 7.21. Chair with side-rails that can be raised.The rails are attached to the chair back with a bolt, on which they swivel vertically.

Falling sideways can be prevented by using a seat with a back and side-rails (Figure 7.19). However, side-rails can be an obstacle to sideways transfer from a wheelchair. Side-rails that can be removed or raised are therefore useful (Figures 7.20 and 7.21). Falling forwards can be prevented by using a horizontal bar which attaches to the sides of the chair (Figure 7.22).

For greater support and comfort, straps can be used. These can be passed round the back of the chair and around the person's waist or chest. Shoulder straps can be attached to the top of the chair back, and passed over the user's shoulders and either crossed and tied at the back, or fastened to a waist strap. These can be made of wide elastic, or strips of fabric or rubber (Figures 7.45, 7.46 and 7.47) or a scarf can be used (Figure 7.23).

Even if these safety measures are taken, there may still be risks to leaving the disabled person alone, especially someone who has epileptic fits or is confused. Disabled people who are unable to walk should not be left sitting on a hard surface for any longer than necessary, as this increases their risk of developing pressure sores.

Seats can be either fixed or movable.

Fixed raised seats (pedestals)

Fixed seats can be made from a variety of materials.

- **Ceramic** is the most durable and easiest to clean, but also the most expensive. It is not always available in rural areas. It also depends on water to flush it, making it unsuitable in areas where water is scarce.

- **Cement-plastered brick** is durable and, when painted, repels urine and is easy to clean (Figures 7.24 and 7.27). Materials are widely available. An alternative is twin cement-plastered brick blocks, one on each side of the toilet hole (Figure 7.26). This uses fewer bricks than a seat, making it cheaper, and has the advantage of being more convenient for anal cleansing.

7

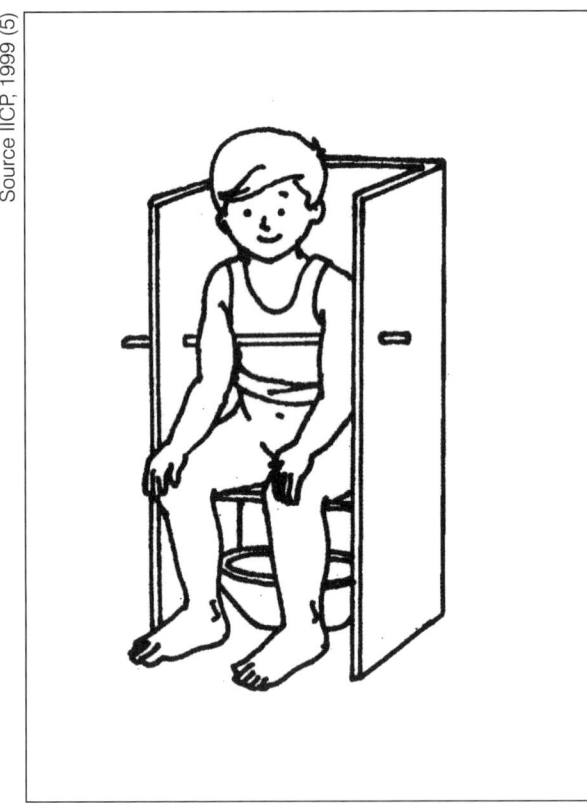

Source IICP, 1999 (5)

Figure 7.22. Toilet chair with removable horizontal bar to prevent user falling forwards.

Both ceramic and concrete can be cold to sit on, but if this is a problem a wooden seat could be placed on the structure (e.g. Figure 7.28).

- **A wooden seat** is less durable than cement or ceramic, but may be cheaper. It can be placed over the latrine pit and dug into the ground for stability (Figure 7.29). The seat has the flexibility to be moved to a new location if needed – when the pit is full, for example, or to avoid flooding in the rainy season. To increase the durability of wood it can be painted or varnished to make it moisture resistant, easier to clean and therefore also hygienic (Figure 7.36).

- **Mud** (air-dried clay): In communities with the skills to make robust structures out of mud and/or dung, a low-cost toilet seat can be made of mud-plastered bricks (Figures 7.30 and 7.33). This is the least durable, especially if it is often wet, but costs little to replace.

- **Adapting existing materials**: where a commercially available PVC toilet pan is used, it can be installed at a height suitable for the user, such as level with a wheelchair seat. This could be on a raised platform of cement-plastered brick (Figure 7.31). Sitting blocks can be added on each side of the toilet pan.

The toilet hole
The hole in the seat needs to be large enough, and set near the front of the seat, to reduce the risk of the user fouling the seat (Figure 7.29). A distance of 10cm between the front of the seat and the front of the hole is suitable, otherwise small children cannot sit far enough back on the seat to defecate directly into the hole.

Hole dimensions: for adults, a width of 20 – 27cm, with a minimum length from front to back of 20cm. For a child, the width of the hole may need to be less (Figure 7.32).

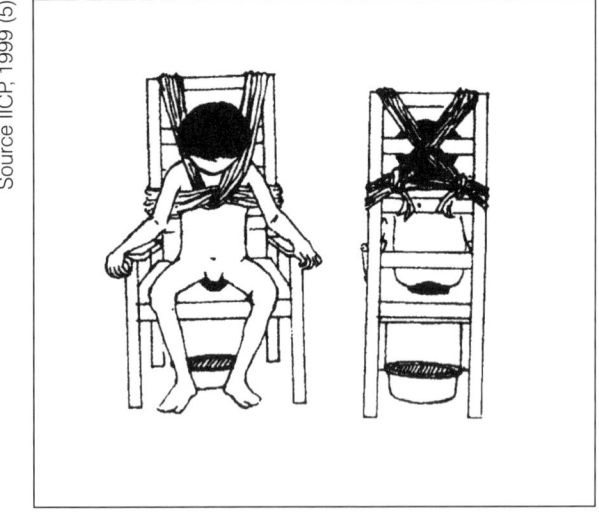

Source IICP, 1999 (5)

Figure 7.23. Child supported with a scarf.

Examples of fixed raised seats

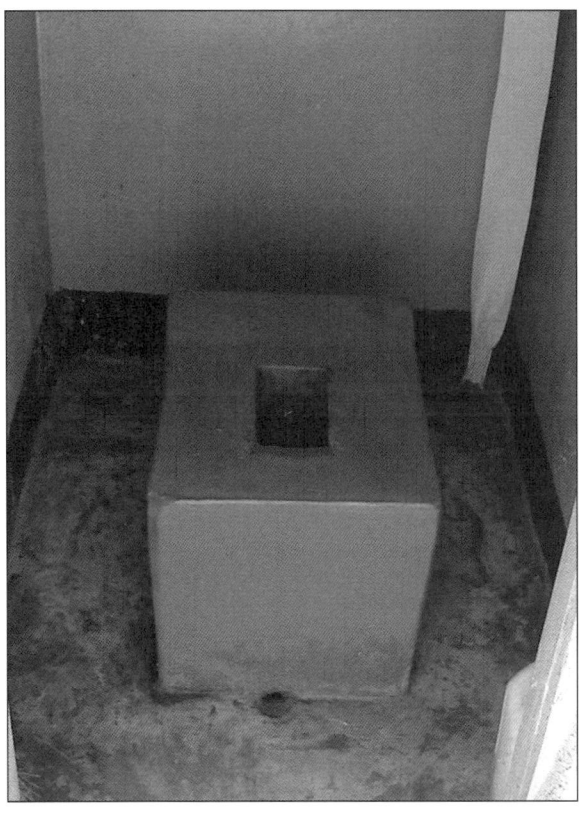

Figure 7.24. Toilet seat made of bricks, plastered with cement mortar and painted. Raised at the back for extra support.
(Case-study 9.24, page 224)

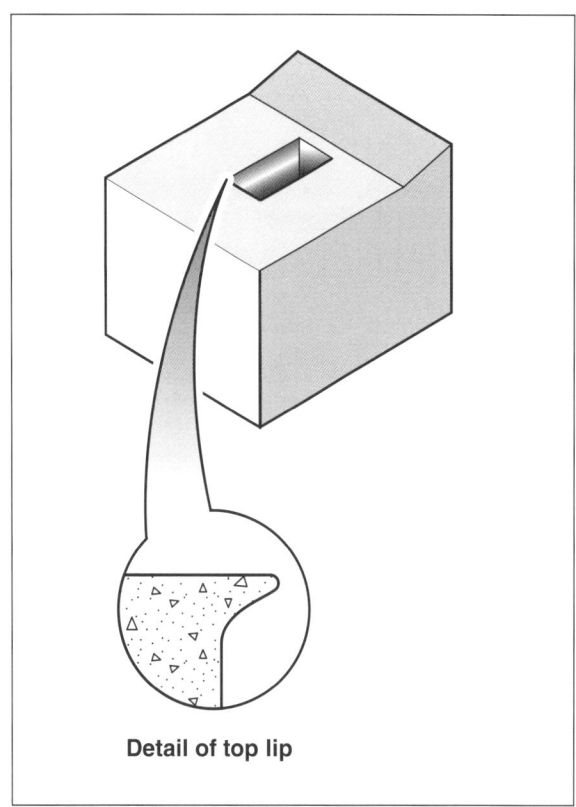

Detail of top lip

Figure 7.25. A 'lip' around the top of the toilet hole.

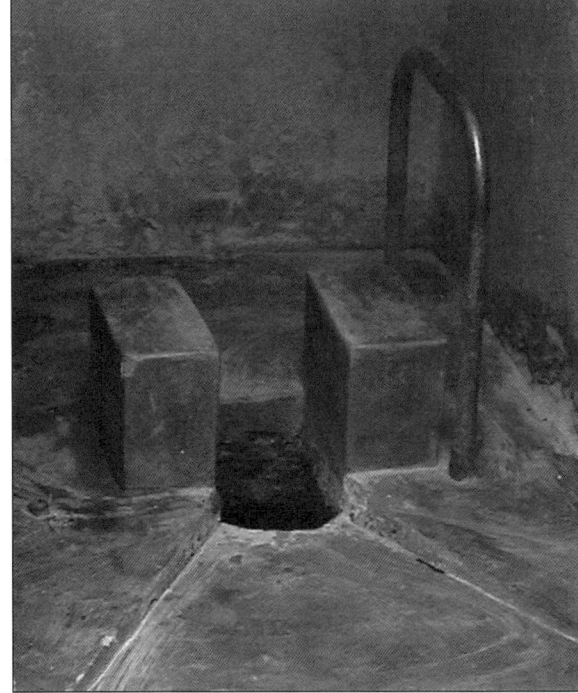

Figure 7.26. Twin cement-plastered brick sitting blocks. Height: 25cm; gap: 14cm. The gap makes anal cleansing easier than on an ordinary seat.
(Case-study 9.26, page 232)

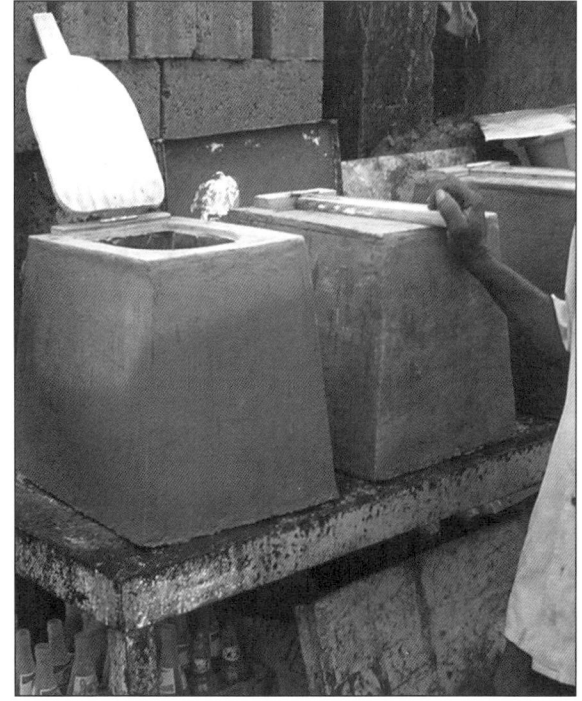

Figure 7.27. Concrete toilet seats on sale, with hinged wooden lid to reduce flies and smells.

Sarah House

7

Toilets – access and use

Examples of fixed raised seats (continued)

Source Werner, 1998 (6)

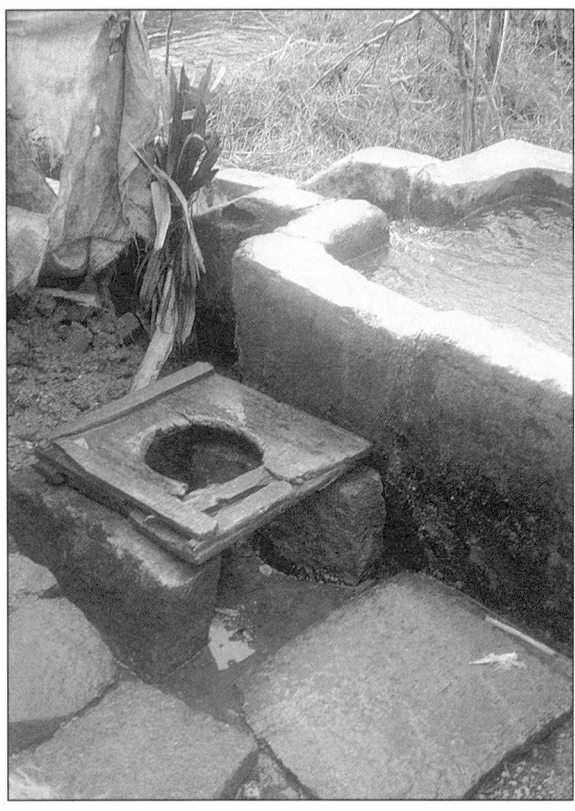

Figure 7.28. Wooden toilet seat supported on two brick blocks over a pit latrine. The pit was dug more than 2m deep to avoid contaminating the water source. Location next to the water trough makes water for anal cleansing and handwashing easily accessible.

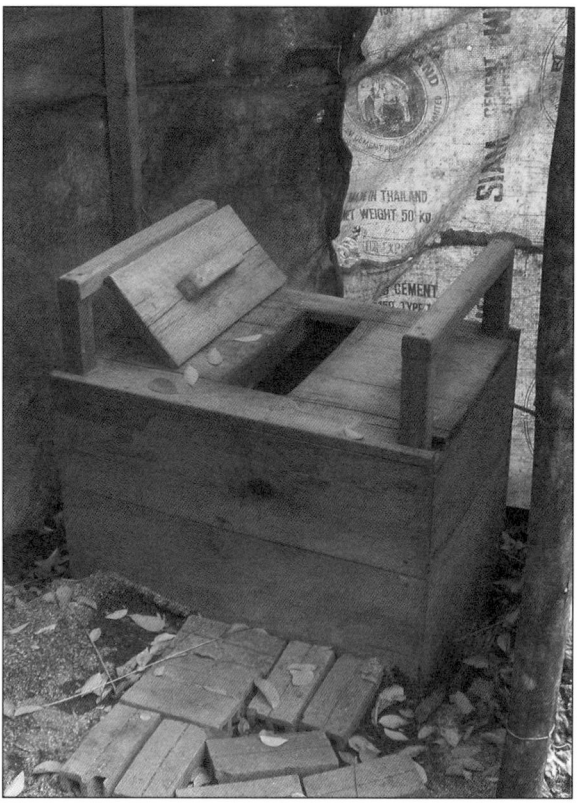

Figure 7.29. Wooden box toilet seat installed over a pit latrine. A cover prevents flies and smells when the toilet is not in use.
(Case-study 9.17, page 209)

Source IICP, 1999 (5)

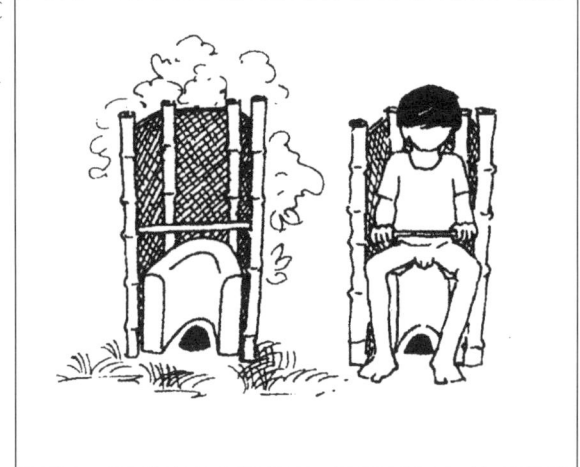

Figure 7.30. Mud toilet seat.

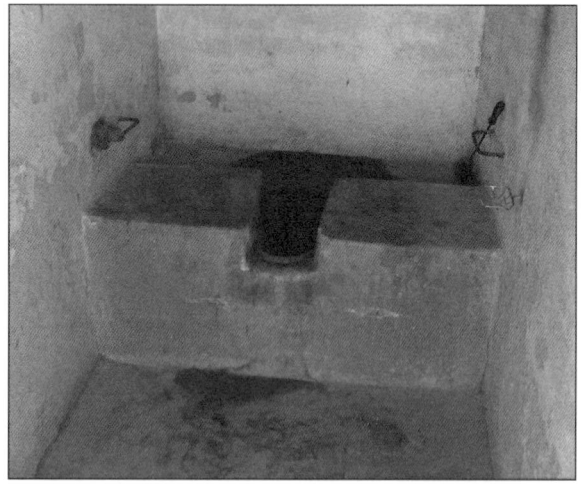

Figure 7.31. Cement-plastered brick platform with commercially available PVC toilet pan inset. Sitting blocks at height for easy wheelchair transfer.
(Case-study 9.1, page 154)

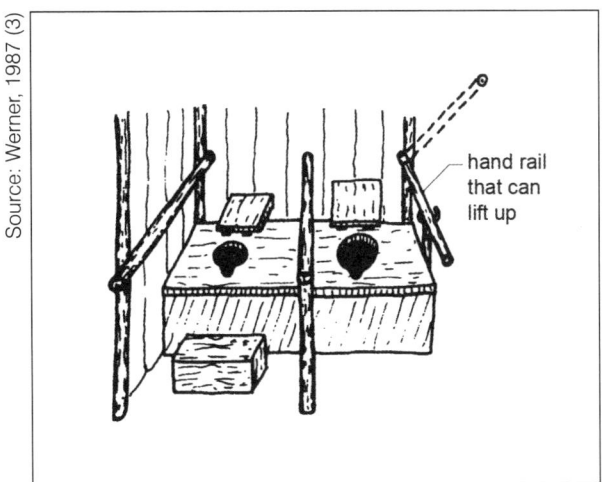

Source: Werner, 1987 (3)

— hand rail that can lift up

Figure 7.32. Two-seater latrine seat with child-sized hole (on the left) with a step.

Twin sitting blocks used by a child (Figure 7.26) should have a gap of 10 – 15cm wide. If the gap is too wide it will be unsafe and off-putting for a small child to use.

A 'lip' around the edge of the hole can help minimise fouling of the sides of the drop hole (Figure 7.25).

Movable toilet seats

These are chairs or stools with a hole in the seat, which are designed to be placed over the toilet pan so that urine and faeces drop directly into the hole. They can be moved off the toilet and placed to one side when not in use, allowing the disabled person to use the same toilet as the rest of the family, with the same amount of privacy.

They come in a range of designs and materials – bamboo, wood, metal or plastic. Often an ordinary wooden household chair with a hole cut in the seat can be used (Figure 7.19). Plastic is more durable but, generally,

Box 7.1. Mud seat for a child unable to sit without support

An NGO was running workshops on how to make cooking stoves out of mud in Pakistan. We showed one of the trainers a picture of a mud chair (from Disabled Village Children) (5), and she constructed several. They were used in the family compound; they were quite heavy, but the families placed them on a piece of tarpaulin and moved them short distances when needed. The chair worked well in the dry climate of Baluchistan, so I am not sure of the effect water/rain might have on it. The people there made their houses, compound walls etc, from mud, so the skills were there, we just provided the idea. The cost was about 10 rupees (20 US cents). We didn't adapt the technique for toileting, but it could easily be tried, either as a commode chair with a removable pot, or a fixed seat over the toilet. *(Sudha Rahman, physiotherapist, Handicap International Belgium)*

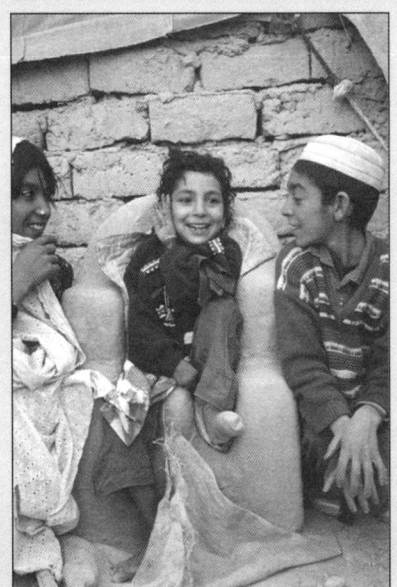

Sudha Rahman

Figure 7.33. Child seated in a mud seat.

7

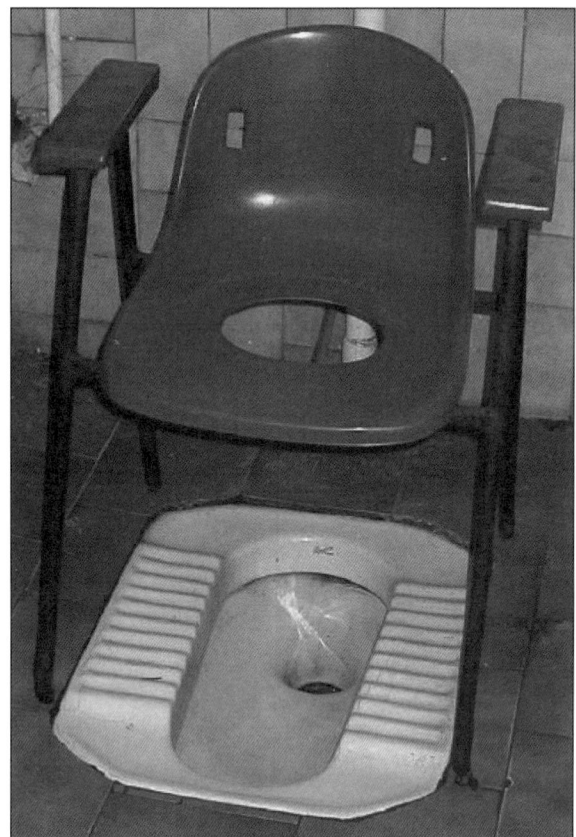

Figure 7.34. Moulded plastic toilet seat: durable, easy to clean, hygienic. High cost. Hole quite far back in seat. No splash-guard.

Angela Martin

Figure 7.35. Wooden toilet stool for use over the family pit latrine. Gap between planks: 10cm – suitable for a child. Front plank acts as splash-guard.
(Case-study 9.30, page 245)

the more durable the material, the higher the cost (Figure 7.34).

A wood or bamboo seat is generally cheaper than brick and concrete, as locally available materials can be used (Figure 7.35). Both can be varnished or painted to make them more moisture resistant, durable, easy to clean and hygienic (Figure 7.36).

On a squat toilet, raised concrete or ceramic footplates need not be an obstacle to using a toilet seat over it, as long as the legs of the seat fit in front of and behind the footplates (Figure 7.36). This can even be an advantage, by serving to position and stabilise the seat directly over the hole.

Drawbacks:

- If the seat is left in place, it may get dirty from others using it inappropriately. Enough space is needed inside the latrine to move the seat off the toilet to one side when not in use.

- If there is not enough room, the seat needs to be carried in and out of the latrine. A support person may need to do this for the user.

- The latrine floor must be firm enough to bear the weight of the seat. Wooden or bamboo bars, or 'runners', can be attached between the front and back legs on each side of the chair at floor level (Figure 7.37). These help spread the weight of the chair more evenly, and minimise the risk of breaking through an earth floor. They also help improve the chair's stability, and on a smooth floor can make the chair easier to move around by sliding it rather than lifting it.

- There is a risk of urine splashing the user's legs or clothing between the seat and the toilet hole. A **splash-guard** – a board or plastic sheet covering the space between the front chair legs – can prevent this.

Examples of movable seats

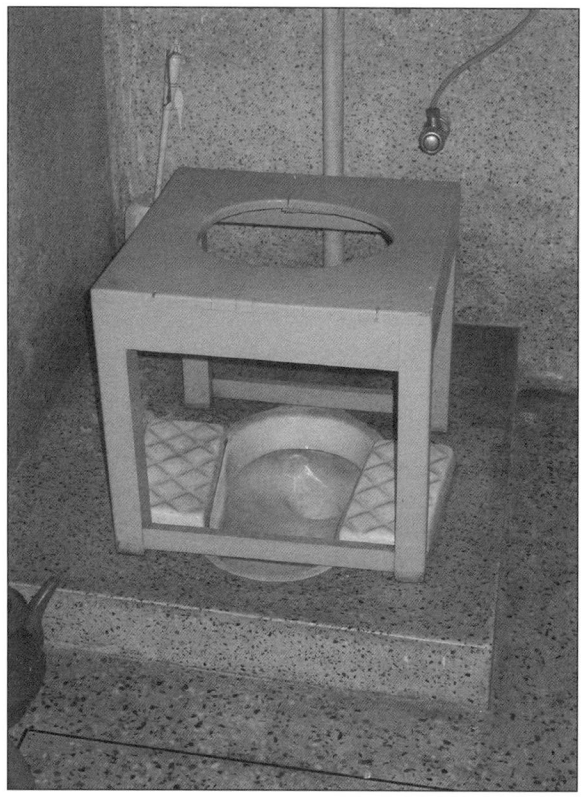

Figure 7.36. Toilet stool used over a squat toilet. Painted wood resists moisture. No splash-guard.

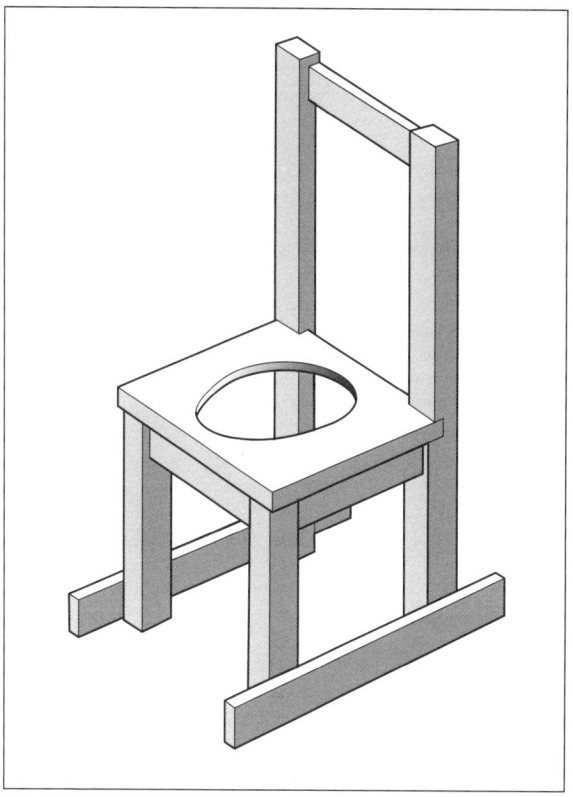

Figure 7.37. Toilet chair with side runners.These spread the weight of the chair and improve stability.

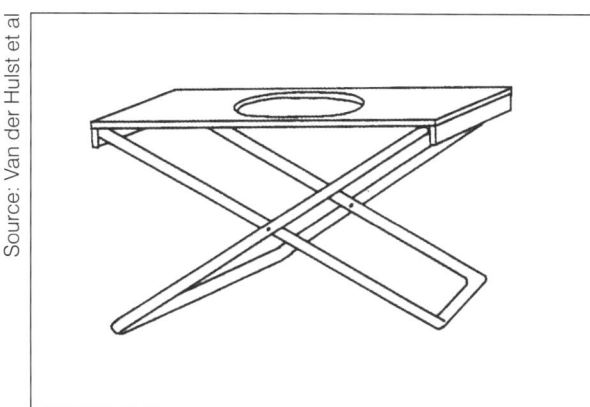

Source: Van der Hulst et al

Figure 7.38. The principle of a foldable toilet seat. Can be stored out of the way when not in use. May lack stability.

7

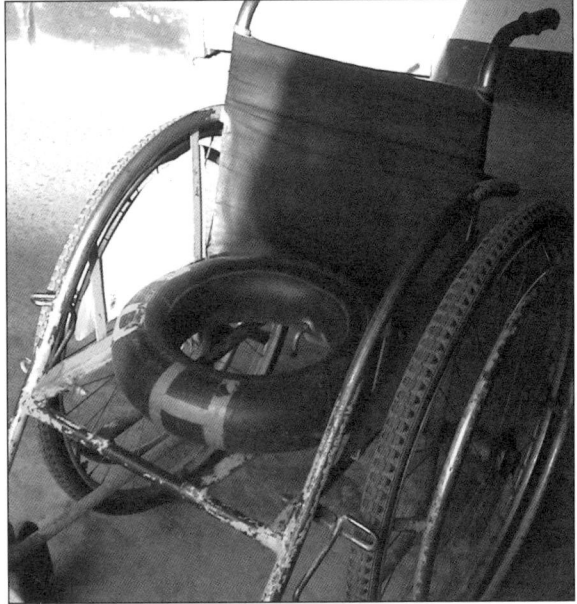

Figure 7.39. Wheelchair with small tyre inner tube in place of seat. Inner tube is durable, easy to clean, widely available at reasonable cost. Suitable for persons with poor sitting balance, so long as it is fully inflated.
(Case-study 9.5, page 174)

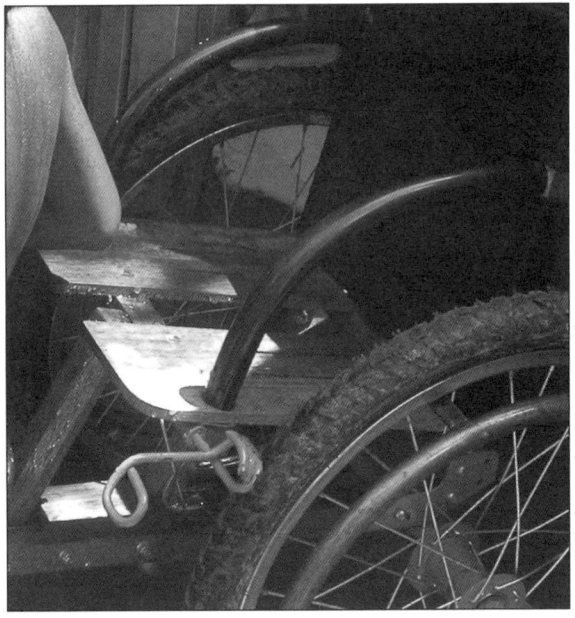

Figure 7.40. Wheelchair with a centre plank removed to leave a gap in the seat for toileting.*
(Case-study 9.15, page 201)

---

* This wheelchair is not designed for this adaptation. The frame directly under the seat means it inevitably gets fouled.

Wheelchair or trolley as a toilet seat

To avoid the need to transfer on and off a wheelchair, low trolley or other mobility device, a wheelchair can be designed or adapted for use as a toilet seat. Users enter the latrine in their wheelchair or trolley, which they position over the toilet hole. They remain seated in the chair to urinate or defecate, so that faeces and urine fall directly into the toilet hole. Here are examples of how this may be done:

- The user removes the seat cushion and board, revealing two metal struts which support the seat but are wide enough apart to leave a gap in the middle. He replaces the seat with a small tyre inner tube, on which he sits to use the toilet (Figure 7.39).

- The user removes the seat cushion and a central plank of the seat, which creates a gap about 10cm wide in the seat (Figure 7.40).

- A small cloth step is added to the wheelchair halfway between the seat and the ground. This makes it easier to transfer into the chair from the ground. This 'transfer' seat has a hole in it, which the user sits on to use the toilet (Figure 7.41).

To ensure that the wheelchair is positioned directly over the toilet hole, some type of guide is useful. This could be marks on the floor or wall, or concrete (or other material) mouldings for the wheels to slot into (Figure 7.42).

Advantages of a wheelchair toilet seat:

- The disabled person uses the same toilet facilities as the rest of the family.

- There is no need to leave a seat in the toilet that may obstruct other users.

- No extra space is needed to park a wheelchair beside the toilet.

7

Example of a transfer seat

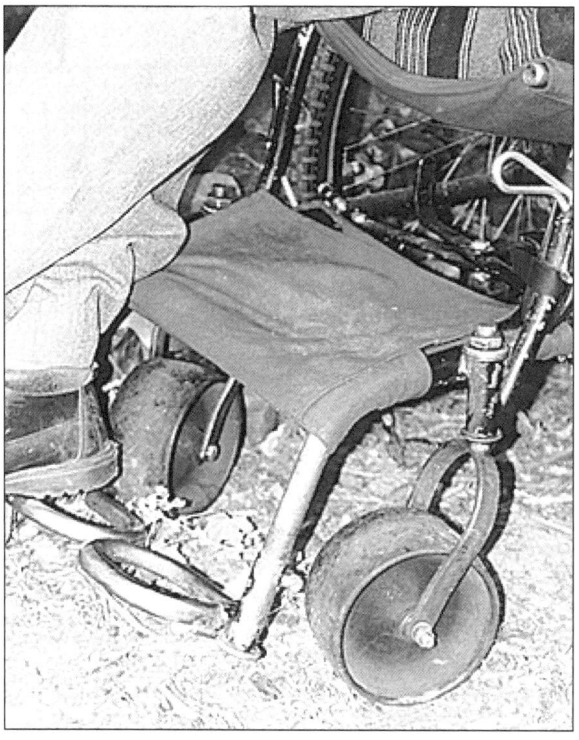

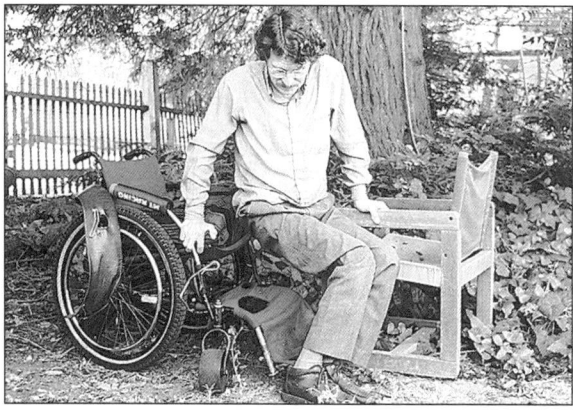

Figure 7.41. 'Transfer' seat as toilet seat (6). The seat has a hole which is covered by a flap fastened into place when not in use. For toileting, the flap is opened and folds out of the way. It could be difficult to keep the cloth seat clean.

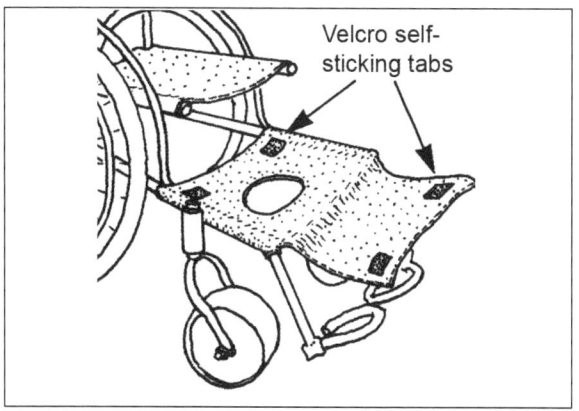

Velcro self-sticking tabs

Drawbacks to the wheelchair toilet approach:

· It is not suitable for all designs of wheelchair. If the frame underneath is not designed so that the central section is kept clear, then the frame can become fouled.

• It can only be used where the toilet pan is set level with the floor, otherwise the wheelchair cannot be wheeled over it.

• The latrine floor must be strong enough to bear the weight of the wheelchair, otherwise there is a risk of the floor collapsing.

• Some users might need help to lift their own weight off the seat in order to swap the cushion for the inner tube.

• Because of the long drop between the seat and toilet hole, there is a high risk of fouling the chair frame. This is not a problem for low-trolley users, who are the most common users of this method (Figure 7.48). For this reason, many wheelchair users prefer to use the commode chair option (see Section 7.6 on Commode seats).

• The inner tube may still be too expensive for the poorest. However, alternatives can be made using cheaper materials, e.g. a plastic ring padded with straw (Figure 7.47).

7.5 Squat latrines

For a person who can squat, but has poor balance, a handrail is often enough to make a squat toilet usable (see page 103 on Types of support rails). Alternatively, a movable toilet seat may be used over the toilet pan, as described above.

For people who use a low trolley (Figure 7.48) or who crawl, the toilet pan should be installed as level as possible with the surrounding floor (Figure 7.43). It is generally recommended that a latrine slab is installed slightly higher

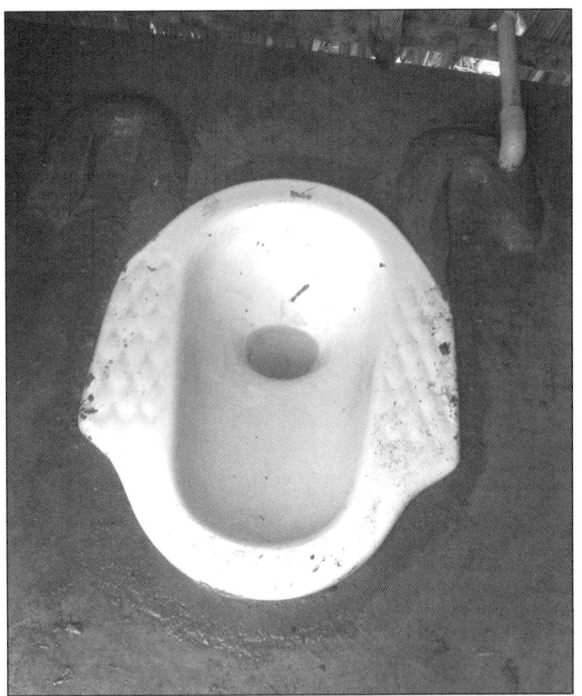

Figure 7.42. Cement mortar mouldings next to toilet pan for wheels of wheelchair to slot into for accurate positioning.
(Case-study 9.15, page 201)

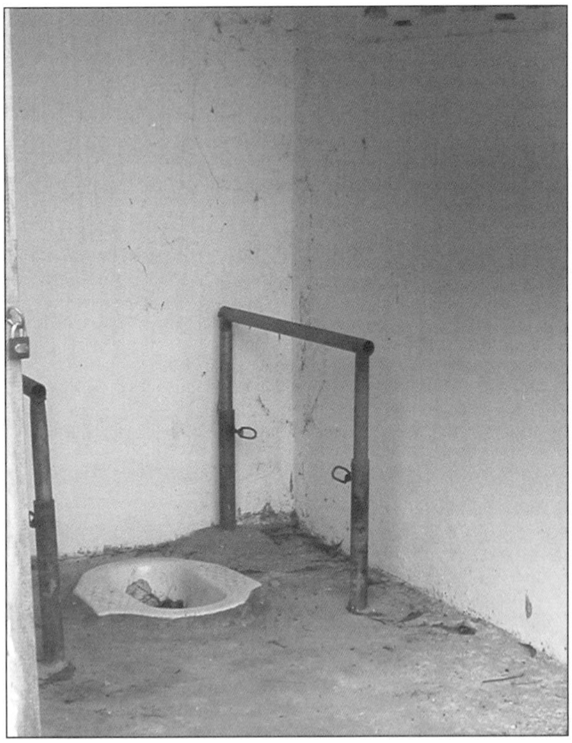

than ground level, to reduce the amount of debris falling in, and to improve the flow of water away from the slab. The earth around the slab should be banked up to finish level with the slab, so that there is no step.

7.6 Commode seats

If reaching or using the latrine is a problem, for whatever reason, a commode seat is another option. This is a toilet seat with a hole, used with a container underneath, such as a bucket, bowl, tin can or piece of plastic or paper. The contents of the container are then disposed of in the toilet or elsewhere by a helper.

Advantages:

- The seat can be placed in the most convenient location for the user or family member, either inside or outside the house. For example, the seat can be placed near the kitchen, so that a mother can keep an eye on her disabled child while she continues with other tasks.

- Proximity: The problem of distance or an inaccessible path to the toilet can be avoided.

- A commode seat is less likely than a toilet seat to become dirty or damaged by other users, or by being repeatedly moved on and off the toilet.

Drawbacks:

- The container needs to be emptied and cleaned after use by a family member.

- A separate private toilet area may need to be created.

- The disabled person risks becoming isolated if left sitting alone for longer than necessary.

Figure 7.43. Squat toilet installed level with the surrounding floor.
(Case-study 9.16, page 207)

Toilets – access and use

Examples of commode seats

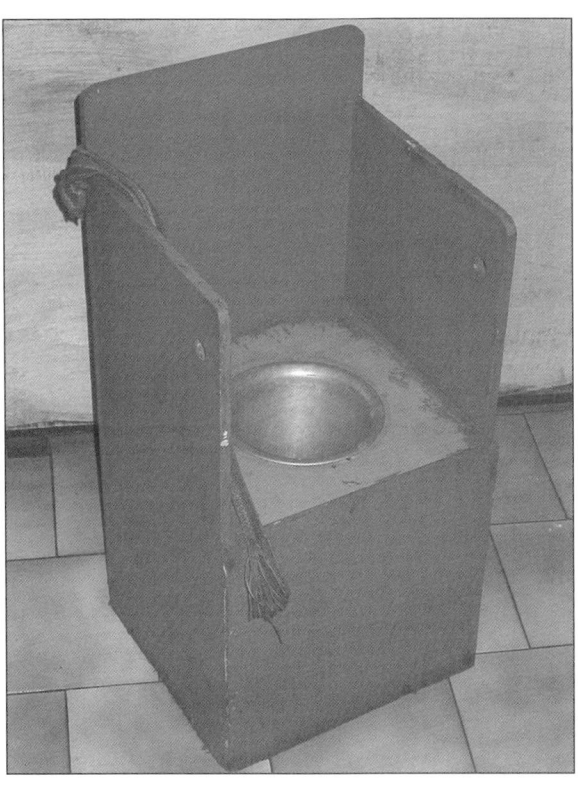

Figure 7.44. Child's wooden commode chair. Note the holes in the sides to insert a wooden bar to prevent child falling forwards.

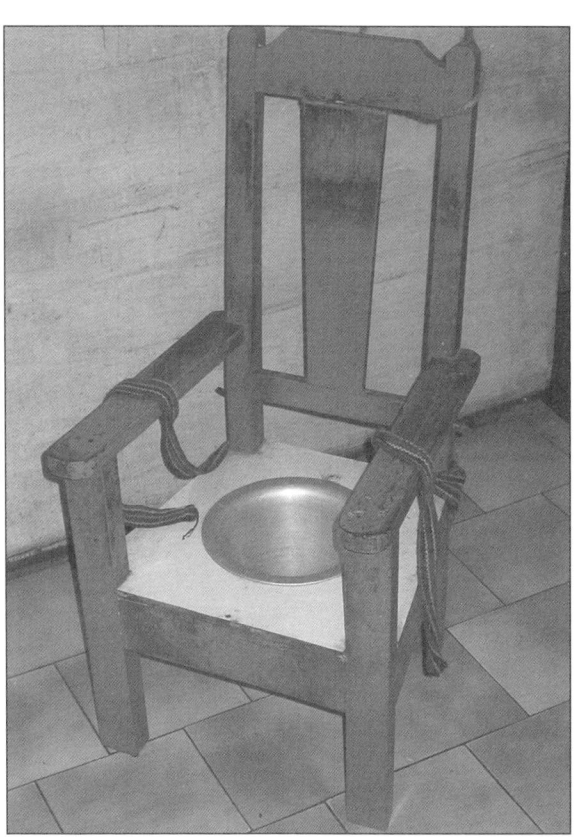

Figure 7.45. Wooden commode chair. Note fabric straps to support the user.

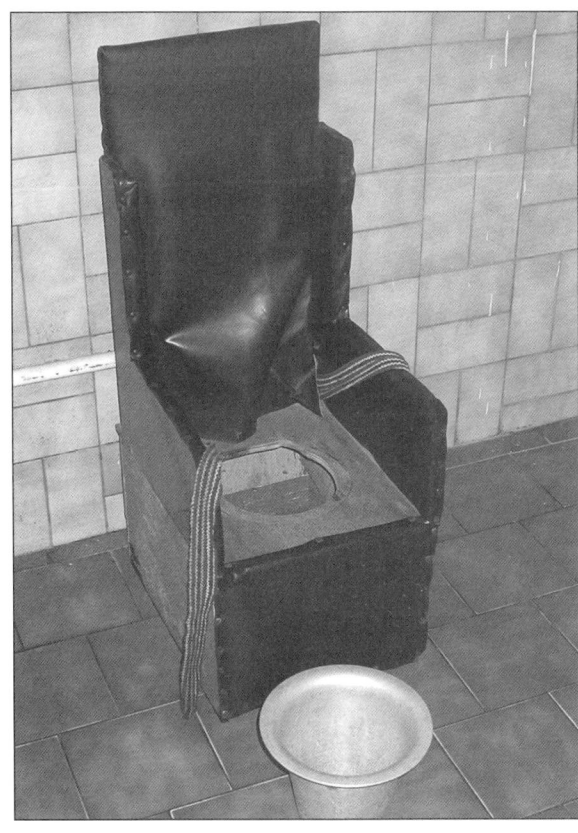

Figure 7.46. Padded wooden commode chair. (Shown with pot removed). Washable plastic covering is hygienic but comfortable.

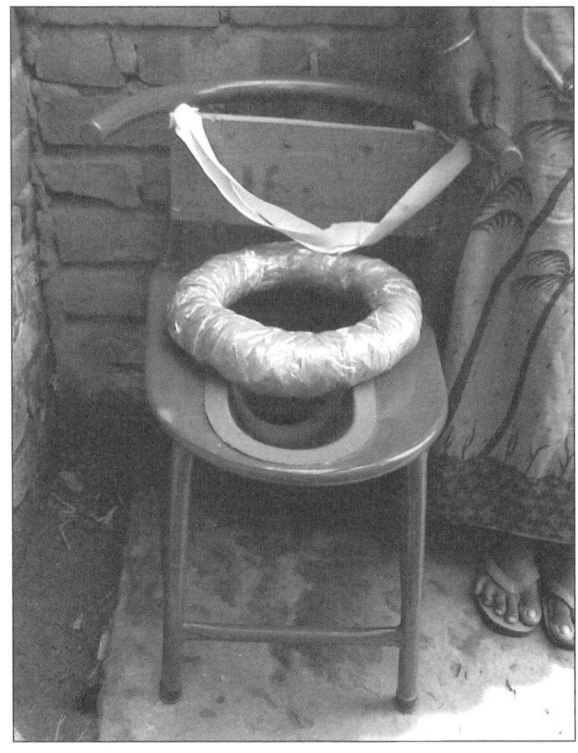

Figure 7.47. Metal commode chair with plastic inset toilet pan. Bought locally and adapted. Note sitting ring padded with straw for extra comfort, wooden plank and waist belt for extra support. *(Case-study 9.8, page 181)*

7

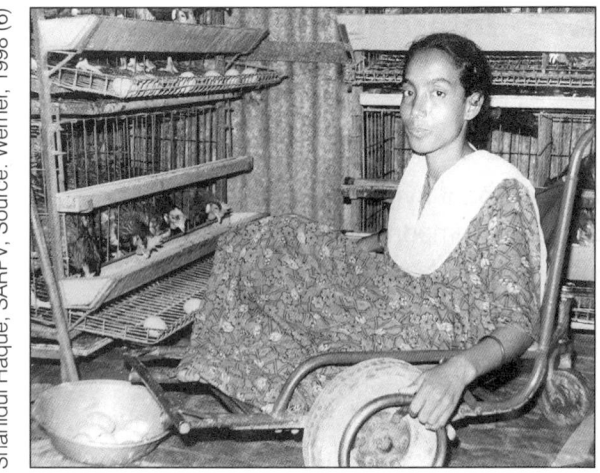

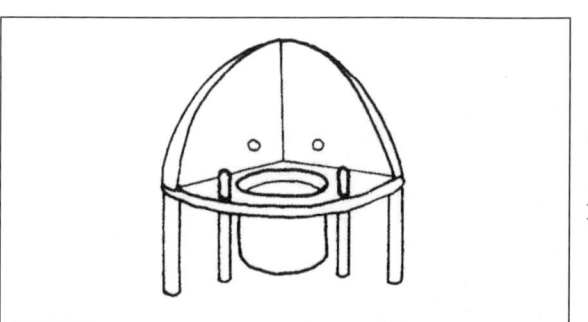

Figure 7.50. Corner seat with potty insert for child with poor sitting balance.

Figure 7.48. Low trolleys in Bangladesh are used mainly by disabled women as they are suitable for floor level activities.

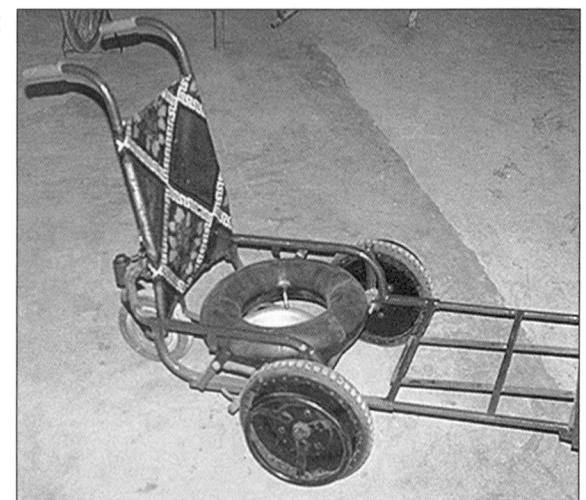

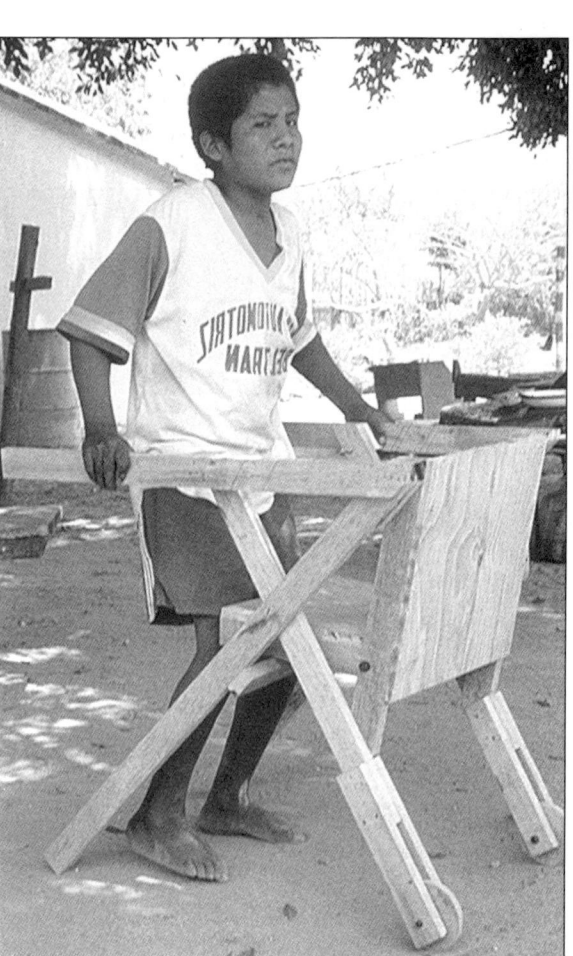

Figure 7.51. This child uses walking frame that converts to a toilet seat (below).The fold-down seat has a potty insert which he can use, wherever he is at the time.

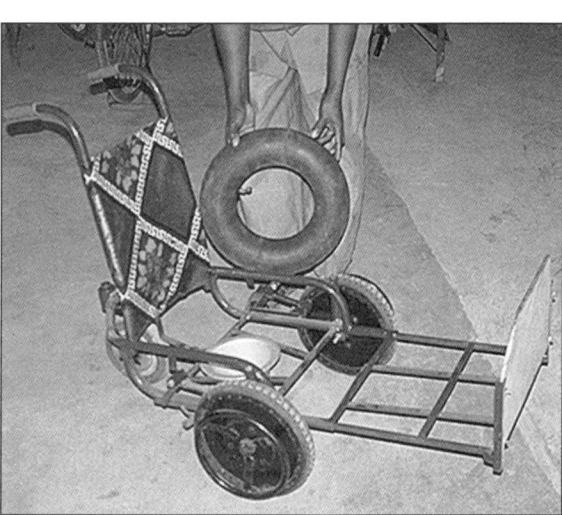

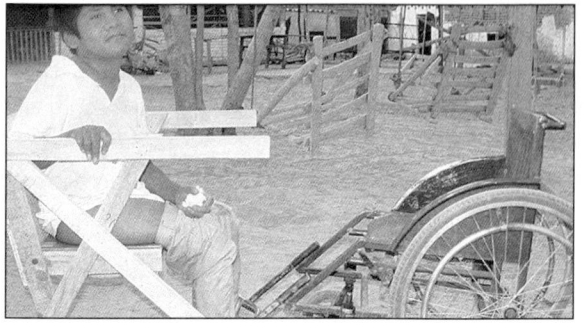

Figure 7.49. The low trolley has a pot that fits into the frame under an inner tube, which functions both as a cushion and as a toilet seat. For general use, the inner tube is covered with a mat.

7

Toilets – access and use

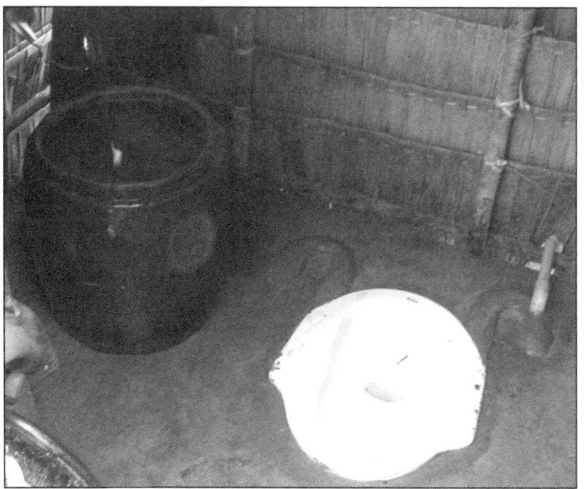

Figure 7.52. Water storage jar beside the toilet.
(Case-study 9.15, page 201)

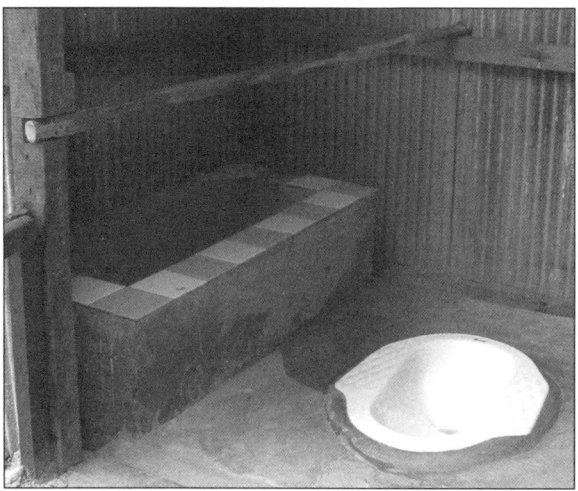

Figure 7.53. Water trough inside toilet cubicle.
(Case-study 9.19, page 215)

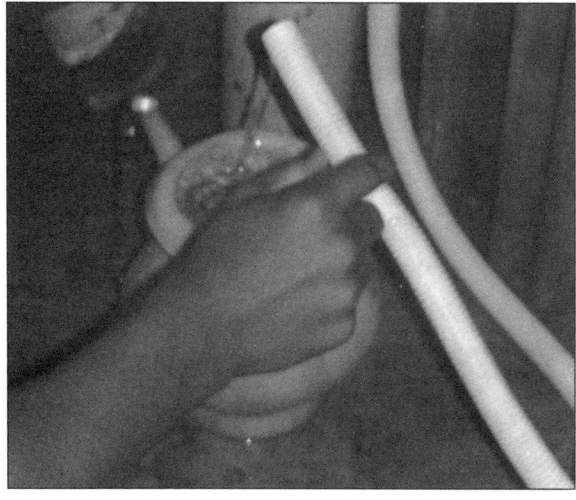

Figure 7.54. Flexible hose attached to a tap allows
the user to fill a container with water using only
one hand.
(Case-study 9.6, page 177)

7.7   Internal water source

A water point inside the latrine cubicle is very important:

For personal hygiene Anal cleansing is particularly important for a number of groups, including adolescent girls and women when menstruating (whether disabled or non-disabled), people who use catheters, or use manual bowel evacuation. Handwashing with soap and/or ash and water is important for everyone after using the toilet.

For toilet flushing Pour-flush toilets need to be flushed with water in order to function.

Many disabled people are unable to fetch water for themselves each time they need it. The water should be within reach of the user when squatting or sitting on the toilet.

If piped water is available, a tap should be provided inside the toilet cubicle.
Tap height for wheelchair users/those using a toilet seat: 80 – 100cm.
Tap height for people using a low trolley, or squatting: ~40cm.
For more details on Taps and tapstands, see page 71.

If there is no piped water, a container should be provided from which water can be scooped, or drawn via a tap. This may be a bucket, or storage jar (Figure 7.52), or a water trough constructed as part of the facility (Figure 7.53). For more details of water storage options, see Section 6.5 on page 80.

A flexible hose attached to a tap allows users to fill a container with water using only one hand (Figure 7.54) or to wash themselves easily (Figure 7.55). The end of the hose should be stored off the ground when not in use, to avoid contamination from the toilet floor.

7

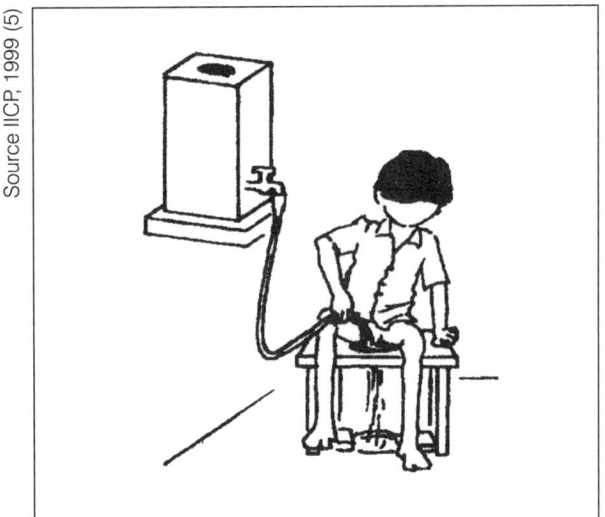

Source: IICP, 1999 (5)

Figure 7.55. Child using a hose to wash himself.

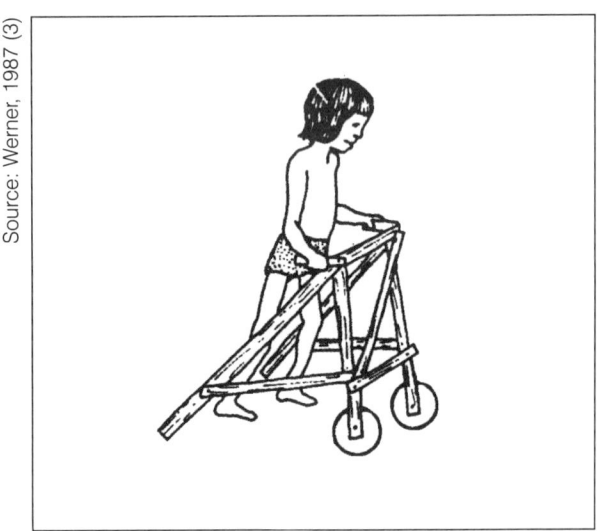

Source: Werner, 1987 (3)

Figure 7.56. Example of a walking frame.

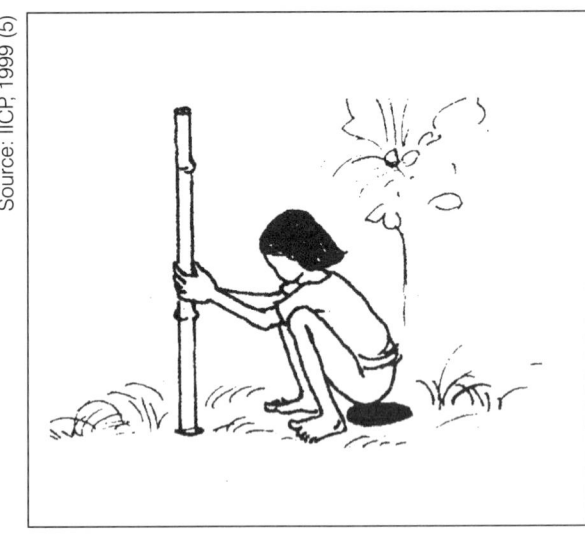

Source: IICP, 1999 (5)

Figure 7.57. Squatting holding a single vertical pole for support.

7.8   Open defecation – support options

Where defecation 'in the open' is the usual practice, support options are still possible. This will depend on factors such as the level of independent mobility, personal preference, and whether the device needs to be mobile or can be fixed in one place. Examples of options include:

*   Walking stick or bamboo pole for the user to lean on while walking to their choice of location, and to lean on while squatting – flexible option, providing minimal support.

*   Walking frame, which supports the user to walk to their chosen location, and provides support while squatting (Figure 7.56) – a flexible option, providing medium support.

*   One or two vertical poles fixed in the ground, at user's arm-length apart – semi-fixed option, providing medium support (Figure 7.57).

*   Horizontal bar tied to two vertical poles fixed in the ground, at a suitable height for the user to hold when squatting (Figure 7.58) – semi-fixed option, providing medium support.

*   A pair of bricks, placed at the desired location, about 10 – 15cm apart depending on the size of the user, to sit on while defecating. Semi-fixed option, providing high level of support. Can be used together with any of the above options.

*   A tree-trunk or branch, or a rope hanging from a branch (Figure 7.59).

7.9   Assistive toilet devices

Anal cleansing devices

Quite a number of disabled and elderly people have problems with anal cleansing after defecation, because of stiff joints or poor co-ordination.

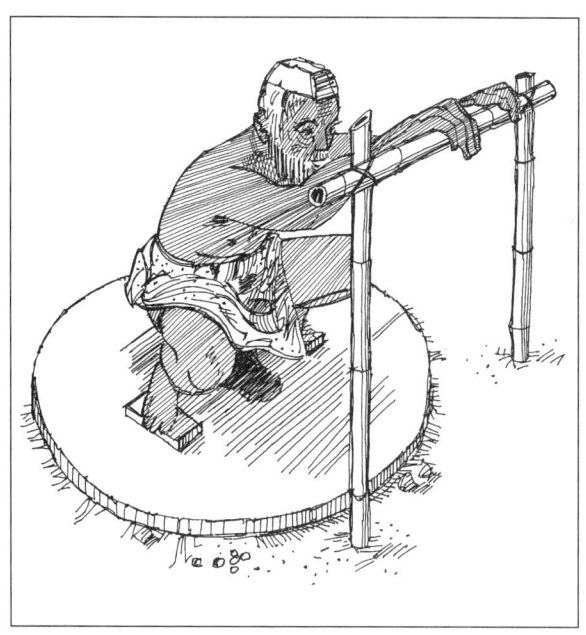

Figure 7.58. Support bar for use when squatting. *(Case-study 9.10, page 185)*

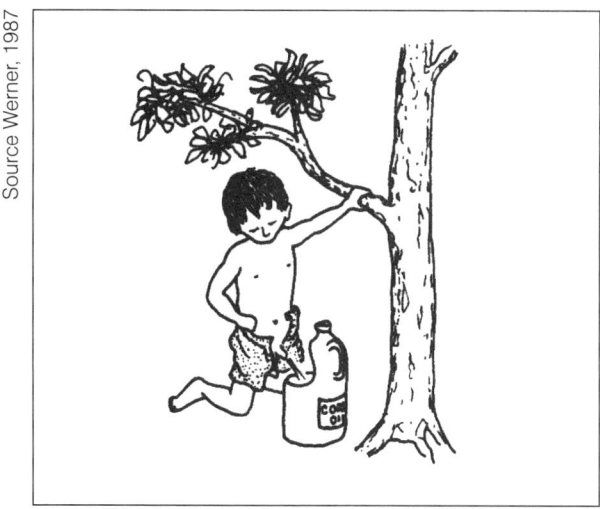

Figure 7.59. Child holding onto a tree branch for support while urinating.

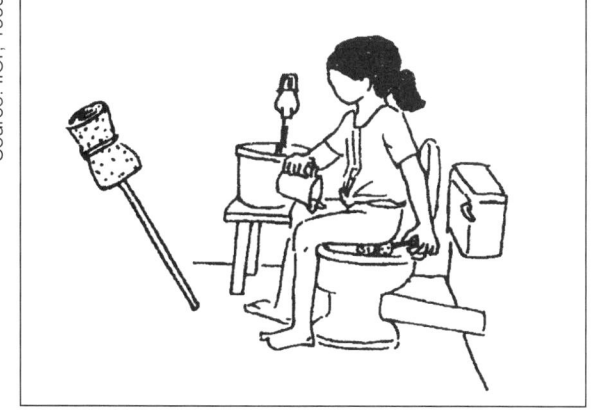

Figure 7.60. Child washing using a long-handled sponge.

Different kinds of cleaning device can be useful to compensate for the user's lack of reach. All have an extended arm or nozzle. Some are sponges with a long handle (Figure 7.60). Some are designed to grip paper or other wiping materials: Figure 7.61 shows a high-cost version, but similar 'pincers' could be made from bamboo or wood for a fraction of the cost (Figure 7.62). Where anal cleansing with water is the custom, a device that pours water and wipes at the same time is useful (Figure 7.63).

All implements need to be washed after use, and replaced regularly, to keep them as hygienic as possible.

The benefits include increased dignity for the disabled person, and personal hygiene tasks are made more pleasant for other family members to carry out.

Knee and hand protectors
For disabled people who move around on their hands and knees, unsanitary areas such as latrines are a terrible health hazard. Their hands and knees are more likely to have abrasions and open wounds, which are regularly in contact with stagnant water, urine and faeces. The result is frequent infections for disabled people. They need to protect their hands and knees from contamination.

Rubber slippers (sandals, flip-flops) can be used on the hands. Wooden 'hand walkers' have the advantage of keeping the hands higher off the ground (Figures 7.64 and 7.65), but the handle may need padding for comfort. Recycled tyres can be made into rubber pads to protect knees and leg stumps (Figures 7.66 and 7.67). Materials are low-cost, durable and easy to clean.

7

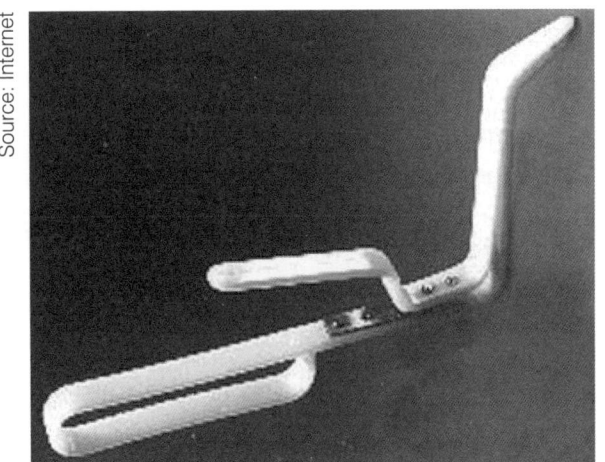

Figure 7.61. Toilet paper tongs with a spring loaded gripping device. Made of hard plastic that can be boiled. High cost.

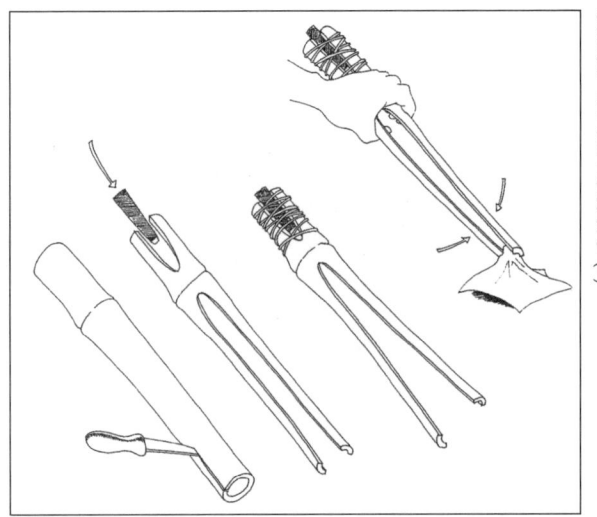

Figure 7.62. Bamboo pincers – low-cost.

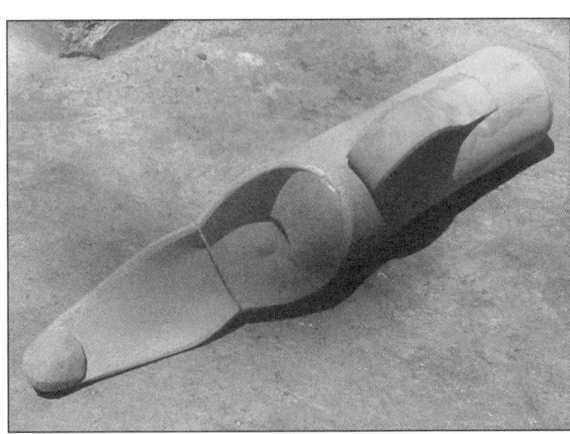

Figure 7.63. Anal cleansing device. The cylinder is filled with water, then the soft rubber 'finger' is used to clean the anal area, letting water slowly trickle out of the tiny opening.
(Case-study 9.15, page 201)

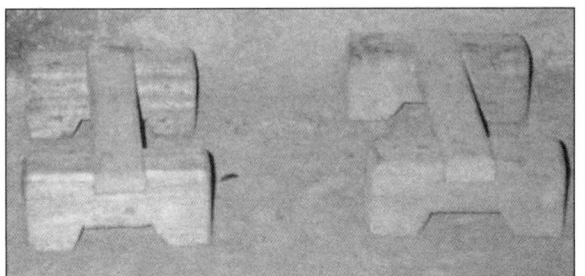

Figure 7.64. Wooden hand walkers.
(Case-study 9.31, page 247)

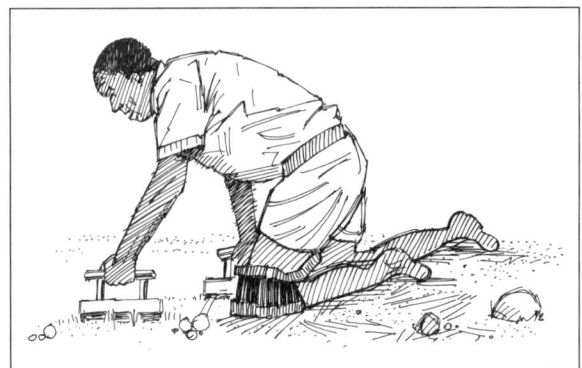

Figure 7.65. Knee protectors and hand walkers in use.
(Case-study 9.31, page 247)

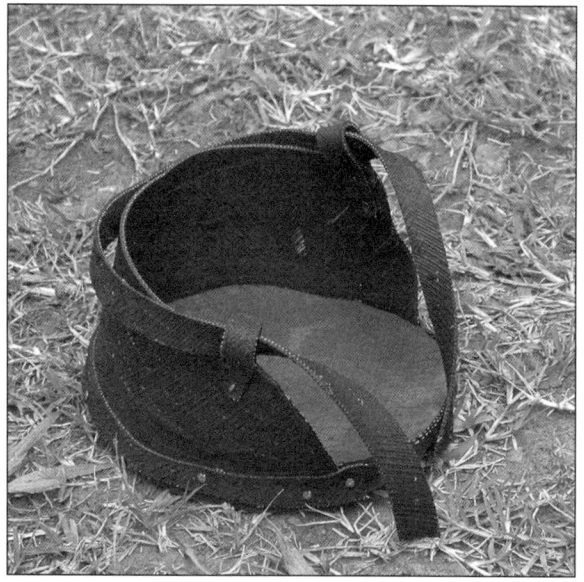

Figure 7.66. Knee protector made from recycled car tyres. Rubber laces run through loops and tie around the leg to hold the pad in place. *(Case-study 9.31, page 247)*

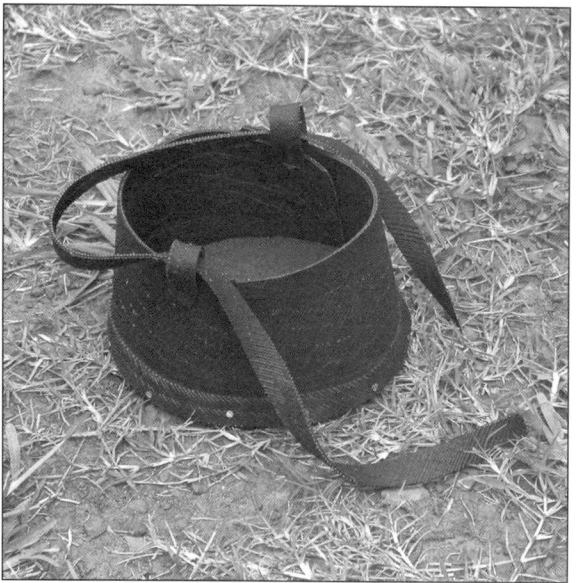

Figure 7.67. Stump protector. *(Case-study 9.31, page 247)*

References

1. WHO (1999) *Promoting Independence Following a Stroke*: A guide for therapists and professionals working in Primary Health Care. World Health Organization. Geneva.

2. WHO (1993) *Promoting the Development of Young Children with Cerebral Palsy*. A guide for mid-level rehabilitation workers. World Health Organization: Geneva.

3. Werner, D. (1987) *Disabled Village Children. A guide for community health workers, rehabilitation workers, and families*. Hesperian Foundation: USA. Available on Healthwrights website.

4. Dacheux, Gilles avec Sophie Ferneeuw (2003) *Infrastructure et post-crise: Reconstruction attentive aux situations de handicap*. Prévention des risques, et construction dans les situations exceptionnelles. Handicap International: Lyon, France.

5. IICP (1999) Series of booklets: *Cleanliness for the Child with Cerebral Palsy, Special Furniture, Toileting for the Child with Cerebral Palsy*. Indian Institute of Cerebral Palsy: Kolkata, India.

6. Werner, D. (1998) *Nothing About Us Without Us: developing innovative technologies for, by and with disabled persons*. Healthwrights: Palo Alto, CA, USA.

7. Van der Hulst, G., Velthuys, M. and de Haan, G. (1993) *More with Less: Aids for disabled people in daily life*. TOOL: Amsterdam.

8. Website: Abledata: your source for assistive technology information. http://test.abledata.com

7

7

Toilets – access and use

Chapter 8

Implementation in practice

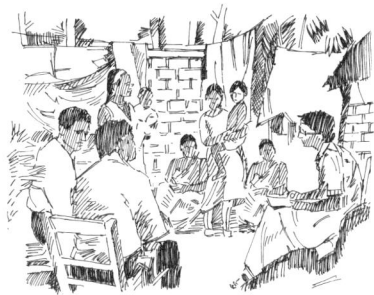

This chapter presents a range of ideas for where and how to start doing something in practice. It is mainly for planners and implementers of services that are relevant to disabled people, including:

- WATSAN professionals who would like to include a disability perspective in their projects and programmes.

- Professionals providing services to disabled people, such as CBR workers or social welfare officials, who would like to include a WATSAN perspective in their work.

- Members of DPOs who, although not service providers, have a consultation and advocacy role.

Each of these groups works in different ways when it comes to practical service delivery. For the WATSAN sector, the lowest 'unit' of implementation tends to be the community level, such as a village or subdivision of a peri-urban area.

Disability service providers work most commonly at household level, with individual disabled people and their families, and less commonly with communities. There are exceptions, such as on issues of educational inclusion, and attitudes, but this is generally the picture.

All approaches are needed, but all don't have to do everything. Their different ways of working complement each other. The majority of disabled people could be catered for with more inclusive WATSAN services. For a minority with complex individual needs an individualised approach is required, which is more likely to be undertaken by the disability sector. There will always be the need for some level of individualised approach, but in the long-term, as WATSAN facilities become more inclusive, this need will reduce.

8.1   Taking a learning approach

Very little is currently known about the best ways to include disabled people in WATSAN, so learning needs to be built into any development of practice. This can be done by collecting

8

information, and carrying out action-research to pilot practical solutions.

Pilot projects can provide the opportunity for agencies to try out new activities and approaches on a small scale that are within their existing programme framework and capacity, requiring minimal external input. If pilot projects are implemented collaboratively between WATSAN and disability sectors, they can also be a way of learning about collaboration with an unfamiliar sector.

Information and learning from pilot activities should be shared. This can help draw attention to disability-related issues, encourage more agencies to undertake similar activities, and stimulate further planned implementation.

If several agencies are involved, there is a risk that pilot activities remain small and undocumented, and any learning from them is lost. Co-ordination is therefore needed to ensure that experience and learning are documented and shared, and can be applied and built on by other agencies.

The primary responsibility for taking a lead on this issue clearly lies with the WATSAN sector. However, DPOs have a key role in advocacy, information dissemination, and consultation on WATSAN issues that affect them. DPOs therefore need to learn from each other about effective ways to advocate for accessible service provision.

- Establish a lead agency – preferably WATSAN – with responsibility for co-ordination, monitoring and dissemination of information about the work.

- Establish the involvement of a major representative DPO, with an advisory/ consultation role.

- Collaborate to develop strategies for piloting and action-research.

8.2 Implementation by the water supply and sanitation sector

It is not necessary to wait for policy and strategy to be in place before starting practical activities. Implementation can begin from any starting point, depending on the interests and skills of the agency involved.

National level policy and strategy
Disability must be recognised and included at national strategy and project design levels, otherwise no resources

will be allocated to it (1). So far there is no model strategy for including a disability perspective in WATSAN. However, several key principles should be considered.

Inter-sectoral collaboration

Discussion and collaboration with the disability sector, i.e. DPOs and disability service providers, are likely to be a challenge, as there may have been little or no previous contact. However, it is essential to any effective development in this area.

Each sector needs to see how their own work fits into a broader context, to recognise different perspectives on an issue, and to value the knowledge and expertise of other sectors. It is useful for the WATSAN sector to gain an understanding of disabled people's issues and needs.

Discussions on the development of strategies that affect disabled people should involve disabled people and their representatives from the outset.

- Develop contacts with DPOs at national level.

- Organise a forum or workshop to bring both sectors together, to exchange information and discuss issues raised.

- Ensure that an organisation with a focus on disabled people, preferably controlled and managed by disabled people (i.e. a DPO), is represented in any consultation process, committee or advisory board. Where possible, involve representatives of disabled women in their own right.

Planning for success

It is not necessary to wait until all relevant agencies are involved before starting practical initiatives. Begin with agencies that are interested, however few, with representation from as many relevant sectors and stakeholders as possible, including government, NGOs and private sector. The involvement of a respected organisation from each sector will provide a 'stamp of approval' that will attract other agencies later.

The process of practical implementation will generate interest and participation from a wider audience, as they recognise its relevance and benefit to their own work. It will show what is (and is not) possible, and provide starting points for action.

- Create opportunities at all stages of the development of pilot implementation for more agencies to become involved.

8

- Share information about practical implementation at regular intervals to generate interest among relevant agencies.

Tap into relevant initiatives and opportunities

Disability inclusion needs to be seen as an integral part of WATSAN service provision, and not develop as a separate and distinct set of projects. In order to avoid this separation, relevant initiatives and trends need to be identified that provide an opportunity to include the issue of disability. For example:

At national level
- Poverty Reduction Strategy Processes: DPOs and disability agencies need representation not only on Task groups dealing with social welfare and social protection, but on all Task groups, including WATSAN.

- Country targets on sanitation, such as the one in Bangladesh, which has recently agreed a target of 100 per cent sanitation by 2010.

- Encourage alliances over common issues of access and equity among representatives of different marginalised groups, such as DPOs, Gender Water Alliance, Associations of the Elderly and others.

At institutional level
- International and national organisations that are increasing their focus on issues of equity and access, including reaching people living in chronic poverty.

- International and national organisations carrying out policy/strategy planning and development activities at organisational level.

- Data collection activities, such as community baseline surveys.

Organisational issues

For individual organisations, a logical starting point is to look at one's own organisation and identify the current capacity and status of disability within it*. Staff at all levels of the organisation may have little understanding or experience of disability, and may therefore be unaware of possible solutions to accessibility. Misinformation and fears about disabled people may be widespread, which can also contribute to negative attitudes among staff.

However, the institutionalised practices of organisations can contribute to discrimination and exclusion, as much as the behaviour of individuals. If the way an organisation is

* See examples of how this has been done on an international scale by the World Bank (2), or DFID (3), or at a local project level (4).

run excludes disability issues, the actions of individuals are unlikely to lead to lasting change.

Suggestions

*   Appoint a person with responsibility for taking a lead on disability (this does not mean that s/he has to do everything). This person must be senior enough to be able to make decisions, including planning and budget allocation.

*   Carry out a disability 'audit': Invite someone from a DPO or disability service provider, or a disabled person from the local community, to help look at the issue of disability in the organisation. This might include looking at policy/ strategy, office practices, physical facilities, or a specific project. For example, go round the office or project site, look at which existing facilities and activities are accessible to disabled people and which are not. Identify how facilities could be upgraded or adapted, and how activities could be made more inclusive. (The questions in Box 8.4, and in Appendix 3 could provide a framework for issues to look at).

*   Learn and implement the disability policy of the organisation or donor agency.

*   Make contact with agencies that can provide Disability Equality Training for staff, ideally by disabled people. In countries where disabled people have not yet developed this capacity, this should be an organisation that has a rights-based or socially inclusive perspective, rather than a medical or welfare focus.

*   Initially, existing training materials could be used. In the long-term, training should be developed which would incorporate the practical expertise of the engineers with a rights-based approach from the disability equality trainers.

*   Develop accessible and inclusive standard designs in collaboration with disabled people: adapt existing designs, construct and pilot their use.

*   Organise an access audit of your office and training facilities, *including the toilets*. This should be done in consultation with disabled people locally, using a locally devised audit framework.

*   Hire qualified disabled people into your organisation as field staff, consultants, trainers, and administrators.

*   Provide ongoing opportunities for staff to build relationships with disabled people that will lead to changed attitudes and real partnerships.

For a list of disability policies of major donor agencies, see Appendix A1.5, page 260.

For examples of training materials on disability inclusion, see Appendix A1.6, page 262.

For examples of access audits see Appendix 4 on page 281 and UNESCAP Community Accessibility Checklist (5).

Project/ programme cycle

At a project or programme level, it may not be clear what steps to take first, what information and skills are needed, and who needs to be involved. It is better to try something, even if it is not perfect, than to do nothing.

There are different models and frameworks for the implementation of infrastructure projects, but all are likely to involve a series of stages: feasibility, design (i.e. preparation and planning), implementation (mainly construction of facilities), operation and maintenance, monitoring and evaluation.

Project design is when it is most crucial to consider disability. This is the stage which provides an opportunity to incorporate a range of proactive measures into the project/ programme to address disability issues (6). The monitoring and evaluation stages are also important, to eventually assess the impact of those measures on disabled people.

Project design stage

The design stage of a WATSAN project involves deciding what the project will do, and how it will do it. Project design is based partly on technical considerations, and partly on communication and negotiation with the community the service is intended to benefit.

Making alliances for inclusive approaches

1. Identify and get to know relevant local and national agencies with an interest in inclusive and accessible services, including DPOs, parents' and elderly people's associations, and agencies that work with disabled children, adults and the elderly, including relevant government departments.

2. Identify issues of common interest, and areas for potential collaboration and exchange.

3. Where a local DPO exists, ensure that it is represented during any planning and project design, and participates in decision-making wherever appropriate. This should ideally be a cross-impairment DPO, whose members include people with different impairments*. Disability service providers and social welfare organisations can also provide useful input.

Review existing information

1. Before embarking on a large information-gathering exercise, it is worth checking with other organisations,

* Like many NGOs, DPOs vary in their capacity, and how far they represent the views of all disabled people. You may need to make an extra effort to contact more marginalised disabled people, such as disabled women, children, those in rural areas, and people with communication difficulties.

8

such as relevant government agencies, DPOs, or disability service providers, whether some of the information needed for project design already exists. This will save time and resources, and large surveys, which may not be the best option (Box 8.1). It will also help to promote inter-sectoral communication.

2. Make reference to relevant government policy and strategy, such as:

    • WATSAN policy and strategy, and the status of vulnerable and underserved groups in those strategies;

    • Relevant disability legislation and policy where it exists;

    • The UN Standard Rules should also be referred to, as they provide a useful framework for disability rights (7)

3. Establish the size of the problem. Accurate information is useful for planning and programme development. Where background data on demographic, social, economic, cultural and institutional aspects are being collected, these should also include information related to disabled people, the elderly, and other marginalised groups in the project area/s. First check whether this information already exists elsewhere (see point 1 above).

4. Include disability-related data as part of each relevant area. For example, data on women should identify the number of disabled women, data on households should identify the number with a disabled person, data on poor households should identify the number of poor households with a disabled person, and so on.

5. Disabled people are not all identical, so disability data needs to be differentiated to identify disabled women, disabled girls and boys, disabled elderly women and men, people with different types of impairment, and levels of poverty.

8

Box 8.1. The problem with surveys

Large surveys tend to be costly, and bring only minimal benefits to the people surveyed. Disabled people have long experience of being surveyed and counted, but then seeing no benefits (8).

At the same time, official statistics on disability are often inadequate. In Bangladesh, the 2001 National Census found that the prevalence of disability is 0.8 per cent*, and that less than 0.4% of children are disabled (9). But a recent Actionaid survey found that this figure was nearer 14% (10).

Until more accurate and reliable data are produced, the official low figure will continue to reinforce the assumption by service providers that disability is an insignificant minority issue.

The challenge is to produce data that present an accurate picture of the size and nature of the problems facing disabled people, that are useful for advocacy, and for practical planning and strategy. In order to produce data that will be accepted by all key stakeholders, agencies need to collaborate and share, not only the results of data collection, but also criteria and methodologies used.

Frameworks such as WHO's 'ICF – International Classification of Functioning, Disability and Health' (11) can be useful in developing accurate and consistent data collection.

* Figures not yet published.

Consultation and assessment
A community-level baseline survey is commonly carried out, often followed by a community consultation exercise, to identify local problems and priorities, vulnerable households and the level and type of demand for services. This should involve participation from community members. The following suggestions could help to make this more inclusive and enable the views of disabled people to be heard.

1. Develop collaboration with DPOs and disability/social welfare organisations: contact them when recruiting project staff or volunteers, for example, or consult them on the design of needs assessments.

2. Include representatives of disabled and elderly people in training for community members on how to conduct community and household needs surveys and assessments.

3. Draw on existing informal and formal support networks of disabled and elderly people at community level to gather information. Other useful networks could be parents' groups, health clinics, social centres, schools for disabled children, places of worship and community programmes.

4. Include questions in baseline surveys to find out the prevalence and types of impairments, level of isolation, vulnerability and functional limitations. Use or adapt available checklists or assessments (see page 137, Household level assessments, and Appendix 5, page 283).

5. When carrying out participatory consultation activities, such as focus group discussions, give elderly and disabled people the opportunity to discuss in small groups. Where appropriate, organise groups of disabled women separately from disabled men, elderly women separately from elderly men, and encourage older disabled children to speak on their own behalf. In this way, they can gain confidence before sharing with the wider community. Mixed discussion groups should also be held, so that others are also made aware of the problems and views of vulnerable groups.

6. Participatory processes and tools can be modified to make them accessible to people with a wide range of impairments. Use simple ranking and mapping tools to identify disabled and other vulnerable people in a community, and to enable vulnerable groups to identify and prioritise their own needs.

7. When presenting information, use a range of formats: verbal, written and tactile. Written materials should be clear (large black lettering on pale background) and use straightforward concise language, such as key words and phrases. These should be read out for the benefit of visually impaired people. Use objects that blind people can touch, such as a relief map of a village, or pebbles, beans or shells for ranking exercises.

8. Consider disability issues when assessing resource requirements and availability. (Disabled people themselves should be seen as a resource).

9. Set realistic time-frames to allow for a participatory process.

10. Check whether or not disabled women, children and men are present, included and actively participating in consultation and assessment activities. If not, find out what is preventing them, and try different solutions.

Solutions to physical barriers to mobility
11. Make meeting places as accessible as possible: use ground floor rooms, or open areas without steps, or add a mobile ramp for temporary access; provide enough space for a wheelchair or other mobility aids to enter and turn.

8

12. Consider locating meetings and other events near the homes of the least mobile participants, or in locations where disabled people meet.

13. Make sure accessible toilets are available, or an acceptable alternative.

14. Find solutions to transport problems: engage neighbours, other disabled people, volunteers to assist disabled people – to push a wheelchair, help carry a child, offer the use of a bicycle, etc.

15. Allocate a volunteer to represent the views of the disabled person who cannot be present, and to feed back information from meetings.

Creating demand among disabled people and their families

If disabled people and their families are going to participate in consultations about WATSAN, they first need to know that it worth their while doing so. The experience of many disabled people is that fine words are often spoken, but in reality nothing changes. Family members need to be made aware of what accessible options might be possible, and how these might benefit the whole family, including carers. Families may feel more inclined to consider inclusive options if they are seen as a modern innovation that benefits the whole community (see next section).

- Provide information to disabled people and their families about accessible/ inclusive designs of facilities, using drawings, photos, and actual demonstration facilities and equipment where available.

- Tell stories of the benefits of inclusive facilities for the whole family, using local examples, or case-studies from Chapter 9.

Working with communities

Communities can play a significant role in promoting services and approaches that either include or exclude disabled and other vulnerable people. Technical solutions to physical barriers need to be accompanied by creative solutions that address social barriers, such as attitudes and behaviour of people in the community.

The most positive way of promoting inclusive facilities may be to show how they meet such universal needs as comfort, convenience and privacy.

8

For further resources on problem-solving approaches to disabled people's participation, see Appendix A1.6, page 262.

- Consult agencies with experience of disability awareness-raising activities, which could provide information and training to implementing staff and local partners. Activities should address attitudes and behaviour, emphasising practical problem-solving approaches to disabled people's participation (Box 8.2).

- Engage the support of local women's groups. Point out the benefits of inclusive facilities for all, especially for women, children and elderly people, in terms of reduced workload, reduced accidents, improved health and family well-being.

- Include disabled people's representatives (especially disabled women and female carers) on community development committees and advisory councils at all levels.

For a list of further resources on needs assessment, see Appendix A1.8, page 264.

Household level - working with disabled people and their families

Some disabled people and their families have complex needs that may require a detailed understanding and assessment, which is beyond the scope of a community-level consultation.

Guidance on assessing the needs of disabled people and their families is covered comprehensively elsewhere, and a number of checklists and frameworks are available (for one example, see Appendix 5, page 283). These can provide guidance, but should not be used rigidly.

Some initial guidance is provided here.

Who can do this?

Individual and household needs assessment can be a time-consuming process, and should be carried out by someone prepared to spend time and make several visits. Such a role is suited to the skills and experience of many disability sector agencies, particularly those providing community-based support, such as CBR workers.

Disabled people themselves can be an excellent resource in supporting each other, although it should not be assumed that they would want to take on this role. Elderly people may have limited physical strength, but usually have more patience and tenacity than younger people, and in many cultures are listened to with respect.

Community development or health workers, youth volunteers, local women's or church groups can all play a valuable role.

8

Household needs assessment

The main source of care and support for disabled people who need it is usually the family. The aim of any intervention should therefore be to strengthen the capacity of the family to provide this support, within the context of the family and community, rather than replace the family by supporting the disabled person directly.

The long-term aim should be to improve the well-being of the whole family, not only of the individual disabled person. This may be by increasing the disabled person's capacity to contribute more to the family, or by reducing the workload of the family, or by making their support tasks easier.

For example, a mother who supports her disabled child to use the toilet may find her task gets more difficult and time-consuming as the child grows heavier; she may develop back pains and risk injuring her child and herself. A simple toilet seat could enable her to support her child more safely, reduce her back pain and also her risk of injury.

A few basic principles need to be borne in mind:

1. It is important that the disabled person and their family are partners in problem-solving. It is a waste of time for an 'expert' outsider to identify the 'perfect solution', if the disabled person and their family do not agree with it.

2. Look at the issue of WATSAN in the context of the whole family situation, not in isolation.

3. Do not make assumptions about a disabled person and what they can and cannot do, and what they need. Each person is different.

4. Find out what solutions the disabled person has already tried – what worked, what didn't? Why didn't it work? They may have their own ideas about how they could adapt their environment. Listen to their ideas and find ways to build on them.

5. Look at the whole family situation: economic, social, skills, resourcefulness, their attitude and behaviour towards the disabled person. What are they already doing to support the disabled person? What else would they like to be able to do?

6. Many people are not aware of what solutions are possible, and cannot imagine how life might be different. In this case, provide information and examples, show pictures of different solutions, and let them ask questions. Tell stories of disabled people you know who have benefited from different solutions (or use selected case-studies from Chapter 9).

7. Take a realistic look at the current situation and identify goals that disabled people would like to achieve. If a goal is difficult to achieve, help the disabled person to break it down into small achievable steps, which gradually progress towards the final goal.

8. Practical trial and error is essential, instead of only talking about a solution. Ask the person to demonstrate how they carry out the activity now. Improvise different solutions, or try out different equipment, if it is available, and see what difference it makes. Be prepared to adapt, adjust and, if necessary, start again. Figure 8.1 provides a guide to the problem-solving process.

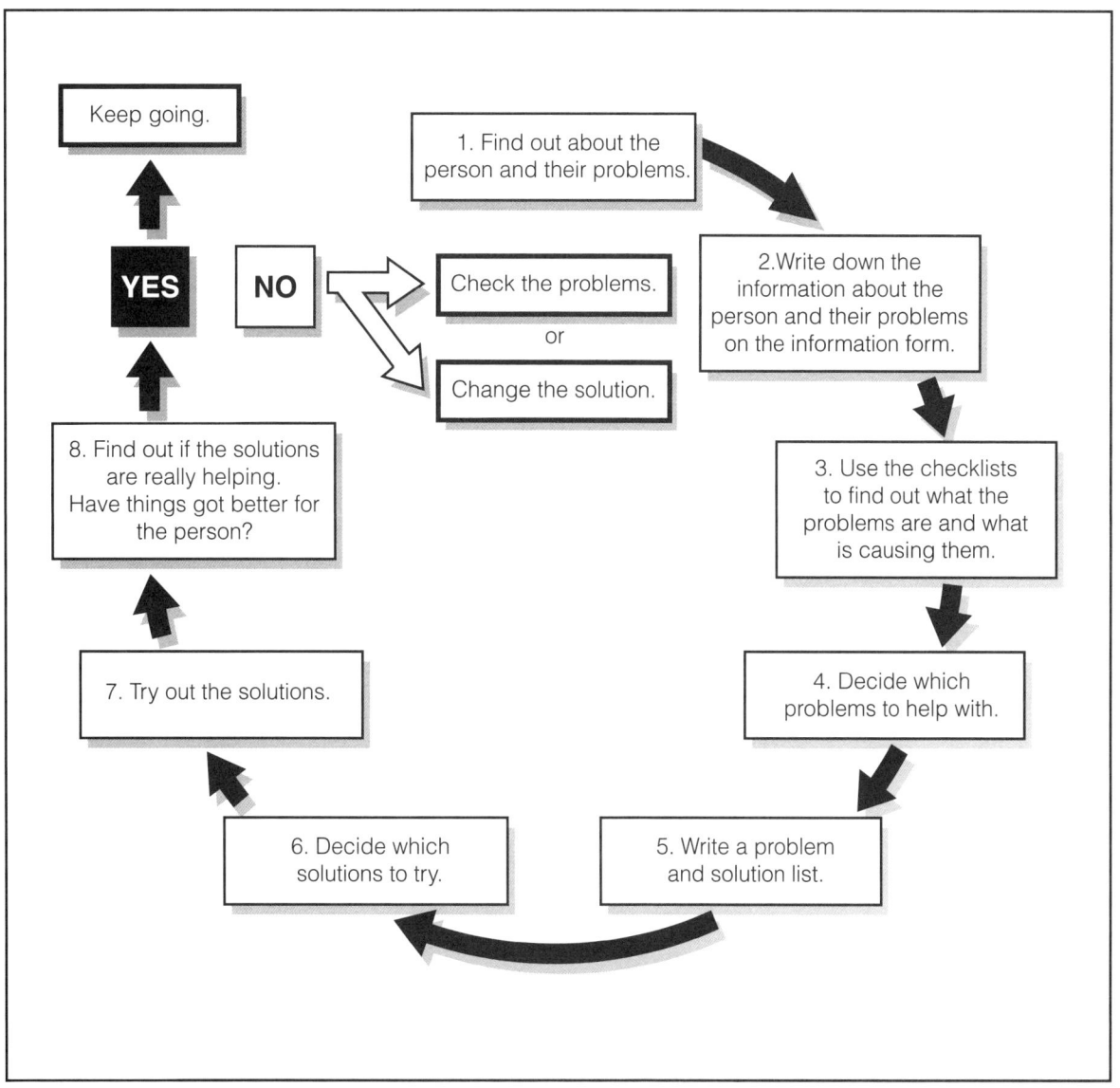

Figure 8.1. Problem solving process. (12)

Common constraints

Many families would like to help their disabled member, but may be too busy. It is often quicker for a helper to do a task, such as bathing or taking a disabled person to the toilet, than to spend time supporting her to do it by herself. If this is an issue, it is important that initial solutions are aimed at reducing the family's workload, and produce quickly visible results. For example, tangible results could be achieved by making or lending a piece of low-cost equipment, and asking a family member to spend 10 minutes a day supporting the disabled person to use it. This could show that it is worth spending time now in order to save time in the future.

Access to water and sanitation may not be a priority for the disabled person and their family, who may have more urgent concerns, such as getting the harvest in, or the roof mended before the rainy season, which cannot be ignored.

8.3 Implementation by the disability sector

This section deals with issues relevant to DPOs and to disability service providers, although we recognise that some agencies, especially NGOs, have programmes that provide both WATSAN and disability services. Likewise, some DPOs are known to provide WATSAN services.

It is not necessary to wait for policy and strategy to be in place before starting practical activities. Implementation can begin from any starting point, depending on the interests and skills of the agency involved.

National level policy and strategy

Disability needs to move on from stand-alone legislation and policies, and be articulated in policies and strategies of relevant sectors such as the WATSAN sector. No resources will be allocated to disability in the WATSAN sector if it is not recognised and included at national strategy and project design levels (1). A lack of awareness and understanding in the sector means that this has not been done.

At the same time, the disability sector tends to have well-established links with certain sectors, including health, social welfare, education and employment, but rarely with the WATSAN sector.

- Strategies for advocacy and lobbying for disability rights and access need to include access and rights to WATSAN.

- Give disability policy and legislation documents to WATSAN sector planners.

- Get to know WATSAN policy and strategies, identify opportunities for including a disability perspective.

- Identify an agency or group of agencies to take a lead on WATSAN issues.

A twin-track approach is needed by the disability sector:
- Including WATSAN issues in the disability sector;

- Advocacy, lobbying and collaboration for the inclusion of a disability perspective in the WATSAN sector.

On both 'tracks', several key principles should be considered.

Inter-sectoral collaboration

Collaboration with the WATSAN sector is essential to any effective development on both of the above 'tracks'.

Each sector needs to see how their own work fits into a wider context, to recognise different perspectives on an issue, and to value the knowledge and expertise of other sectors. It is useful for the disability sector to be aware of the potential contribution of the WATSAN sector to meeting the needs of disabled people, and what options are possible, but also the constraints under which the sector works.

All initiatives on the part of DPOs and disability service providers to address WATSAN issues for disabled people need to involve the WATSAN sector from the outset. This makes their co-operation more likely at later stages of implementation when technical input is needed, and help avoid expensive failures.

- Develop contacts with the WATSAN sector at national level.

- Organise a discussion forum or workshop to bring both sectors together, to raise issues and to exchange information.

- Invite the WATSAN sector to provide input into disability policy and strategy discussions.

Planning for success

It is not necessary to wait until all relevant agencies are involved before starting practical initiatives. Begin with agencies that are interested, however few, with representation from as many relevant sectors and stakeholders as possible,

8

including government, NGOs and private sector. The involvement of a respected organisation from each sector will provide a 'stamp of approval' that will attract other agencies later.

The process of practical implementation will help generate interest and participation from a wider audience, as agencies recognise its relevance and benefit to their own work. It will show what is (and is not) possible, and provide starting points for action.

- Create opportunities at all stages of the development of implementation for more agencies to become involved.

Tap into relevant initiatives and opportunities (advocacy)
Disability inclusion needs to be seen as an integral part of WATSAN service provision, and not develop as a separate and distinct set of projects. In order to avoid this separation, ensure you identify existing relevant initiatives and trends that provide an opportunity to raise and include the issue of disability. For example:

At national level
- Poverty Reduction Strategy Processes: DPOs and disability agencies need representation not only on Task groups dealing with social welfare and social protection, but on all Task groups, including WATSAN Task group.

- Country targets on sanitation: for example, Bangladesh, which has recently agreed a target of 100 per cent sanitation by 2010.

- Form alliances with representatives of other marginalised groups that have an interest in inclusive and accessible services, such as Gender Water Alliance, Associations of the Elderly, agencies working with people living with HIV/AIDs, and other vulnerable groups. Identify issues of common interest in WATSAN, and areas for potential collaboration and exchange. Presenting a stronger and united voice improves the chances of being listened to, and being included when activities are planned and developed.

At institutional level
- International organisations that are increasing their focus on issues of equity, including reaching people living in chronic poverty.

- International organisations carrying out strategy development and planning activities at organisational level.

- Data collection activities, such as community baseline surveys, vulnerability mapping, poverty analysis.

At project level
In the design of WATSAN programmes, a community-level baseline survey is commonly carried out, often followed by a community consultation exercise, to identify local problems and priorities, vulnerable households and the level and type of demand for WATSAN services. This should involve some level of participation from community members.

- Suggest that groups of disabled people should be consulted in their own right.

- Suggest organisations that can provide advice, training, and technical input as needed.

DPOs, associations of the elderly and other self-help groups often have established networks at many district and village levels. Depending on their capacity and interests, these could participate in a number of ways to help make this more inclusive and enable the views of disabled people to be heard:

- Information gathering – they could be a ready-made entry point to an existing network.

- As project staff or volunteers, as participants in training sessions for community members on how to conduct community and household needs surveys and assessments.

- In consultation on questions to include in baseline surveys (prevalence and types of impairments, functional limitations, level of isolation and vulnerability) and the design of needs assessments. Provide or adapt available checklists or assessments (see page 147, Household level assessments).

- Participate in consultation activities, such as focus group discussions.

- Suggest ways to modify participatory processes and tools (such as ranking and mapping exercises) to enable people with visual/hearing/communication impairments to participate, to (a) identify disabled and other vulnerable people in a community, and (b) enable vulnerable groups to identify and prioritise their own needs.

- Suggest practical ways to address physical and social obstacles to disabled people's participation in meetings and consultations, or to seek the views of those who are unable to leave their houses, socially stigmatised or unaccustomed to being consulted.

8

- Engage with local groups of women, mothers and the elderly: point out the benefits of inclusive facilities for all, especially for women, children and elderly people – reduced accidents, improved health and family well-being.

- Make sure disabled people's representatives (especially women) are included on community development committees, village water committees and advisory councils at all levels.

Practical ideas for engaging with the water supply and sanitation sector

Find a starting point that WATSAN professionals will perceive as relevant (see Section 3.4), and which will engage interest from the outset.

- Provide numbers of people affected, examples of problems of disabled access, the link between disability and poverty, that disabled people are part of the most marginalised and vulnerable groups, and that MDGs will be hard to achieve without addressing disability.

- Emphasise the benefits to the whole community of inclusive access solutions. Give practical examples such as: a handrail beside steps is good for elderly people, children, pregnant women and people living with HIV/AIDS.

Present practical solutions that engineers can see they have the technical expertise to implement:

- Demonstrate that engineers have a crucial role to play in inclusive access, by describing an access problem, and asking them how they would go about solving it. Expose current problems in legislation and building codes.

- Give examples of simple low-tech solutions to improve access for disabled people, e.g. when deciding the location for a communal water source, give priority to installing it near to users with limited mobility.

- Provide practical examples of communal water and sanitation facilities with inclusive features suitable for the whole community. These could be included as part of the range of options for users to choose from in a demand-responsive approach to WATSAN implementation.

Build on the strengths of engineers: a practical problem-solving exercise is guaranteed to engage interest, demonstrate the expertise of engineers and their vital role, and at the same time show that it is not a highly technical issue.

Use formats accessible and useful for WATSAN sector professionals:

- Use diagrams, technical drawings, photos, etc. to illustrate main points.

- Use language that appeals to the interests and skills of engineers, and links in with issues that they perceive are of concern to them. For example, when introducing a presentation, instead of using a title such as 'WATSAN for disabled people – a human rights issue', change the title to 'WATSAN for disabled people – technical solutions', or 'WATSAN for all – the role of the engineer in designing for different needs'.

Organisational issues

Disabled people and disability service providers may have had little previous contact with the WATSAN sector, and may need to develop some understanding of how the sector works, and how it could contribute to their own disability work.

Options for the disability sector can be categorised into two main 'tracks':

- Including WATSAN issues in disability-specific projects/ activities;

- Advocacy and collaboration for the inclusion of a disability perspective in the WATSAN sector.

Suggestions

- Get to know which agencies do what in WATSAN locally.

- Strategies for advocacy and lobbying for disability rights and access need to include access and rights to WATSAN.

- Appoint a person to take a lead on WATSAN issues.

- Carry out a WATSAN 'audit': invite a professional from the WATSAN sector to discuss possible strategies for including WATSAN issues; to visit your organisation, or project locations/homes of disabled people and identify areas for improvement, gaps, issues for discussion and development.

Programme/project cycle

Situation/needs analysis, project planning and implementation, monitoring and evaluation, budget planning and research and development are part of all implementation, some more structured than others. The project planning stage is the most crucial stage for WATSAN to be considered.

8

These suggestions relate to including WATSAN in disability related work. To get a better understanding of ways to advocate for disability inclusion in the WATSAN sector, read the corresponding section for the WATSAN sector on page 132.

Situation/needs analysis
Consider whether WATSAN is an issue that needs to be addressed by the project. If so, include questions about WATSAN in the situation analysis.

Review existing information on WATSAN in the intended project/programme areas, drawing on the expertise of WATSAN agencies to help identify relevant information.

Make reference to WATSAN policy and strategy, and the status of vulnerable, unreached, and under-served groups in those strategies.

Working with communities
Communities can play a significant role in promoting services and approaches that either include or exclude disabled and other vulnerable people. Technical solutions to physical barriers need to be accompanied by creative solutions that address social barriers, such as attitudes and behaviour of people in the community.

- Include issues of access to WATSAN in awareness-raising activities addressing issues of attitudes and behaviour. Look not only at the problems, but focus on the role of community members in improving disabled people's participation (Box 8.2).

Box 8.2. Engaging communities in problem-solving using drama

A Disabled Children's Advocacy Group, supported by CSID in Dhaka, Bangladesh, has found that drama is a powerful tool in changing people's thinking on disability. The group develops dramas based on the children's own experiences of being excluded from school. They then present their drama to groups of teachers in local Primary Schools. After the performance, they invite teachers to discuss the issues raised. In this way they have succeeded in persuading several Primary Schools to accept disabled children.

Group members felt that they could use the same approach to raise awareness about accessible water and sanitation, as this is a problem that many disabled children face on a daily basis, both at home and at school (13).

Household level – working with disabled people and their families

WATSAN service providers tend to work with communities as a whole, rather than with individual households (see Section 3.1 on how the WATSAN sector works). Some disabled people and their families have complex needs that may require a detailed understanding and assessment, beyond the scope of the WATSAN sector, and better suited to the skills and experience of the disability sector.

Household needs assessment

The main source of care and support for disabled people who need it is usually the family. The aim of any intervention should therefore be to strengthen the capacity of the family to provide this support, within the context of the family and community, rather than replace the family by supporting the disabled person directly.

The long-term aim should be not only to enhance the dignity, capacity and opportunities of the individual disabled person, but to improve the well-being of the whole family. This may be by increasing the disabled person's capacity to contribute more to the family (e.g. Box 8.3), or by reducing the workload of the family, or by making their support tasks easier.

For example, a mother who supports her disabled child to use the toilet may find her task gets more difficult and time-consuming as the child grows heavier; she may develop back pains and risk injuring her child and herself. A simple toilet seat could enable her to support her child more safely, reduce her back pain and also her risk of injury.

A few basic principles need to be borne in mind:

Look at the issue of WATSAN in the context of the whole family situation, not in isolation. A number of checklists and frameworks are available for carrying out needs assessment, which can provide guidance, but should not be used rigidly. (See Appendix 4 on page 281 for one example.)

For a list of further resources on needs assessment, see Appendix A1.8, page 264.

8

Box 8.3. Water collection as a group activity

It is usual in many countries to see children and women fetching water in pairs or groups. Often, one person pumps water while the other holds the container. In this context, the contribution of a disabled person to the group activity is often valued, even if he or she can only do one aspect of the task, such as carrying but not drawing water.

For many disabled people, the ability to make a contribution in the family may be a more valid and realistic goal than focusing solely on a goal of individual self-reliance (14).

Common constraints

Many families would like to help their disabled member, but do not feel they have enough time. It is often quicker for a helper to do a task, such as bathing or taking a disabled person to the toilet, than to spend time enabling them to do it by themselves. If this is an issue, it is important that initial suggestions and solutions are aimed at reducing the family's workload, and that results will be quickly visible. For example, tangible results could come from making or lending a piece of low-cost equipment, and asking a family member to spend 10 minutes a day encouraging or teaching the disabled person to use it. This could show that it is worth spending time to save time.

It may be that the issue of access to water and sanitation is not a priority for the disabled person and their family, who may have more urgent concerns such as getting the harvest in, or the roof mended before the rainy season, which cannot be ignored.

Problem solving

It is a waste of time for an 'expert' outsider to identify the 'perfect solution', if the disabled person and their family do not agree with it. For this reason, it is important that the disabled person and their family are partners in problem-solving.

Find out what solutions the disabled person has already tried – what worked, what didn't? Why didn't it work? They may have their own ideas about how they could adapt the environment. Listen to them, and find ways to build on their ideas.

Many people are not aware of what solutions are possible, and cannot imagine how life might be different. In this case, provide information and examples, show pictures of different solutions, and let them ask questions. Tell stories of disabled people you know who have benefited from different solutions (or use selected case-studies from Chapter 9).

Take a realistic look at the current situation and identify goals that disabled people would like to achieve. If a goal is hard to achieve, help the disabled person to break it down into small achievable steps, which gradually progress towards the final goal.

Practical trial and error is essential, instead of only talking about a solution. Ask the person to demonstrate how they carry out the activity now. Improvise different solutions, or try out different equipment, if it is available, and see what difference it makes. Be prepared to adapt, adjust and, if necessary, start again. Figure 8.1 provides a guide to the problem-solving process.

Who should do all this
Individual and household needs assessment can be a time-consuming process, and should be carried out by someone prepared to spend time and make several visits. Such a role is suited to the skills and experience of many disability sector agencies, particularly those providing community-based support, such as CBR workers.

Disabled people themselves can be an excellent resource in supporting each other, although it should not be assumed that they would want to take on this role. Elderly people may have limited physical strength, but usually have more patience and tenacity than younger people, and in many cultures are listened to with respect.

Community development or health workers, youth volunteers, local women's or church groups can all play a valuable role.

8.4   Monitoring and evaluation

Monitoring and evaluation should be built into the project at the design stage, when mechanisms are established to collect information, and to periodically review whether the project is achieving what it set out to do.

The main question for disabled people is 'In terms of the project objectives, have disabled people benefited to the same extent as non-disabled people?' This can be more easily measured if disability-related data is collected from the beginning of the project (see pages 132 and 143). During the project design, indicators should be identified from this data to monitor the impact on disabled people.

It is important that disabled people are not treated as a single identical group. Data on disabled people need to be

8

differentiated to identify disabled women, disabled girls and boys, disabled elderly women and men, people with different types of impairment, and levels of poverty. This will help determine whether disabled women have benefited from the project as much as disabled men, for example, or whether only wheelchair users have benefited, but blind people have been forgotten.

The project may not have included disability-related data from the beginning. This does not automatically mean that disabled people have been excluded. It also does not prevent the issue of disability being included in an evaluation. Box 8.4 provides examples of questions for inclusion in review or evaluation of a WATSAN project or programme.

Evaluation of water supply and sanitation in disability-focused work

It is useful to know what works well and what works less well, especially in a new area of work. In evaluating the WATSAN element of disability work, it is worth considering the use of a framework commonly in use in the WATSAN sector:

Functionality – Does it work properly, in the way it was intended to? Is it reliable? If not, why not?

Utilisation – Are the people using it those who were intended to use it? Are they using it in the way it was expected, to the extent and in the numbers expected? If not, why not?

Impact – Is it having the impact/benefit expected? If not, why not?

> **On the disabled person** – In terms of self-reliance, time spent, range of activities/contribution, expenditure, income.

> **On the family** – In terms of workload, time spent, range of activities, income.

For more detailed information on monitoring and evaluation of WATSAN activities, see selected documents in the list of resources on page 256.

8

Knowledge

- Knowledge/ skills/ disability awareness of project staff/ community on how to include disabled people and other vulnerable groups;
- Increased knowledge/ skills for disabled people and other vulnerable groups on design options and approaches that improve their lives;
- Transfer and dissemination of knowledge and skills on inclusive options that benefit vulnerable groups.

Inclusion

- Numbers of disabled people (women, men, children) benefited;
- Number of households with disabled person benefited;
- Poor households with a disabled person benefited;
- Female-headed households with a disabled person benefited;
- Types of impairment benefited;
- Are inclusive design options part of the range of available design options?
- How has the project monitored the impact on disabled people?

Participation

- Have disabled people participated in consultations on the project design? e.g. focus groups of disabled people, proactive measures to ensure participation of disabled people.

Access

- Have accessible physical environments/ inclusive design options been promoted?
- Have disabled people's livelihoods been improved as a result of the project?

Fulfilling obligation

- Criteria for project proposals that they consider will address disability;
- Mechanisms in place to ensure inclusion of a disability perspective, e.g. DPO representative on programme steering group and local WATSAN committee;
- WATSAN guidelines and training materials include guidance on disability, e.g. design options must include accessible options, community consultations include focus group of disabled people, etc.;
- Is the project working on guidelines or standards that promote equality for disabled people?
- Has the project helped to raise awareness among disabled people at national and local level of their rights and entitlements?

Potential Informants

National level DPOs (find out through DPI* or National Ministry of Social Welfare);

DPOs at local community level (find out through National DPOs or NGOs);

Women's Associations, war veterans associations, Associations of the Elderly.

(See Appendix 3 for further details of this framework.)

* DPI address in Appendix 2.3.

8

References

1. ADB (2005) *Disability Brief: Identifying and Addressing the Needs of Disabled People*. Asian Development Bank: Manila. http://www.adb.org/Documents/Reports/Disabled-People-Development/disability-brief.asp

2. Stienstra, D., Fricke, Y. and D'Aubin, A. (2002) *Baseline Assessment: Inclusion and Disability in World Bank Activities*. The World Bank: Washington.

3. Thomas, P. (2004) DFID and Disability. *A Mapping of the Department for International Development and Disability Issues*. Disability KAR: UK.

4. Jones, H. (1999) Integrating a disability perspective into mainstream development programmes: the experience of Save the Children (UK) in East Asia. In E. Stone *Disability and Development: learning from action and research on disability in the majority world*. The Disability Press: Leeds, UK.

5. UNESCAP (1995) *Promotion of Non-handicapping physical environments for Disabled Persons: Guidelines*. United Nations Economic and Social Commission for Asia and the Pacific: UN: New York.

6. Ortiz, I. (2004) *Disability KAR: Assessing Connections to DFID's Poverty Agenda*. Overseas Development Group: UK.

7. United Nations (1993) *Standard Rules on Equalization of Opportunities for Disabled Persons*. United Nations: New York. http://www.independentliving.org/standardrules/StandardRules1.html

8. Saunders, C. and Miles, S. (1990) *The Uses and Abuses of Surveys in Service Development Planning for Disabled People: the Case of Lesotho*. Save the Children/UK: London.

9. Bangladesh Bureau of Statistics (2000) *Statistical Pocketbook*. Dhaka, Bangladesh.

10. Actionaid Bangladesh (1996) *Four Baseline Surveys on Prevalence of Disability*. Disability & AIDS Coordination Unit. Actionaid: Dhaka, Bangladesh.

11. WHO (2001) *The International Classification of Functioning, Disability and Health - ICF*. World Health Organization: Geneva.

12. CBR-DTC (undated) *Finding Out about a Person and Her Problem*. CBR Development Training Centre: Solo, Indonesia.

13. Jones, H.E. and Reed, R.A. (2004) *Water supply and sanitation access and use by physically disabled people: report of second field-work in Bangladesh*. WEDC, Loughborough University and DFID: UK.

14. Jones, H.E. and Reed, R.A. (2003) *Water Supply and Sanitation Access and Use by Physically Disabled People*. Report of field-work in Uganda. WEDC, Loughborough University and DFID: UK.

Chapter 9

Case studies

The case-studies in this section are examples of real life situations. The disabled people concerned found the ideas described helpful for them. However, it is not suggested that they would be suitable for everyone.

Where appropriate, the drawbacks of particular facilities or equipment have been identified, and improvements suggested that would make them more suitable for a wider range of users.

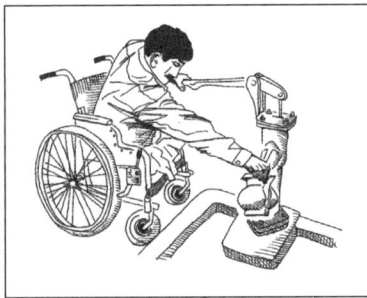

Figure 9.1. Spout and handle at 90° make it easy to pump and hold a water container at the same time.

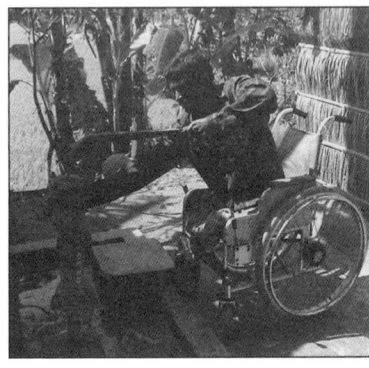

Figure 9.2. Ramizuddin operates the handpump from his wheelchair.

9.1 Wheelchair user's handpump and toilet (Example 1)

Mohammed Ramizuddin Miah is 35 and lives with his wife and children in a rural village in Tangail District, Bangladesh. He was previously an agricultural worker; now he is a poultry trader.

Five years ago both his legs were amputated above the knee. He uses a wheelchair to move around the family compound. He can get in and out of his wheelchair independently.

Accessible handpump apron

Description
- A square concrete apron is bounded by a low concrete wall. The handpump is installed next to the edge of the apron, suitable for use by a person standing or seated near the ground.

- Pump handle and spout are at 90° to each other.

- A low concrete sitting platform is constructed on the apron edge.

Dimensions
- Apron: 135cm x 135cm;

- Height of boundary wall from apron: ~10cm; height from surrounding ground: between 5cm – 20cm (the ground is uneven).

- Platform: L: 38cm x W: 38cm x H: 17cm.

Approach
- Located ~3m from the kitchen. A smooth earth path leads to a level area next to the apron.

- Ramizuddin maintains the path by annually replacing any earth that is eroded by rain.

Use
- Ramizuddin wheels to the edge of the apron in his wheelchair, pumps water with one hand, into a jug held in the other hand.

- He can also get down from his wheelchair onto the low sitting platform and pump water from the platform, especially when water is for use at the pump. He sits on the platform to bathe himself or his children, or to wash clothes or dishes.

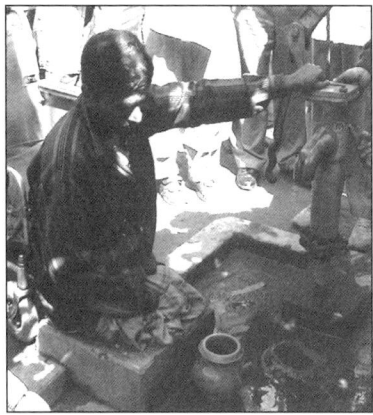

Figure 9.3. Sitting on low concrete platform to bathe.

Key features

- One basic design with minor adaptations for individual households/ users, e.g. the dimension and location of the platform can be changed.

- Proximity of a water source to the house reduces the time spent fetching water by the whole family, and also reduces the need to carry and store water.

- Level ground allows the wheelchair to wheel right up to the edge of the apron.

- Pump spout and handle at 90° allow user to pump and collect water at the same time.

- The pump can be used from a chair or from low concrete platform, i.e. sitting or standing.

- Minimal additional cost compared to a standard concrete apron.

Suitable for

- Users with good sitting balance, but with difficulty squatting or bending, e.g. wheelchair/crutch users, frail elderly people.

- Users with strong enough arms to lower themselves to the sitting platform.

- The whole family, no separate facility is needed. The platform is convenient for other family members, e.g. women washing clothes or bathing children.

Unsuitable for

- People with poor sitting balance. People with weak arms, weak or stiff legs would need help lowering themselves onto the low platform and back.

Case studies

9

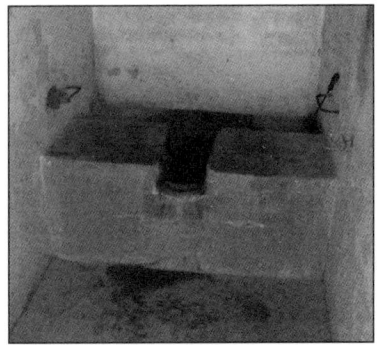

Figure 9.4. Raised brick toilet platform with inset PVC pan.

Pour-flush latrine with raised sitting platform

Description
- Brick built structure with smooth cement- plastered walls and tin roof. Smooth concrete floor. Holes high in the wall for ventilation and light. A tin door on a wood frame opens outwards. A chain on the inside of the door hooks over a nail to keep the door closed.

- A commercially available PVC toilet pan is set into a cement-plastered brick platform, constructed the full width of the cubicle. Two raised concrete blocks on each side of the toilet pan are for sitting on.

Approach
- ~5m from the house via an earth path. There is a level area in front of the door. The toilet floor is only 1-2cm above the surrounding yard. (Ramizuddin regularly replaces any earth washed away by rain).

Support features
- Two horizontal handrails are cemented to the side walls, one on each side of the platform.

Dimensions
- Internal: L: 180cm, W: 106cm.

- Entrance W: 90cm.

- Handles: 20mm Ø g.i. pipe, L: 45cm, H: 74cm.

- Toilet seat: W: 106cm, D: 74cm, H: 42cm (same as wheelchair seat).

- Gap between sitting blocks: 27cm.

Use
- Ramizuddin enters the latrine in his wheelchair, closes the door by turning slightly in the chair (which he finds awkward). With the wheelchair facing the toilet, he moves across onto the sitting blocks, holding the handrails for support. When finished, he transfers back to his chair and reverses out of the toilet.

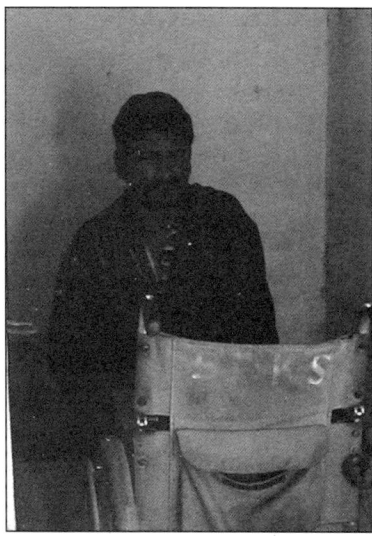

Figure 9.5. Transferring from wheelchair to toilet.

Key features

- Durable. Materials are available locally.

- The basic design is adaptable to suit individual needs, e.g. the location of handrails.

- The entrance is wide enough for a wheelchair to enter.

- Height of platform is suitable for wheelchair transfer.

- Twin sitting blocks are convenient for anal cleansing.

- Handrails provide support for balance while transferring onto toilet.

- Light, well ventilated, easy to keep clean – pleasant for all the family to use.

Drawbacks and comments

- High cost. Reducing the width of the platform would reduce the quantity and cost of materials used.

- The concrete absorbs urine and is unhygienic, so it would be better to paint it for moisture resistance, making it easier to keep clean and hygienic.

- The door is difficult to close from inside in a wheelchair.

- The cubicle is too narrow to turn the wheelchair, so Ramizuddin must reverse out. A wider cubicle would allow space to turn, and to shut the door more easily.

- Handrails on side walls would be too wide apart for many users, and could instead be fixed to the floor, or a rope hung from a roof beam.

- No water for cleansing. User must carry water from the hand pump.

Suitable for

- People with difficulty squatting; wheelchair users; people with some sitting balance.

Unsuitable for

- People who need a support person to help them, as there is not enough space.

Benefits

Self-reliance and independence: According to a neighbour, Ramizuddin used to be very dependent on his wife, which prevented her getting on with her work and caused tension between them. He is now no longer dependent, and tension between them has reduced.

Ability to contribute to the family: Ramizuddin can now contribute to household chores, by washing clothes, dishes, bathing the children.

Time-saving: Before the well was built, his wife spent at least an hour a day collecting water from neighbours' wells. (He didn't contribute to this). She now spends the time saved on other economic activities, including going out to work. The new latrine is also more comfortable and less work – it is easier to keep clean than their old pit latrine.

Status in the community: Not only family members but also neighbours and passers-by (around 15-20 people a day) use the toilet and well (the house is near the road). This means extra cleaning, which he and his wife share, but Ramizuddin not only doesn't mind, but feels proud to provide this community service.

Process for obtaining adaptations/external support

Bangladeshi Protibandhi Kallyan Somity (BPKS), a national cross-impairment DPO in Bangladesh, implemented an Accessible Tube-well and Sanitary Latrine Programme for families with a disabled member. The criteria for selecting beneficiaries were severe disability and poverty. Local disabled people's groups of NDPO (Nagarpur Disabled People's Organization to Development) held discussions among their members to decide who would benefit first from the project. Members in this group agreed that Ramizuddin fitted the criteria, and would benefit the most.

The total cost was 9,000 taka (~ 150 US dollars). BPKS paid 7,000 taka ($117); the family paid 2,000 taka ($33). The family also bears the cost of maintenance. Ramizuddin thinks the money was a good investment, because the family is economically better off than before.

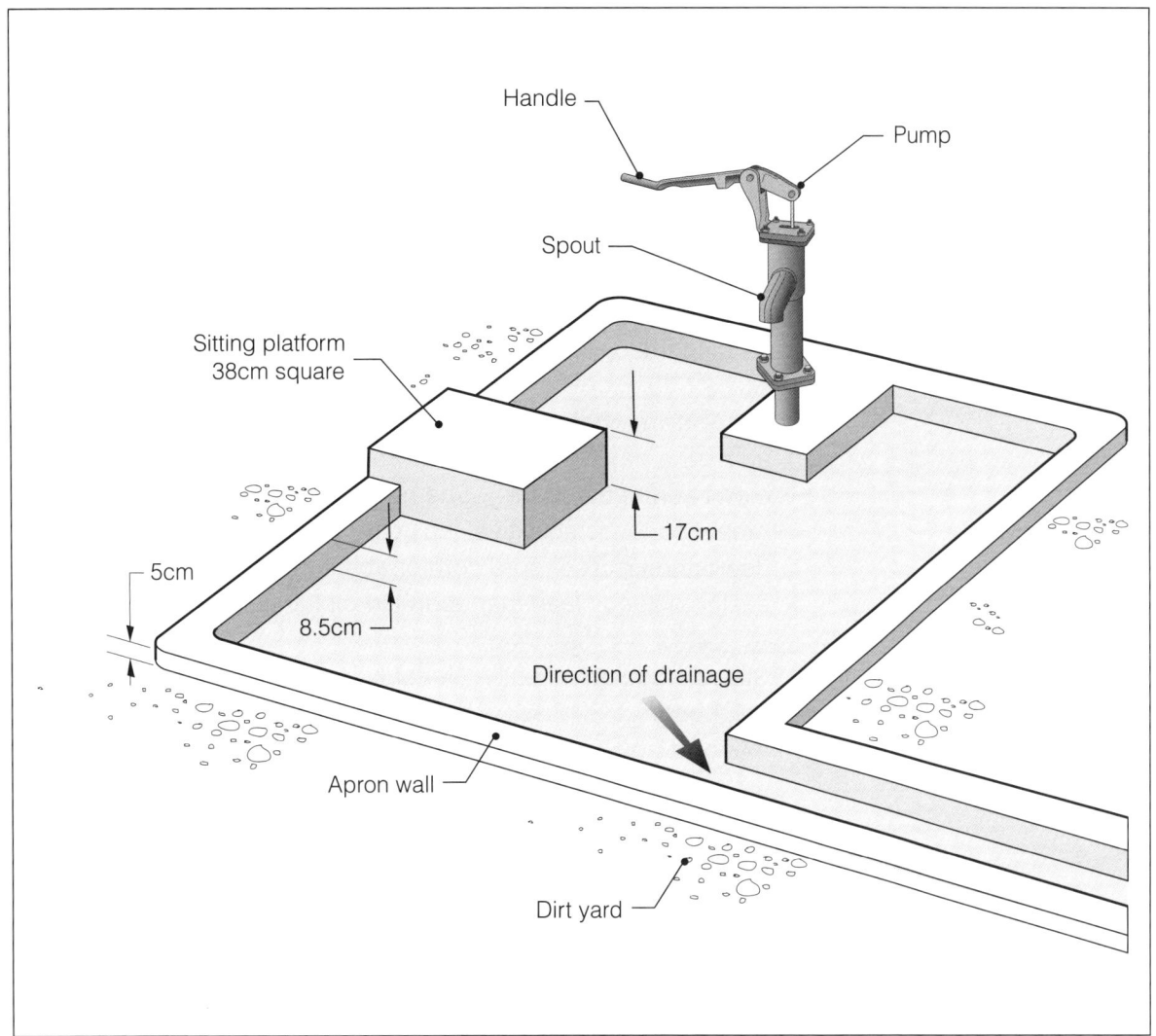

Figure 9.6. Handpump apron with sitting platform.

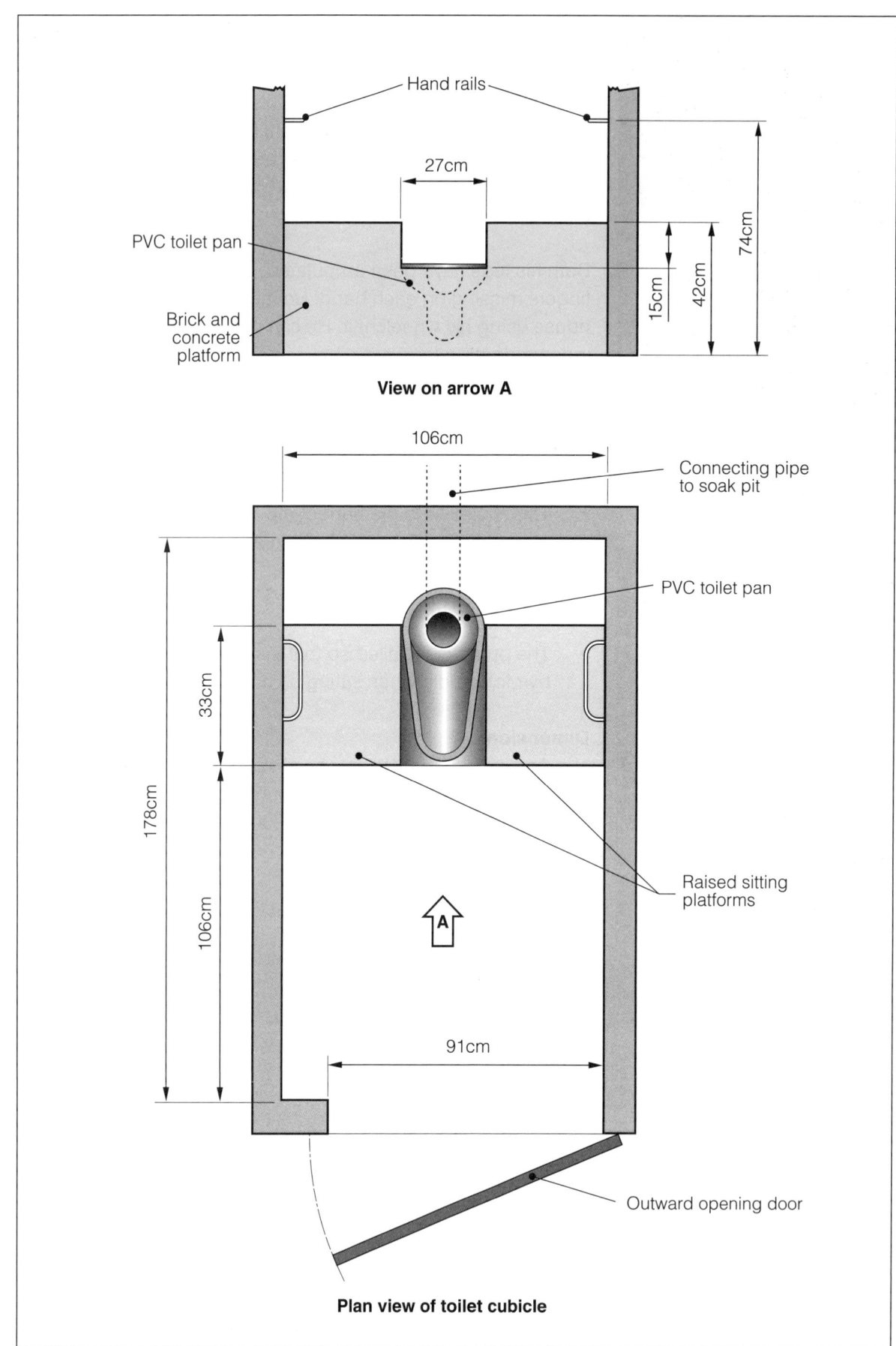

View on arrow A

Hand rails

27cm

74cm

42cm

15cm

PVC toilet pan

Brick and concrete platform

106cm

Connecting pipe to soak pit

PVC toilet pan

33cm

178cm

106cm

Raised sitting platforms

A

91cm

Outward opening door

Plan view of toilet cubicle

Figure 9.7. Pour-flush latrine with raised sitting platform.

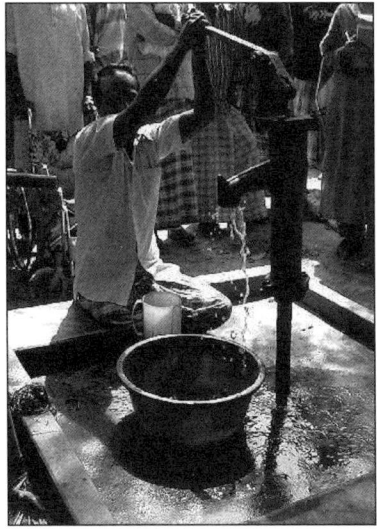

9.2 Wheelchair user's handpump and toilet (Example 2)

Mr Mofizuddin is 45 and lives with his wife Bibi Hawa in a rural area in Tangail District, Bangladesh, in a compound shared by his extended family. The family business is poultry raising, and Mofizuddin makes bamboo household items. He has four children.

Both his legs have been amputated, and he has several fingers missing on each hand. He moves around outside the house using his wheelchair. He can get in and out of his chair independently.

Figures 9.8 and 9.9. Mofizuddin sits on low platform to pump water and bathe or wash clothes.

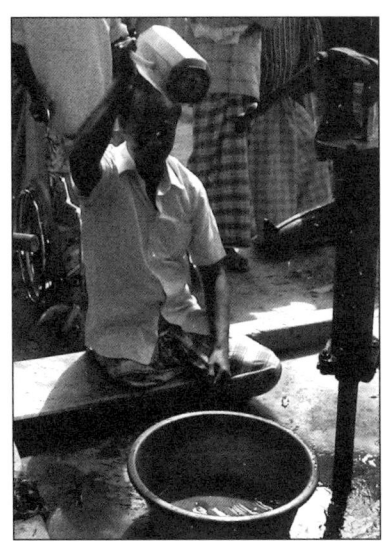

Accessible handpump apron

Description
- This is similar to the handpump apron in 9.1, with some minor differences of dimension and design.
- Two concrete sitting platforms are constructed on the edge of the apron.
- The pump is installed so that the handle can be reached by Mofizuddin when sitting on a low platform.

Dimensions
- Apron: 135cm x 135cm; height of boundary wall from apron: ~10cm; from the surrounding ground: 5cm – 20cm. Sitting platforms: L: ~30cm, W: 80cm, H: 10cm.

Approach
- A smooth earth path leads to a level area next to the pump.

Use
- Mofizuddin parks his wheelchair on the edge of the apron, gets down onto the sitting platform. He pumps water into a container placed on the apron in front of the platform. He bathes in this position.

Key features
- A basic design with minor adaptations to suit individual users, e.g. dimension and location of platform and pump.
- The level ground allows a wheelchair to wheel right up to the edge of the apron.
- Proximity of water source to the house reduces the time spent by the whole family fetching water and reduces the need to fetch and store quantities of water.

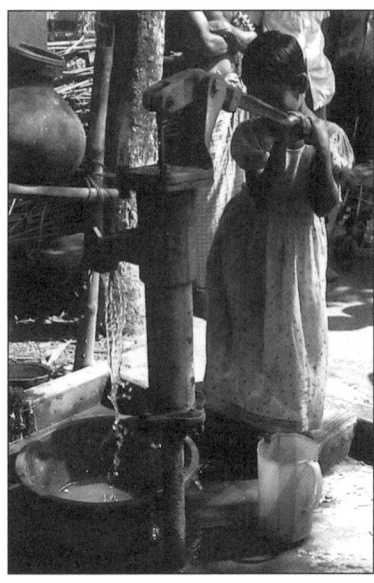

Figure 9.10. The pump is easy for the rest of the family to use.

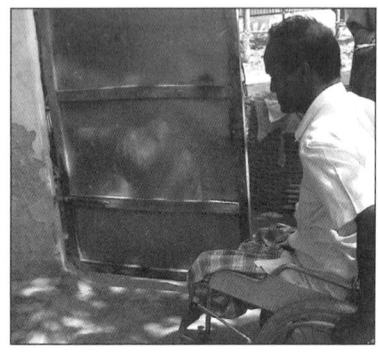

Figure 9.11. Entering the toilet in wheelchair.

- The pump can be operated from sitting on the low platform or from standing.

- Two sitting platforms allow more than one person to use the apron at the same time, e.g. women washing clothes or bathing children.

- Minimal additional cost compared to a standard concrete apron.

Suitable for
- Users with good sitting balance, but with difficulty squatting, bending, e.g. wheelchair/crutch users.

- Users with strong enough arms to transfer from wheelchair to platform.

- Whole family, no separate facility needed. Concrete platform convenient for other family members, e.g. women washing clothes or bathing children.

Unsuitable for
- People unable to sit without support.

- Users with weak arms/legs would need help transferring from wheelchair to low platform.

Pour-flush latrine with raised sitting platform

Description
- Same design as in Section 9.1.

Drawbacks and comments
- Others bring water for Mofizuddin to wash himself. He intends to arrange water storage inside the latrine, e.g. in an overhead tank, so that he would not need to ask others to fetch water for him.

Benefits
Before, Mofizuddin used a bed-pan. The latrine is much more comfortable and convenient to use.

Three people in his immediate family use the latrine. The toilet pan has a water sealed trap, and the latrine is well ventilated, so there is no bad smell, and the latrine is therefore pleasant for all to use.

His wife has benefited in particular. The new latrine is easy to keep clean. It is much less work and more pleasant than emptying and cleaning a bed-pan, which was an unpleasant and tedious job.

Time-saving: Previously his wife spent an hour and a half a day fetching water. The pump has saved her a lot of time.

After the well was found to be arsenic contaminated, his brother installed another tube-well about 5m away. He copied the idea of the low concrete platform for the new apron, because the rest of the family, especially the women, found it comfortable and convenient.

Process for obtaining adaptations
Both latrine and tube-well were provided by a local branch of BPKS. Mofizuddin, his wife and other members of the family were involved in discussion about their requirements from the facilities. For example, the BPKS project officer sat down and discussed step by step his requirements for the tube-well and latrine: How would he move from the chair to the toilet pan? What height should handrails be? etc.

The total cost was 9,000 taka (~150 US dollars*). Mofizuddin paid 2,000 taka ($33); BPKS paid the rest. Maintenance of both facilities are his responsibility, e.g. replacing parts of the pump.

* @ US$1 = 59.49 Bangladesh taka, at time data collected.

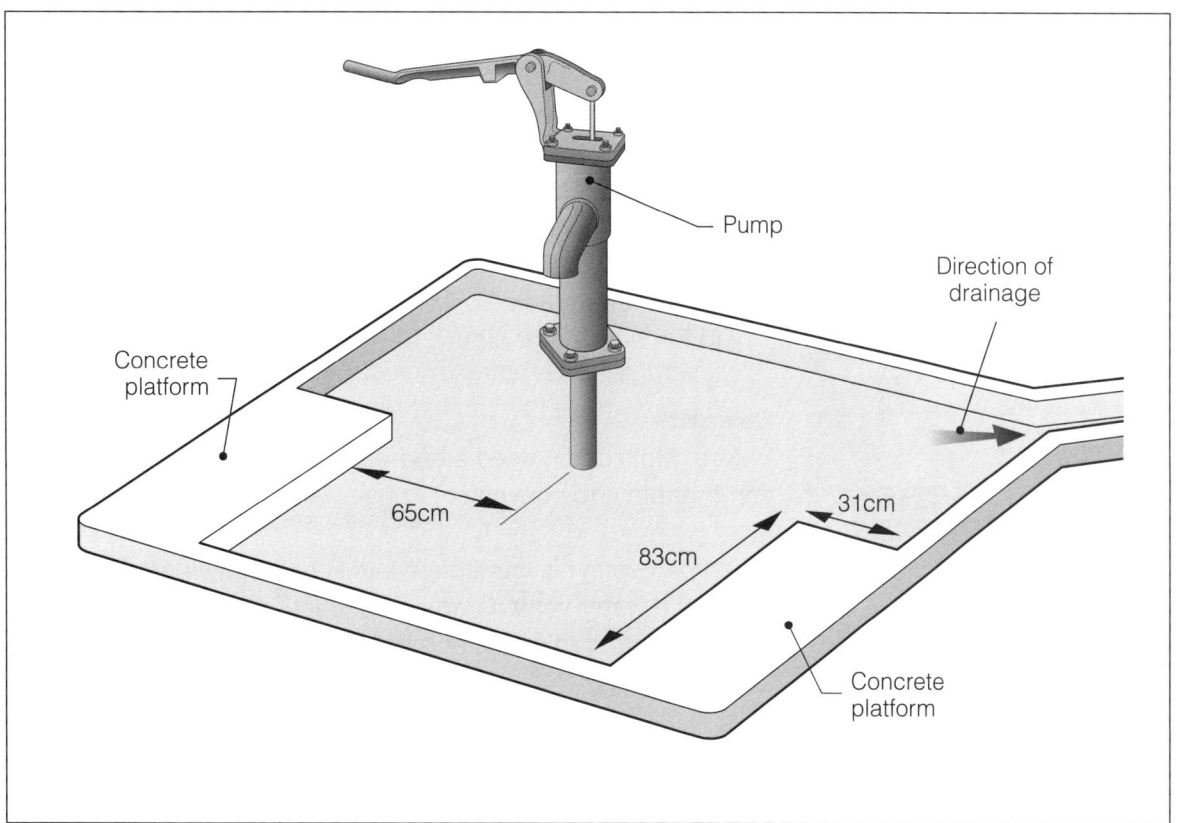

Figure 9.12. Handpump apron with two sitting platforms.

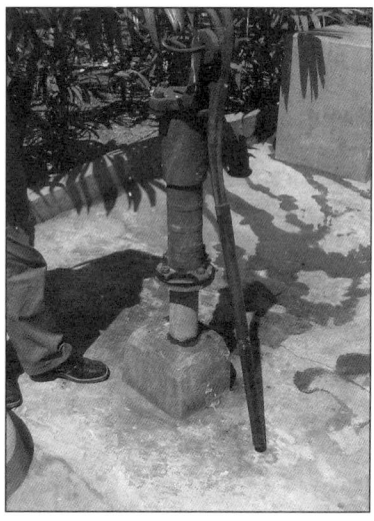

Figure 9.13. Handpump with wide concrete apron for easy wheelchair access on three sides.

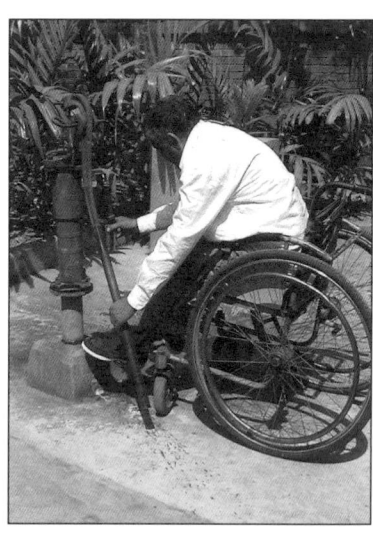

Figure 9.14. Water drains away from the apron.

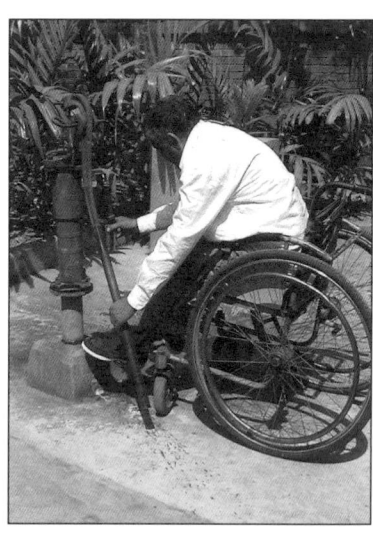

Figure 9.15. A wheelchair user operating the handpump from his wheelchair.

9.3 Handpump, bathroom/laundry and toilet for wheelchair users

The Centre for the Rehabilitation of the Paralysed (CRP) in Dhaka, Bangladesh, provides treatment and rehabilitation mainly for people with spinal cord injuries. After treatment and before returning home, patients spend 15 days at CRP's transit hostel. They practise using the kind of facilities they will use when they go home, with supervision and advice from therapists.

Handpump with wide concrete apron

Description
- The handpump is surrounded by a wide concrete apron, with enough space to allow wheelchair access from three sides. A concrete ramp leads onto the apron. The drainage slope is in the opposite direction to the approach ramp.

- The pump handle has an extension to make it longer than normal.

Dimensions
- Pump handle L: 105cm.

Use
- The user can wheel right up to the pump in a wheelchair, pump water and hold a water container at the same time, whilst sitting in the wheelchair.

Key features
- The pump handle and spout are at 90° to each other, which makes it easy to pump water and hold a container at the same time. The lengthened pump handle gives more leverage for pumping. The concrete ramp onto the apron makes wheelchair access easy.

Suitable for
- All users, especially wheelchair users.

Drawbacks and comments
- The large area of concrete is expensive.

- The longer pump handle means larger action needed when pumping – difficult for those with limited arm movement.

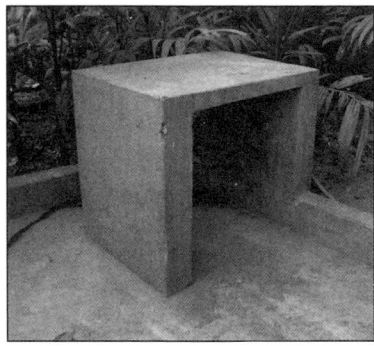

Figure 9.16. Concrete laundry slab located on edge of handpump apron.

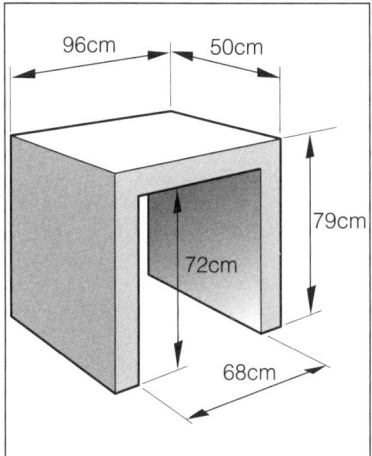

Figure 9.17. Dimensions of laundry slab.

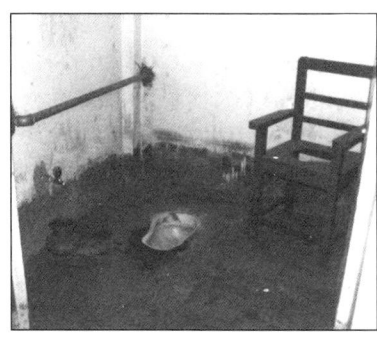

Figure 9.18. Multi-purpose bathroom with toilet in corner.

Concrete slab for washing clothes

Description

- Brick-built, cement-plastered structure. One is located outside near the handpump, another in a bathroom near a tap.

Dimensions

- H from ground to underside of horizontal slab: 72cm. W of knee hole: 68cm.

Use

- A wheelchair user can sit to wash clothes.

Key features

- Users can stay in their wheelchair and get close enough to the slab, with their knees under the shelf.

Drawbacks and comments

- Locating the slab next to a water source would avoid the need to fetch water from the water source.

Suitable for

- Wheelchair users, people who prefer to sit on a chair to wash clothes, crutch users and others with difficulty bending.

Multiple use bathroom

Description

- Brick-built, with cement-plastered walls and a smooth concrete floor.

- A pour-flush toilet is installed in one corner of the room. The ceramic toilet pan is level with the floor. A horizontal handrail is attached to one wall beside the toilet.

- Water is piped to an inside tap.

Approach

- A concrete approach path level with the bathroom entrance. Double doors open inwards.

Dimensions

- 200cm x 184cm; Entrance W: 90cm.

- H of tap: ~50cm.

- Handrail: 35mm o/s Ø g.i. pipe; H: 80cm.

Use

- To bathe: the bather enters the room in his wheelchair, replaces his wheelchair cushion with a tyre inner tube (see below). He fills a bucket with water from the tap and scoops water over himself with a mug.

- To use the toilet, he either transfers from his wheelchair to a toilet chair placed over the toilet hole, or positions his wheelchair over the toilet, and uses it as a toilet chair.

Key features

- The entrance is smooth, level and wide enough for a wheelchair to enter.

- There is enough space inside for a wheelchair to enter and turn, and for a helper. The toilet pan in the corner and the double doors also reduce obstruction.

- There is space beside the toilet to move the toilet chair to one side after use.

- The smooth concrete floor is easy to keep clean.

- The internal water source means there is no need to carry water for bathing.

Drawbacks and comments

- High cost.

- The smooth floor may get slippery and become unsuitable for crutch users and others who are unsteady on their feet.

- A lower or diagonal handrail would provide support for a person squatting on the toilet.

Suitable for

- Whole family.

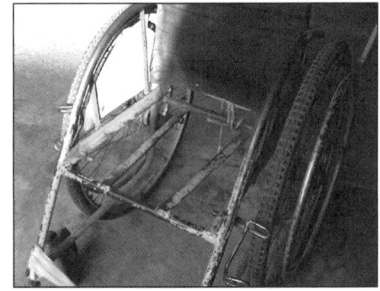

Figure 9.19. Wheelchair with cushion and seat board removed.

Wheelchair convertible to a bathing seat

Description

- The wheelchair has a removable seat board and cushion. These are replaced by a small tyre inner tube, which is supported on two metal struts, but with a wide enough gap for drainage.

Use

- The bather enters the bathroom in the wheelchair, replaces the seat with the inner tube, which he or she sits on while bathing.

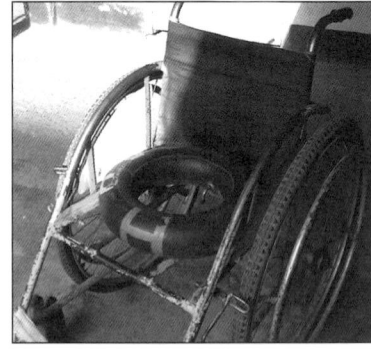

Figure 9.20. Tyre inner tube in place.

Key features

- Inner tubes are durable, easy to clean, and hygienic, and are widely available at reasonable cost.

- The user does not need to transfer out of the wheelchair to bathe.

- The chair back and side-rails help support bathers with poor balance.

Drawbacks and comments

- High cost.

- The wheelchair gets wet, which could contribute to corrosion of the frame.

- The bather needs to move his or her weight off the seat to swap the inner tube, so may need help to do this.

Suitable for

- Users with poor sitting balance, but with some arm strength.

Benefits

Benefits are indirect and long-term. Disabled people who spend time at the transit hostel get ideas to use when they return home, like Mr Bakul (Section 9.5).

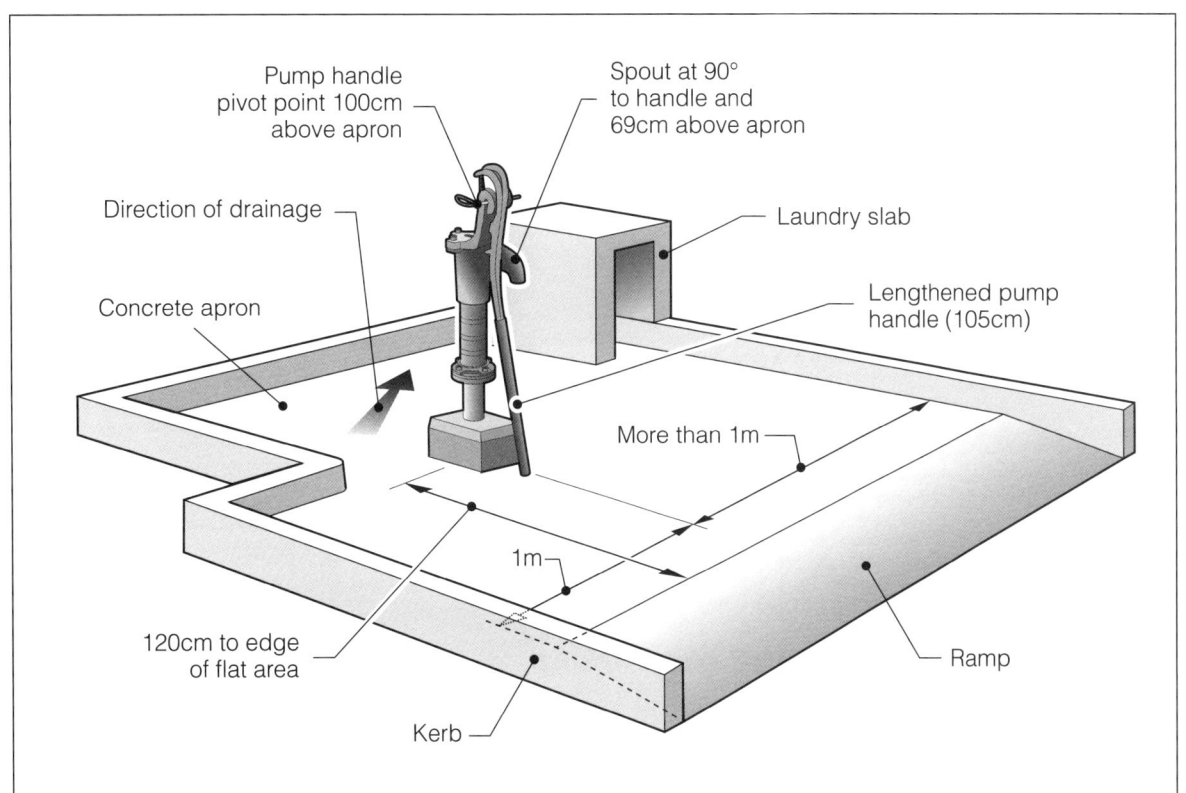

Figure 9.21. Layout of CRP handpump apron.

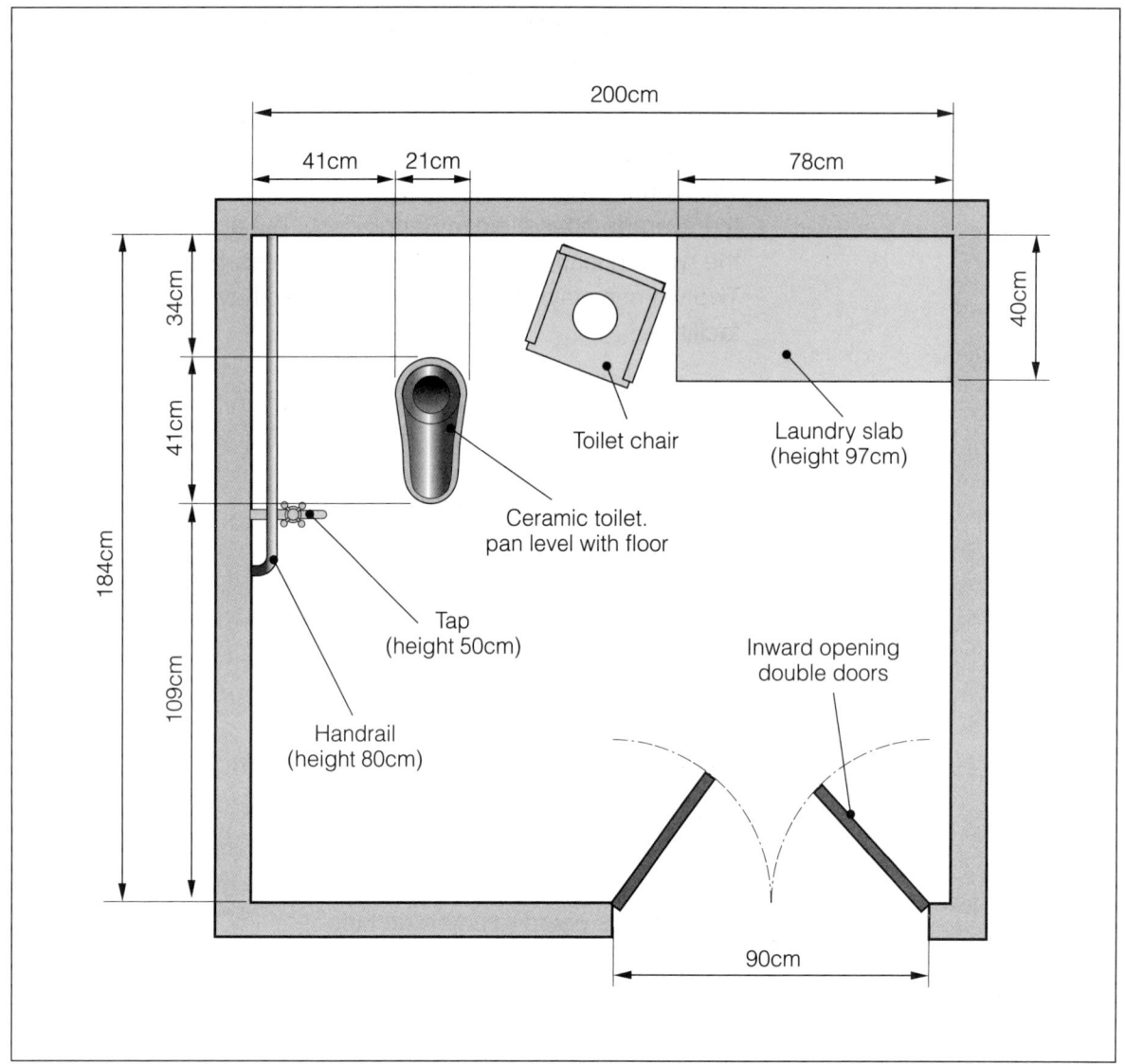

Figure 9.22. Dimensions and layout of CRP multiple use bathroom.

9.4 Bathroom/ laundry and toilet for wheelchair and crutch users

CRP Women's Hostel is in a peri-urban area 30km from the centre of Dhaka city. Disabled women stay here to learn vocational skills. The facilities aim to be of a similar standard to the average household in Bangladesh, but accessible, so that the women learn to cope with such facilities independently. Two women staying at the hostel showed how they used the facilities.

Ms Fatema Akhter Popi is 20 and a trainer in tailoring. Both her legs are weak: she can move around slowly in a squatting position, but mostly uses a wheelchair. She can get from her wheelchair to the floor and back again.

Ms Anwara is 15, and is learning embroidery. She has a mild impairment in her left leg, and walks with a limp. She does not need to use a wheelchair.

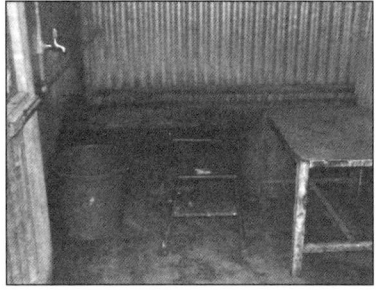

Figure 9.23. Bathing and laundry room

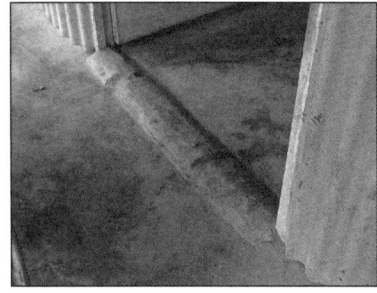

Figure 9.24. Flood prevention threshold has been rounded for easier wheelchair access.

Multiple use bathroom/laundry room

Description
- Corrugated tin walls and roof on a wooden frame. The floor is smooth concrete. The tin door opens inwards. Water is piped to an inside tap.

Dimensions
- Overall: L: 270cm, W: 145cm.

- Door W: ~90cm; Tap H: 1 metre.

Approach
- Along a concrete path level with the bathroom floor. A flood prevention threshold is rounded and minimised to make it wheelchair accessible.

Use
- Popi enters in her wheelchair, and transfers to a low stool in front of the tap and bucket. To bathe, she uses water straight from the tap, or fills the bucket which stands under the tap. She uses a plastic jug with a handle to scoop water over herself.

- She washes clothes directly on the floor.

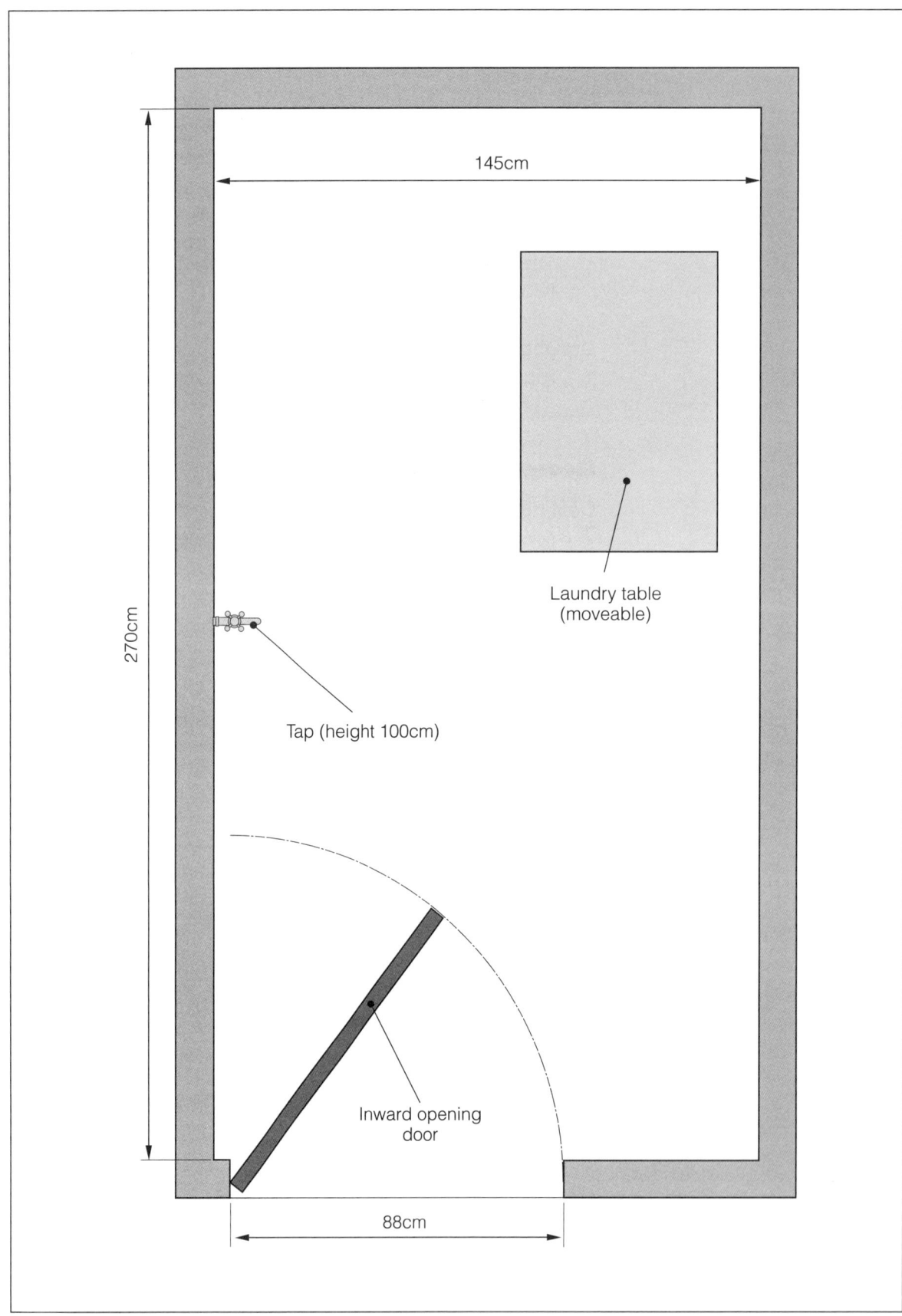

145cm

270cm

Laundry table
(moveable)

Tap (height 100cm)

Inward opening
door

88cm

Figure 9.25. Layout of laundry/bathroom.

Key features

- The entrance is wide and smooth enough for a wheelchair to enter.

- There is space inside for a wheelchair to turn, and for a helper.

- The internal water point means there is no need to fetch water for bathing.

- The tap can be operated either from a wheelchair or from floor level.

Drawbacks

- High cost of piped water and concrete floor.

Floor-level washing up sink

Description

- In one corner of the concrete floored kitchen is a floor-level rectangular trough or sink, formed by a low cement-plastered brick wall. There is a tap over the sink. Water drains to the outside through a hole in one corner of the sink (Figure 9.26).

Dimensions

- Sink area: W: ~ 60cm, D: 40cm.

- Low wall: H: 12cm, W: 12cm.

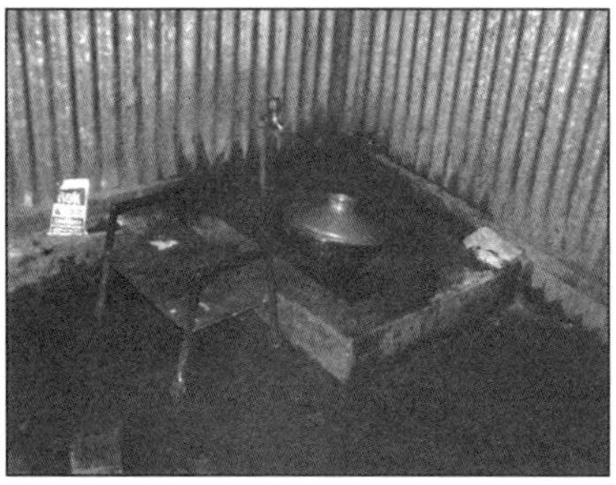

Approach

- Smooth concrete floor level with concrete path outside.

Use

- Popi enters the kitchen in her wheelchair, which she parks near the sink. She transfers to sit next to the sink (Figure 9.27) on a low stool (Figure 9.29).

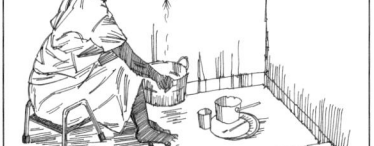

Figure 9.26. Floor level washing up sink with low concrete wall.

Figure 9.27. Popi sits on a low stool to wash dishes.

Key features

- The user is raised off the floor, which prevents her clothes getting wet and dirty.

- Concrete is durable and easy to clean.

- The sink could also be used from a low trolley (Figure 7.54) or other low mobility devices.

- The tap means there is no need to carry water.

Drawbacks

- Many people find it difficult to lower themselves and get up again.

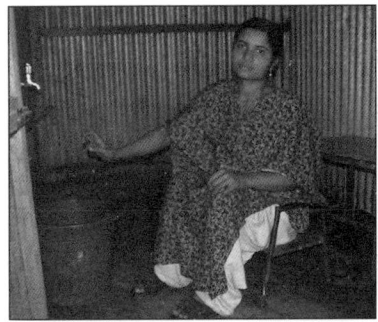

Figure 9.28. Popi sits on metal framed stool to bathe.

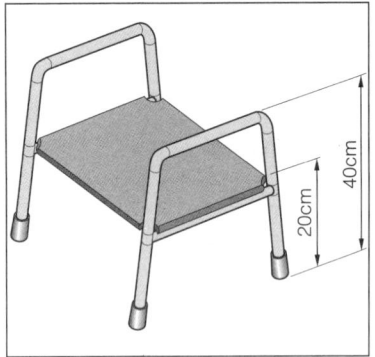

Figure 9.29. Metal-framed low wooden stool.

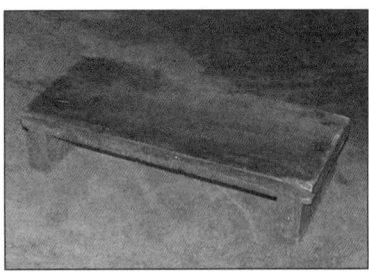

Figure 9.30. Low wooden stool.

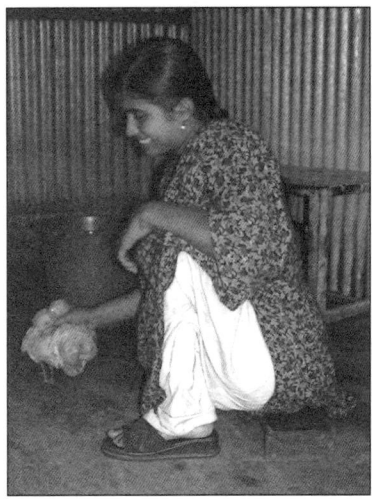

Figure 9.31. Popi sits on a low stool to wash laundry.

Assistive devices - Metal framed stool

Description
- Low metal-framed stool with a wooden seat

Dimensions
- Seat H: ~20cm; side-rails H:~40cm.

Use
- For bathing: bather sits on the stool in front of the tap and bucket. She places her clothes on laundry table to keep them dry while bathing.

- For washing dishes: user sits on the stool on the edge of a floor level washing up sink (Figure 9.27).

Key features
- Durable materials; easy to clean.

- Side-rails provide stability and extra support to the user, and also allow the seat to be easily picked up and moved with one hand.

- The bather is comfortable – not sitting in dirty water.

- The low height is convenient for a wide range of low-level tasks, including using a bucket or bowl on the floor.

Drawbacks and comments
- Metal frame is high-cost.

- Strength and balance are needed to transfer to/from stool.

- The stool is constantly wet, so a painted seat would help resist moisture and slow down deterioration.

Suitable for
- People with good sitting balance.

Low wooden stool

Description
- Low wooden stool which is only slightly higher than if the user were squatting

Dimensions
- L: ~30 x W: ~15 x H: ~10cm.

Use
- Popi sits on the stool to wash clothes at floor level.

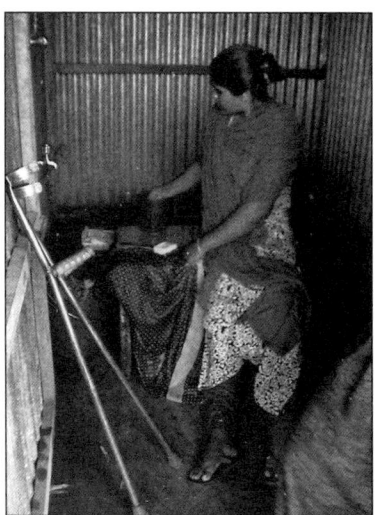

Figure 9.32. Washing clothes on the laundry bench.

Key features
- Durable, low-cost, locally available.
- When washing clothes, the stool prevents the user's clothes getting wet and dirty.

Drawbacks
- Very low - difficult to get up and down from.

Suitable for
- People with good sitting balance, including children.
- Widely used by non-disabled people in Bangladesh to carry out floor-level tasks.

Assistive devices used – laundry table

Description
- Laundry table with metal frame and aluminium top.

Dimensions
- H: ~60cm.

Use
- The user sits on the table and washes clothes on the table beside her. It is also used by bathers to put their clothes on while bathing.

Key features
- Durable, locally made.
- There is enough space on the bench for the user to have all the equipment she needs beside her.
- The user is raised off the floor, which prevents her clothes getting wet and dirty.
- The table could also be used for other tasks.

Drawbacks and comments
- High cost.
- Takes up a lot of space.
- The user has to twist the upper body to one side to wash clothes (Figure 9.32), which may be difficult for some disabled people.

Suitable for
- People with good sitting balance.

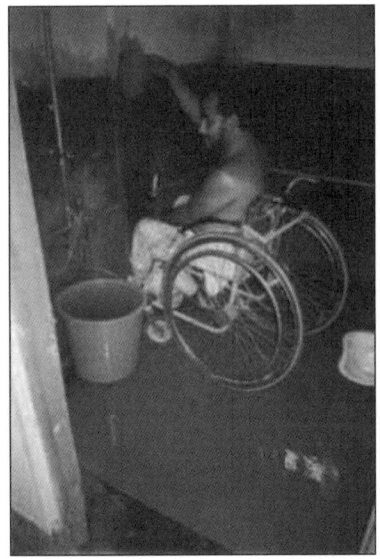

Figure 9.33. Bakul sits in his wheelchair to bathe. Note toilet pan in the corner on the right.

9.5 Wheelchair user's bathroom with toilet

Mr Aziz Ahmed Chowdhury (Bakul) lives in a rural area of Moulavibazar District, Bangladesh. He is 38, unmarried, and economically quite well off.

He is paralysed below the waist due to a spinal cord injury, and cannot walk or stand. He uses a wheelchair for mobility inside and outside the house. His upper body is strong – he can transfer from his wheelchair to bed or bench and back again. He employs a support worker.

Bathroom used with a convertible wheelchair

Description
- Brick-built structure with cement-plastered walls and a smooth concrete cement screed floor which is painted.

- A water flush toilet is located in one corner of the room. The ceramic toilet pan is installed level with the floor. Water is piped to an inside tap.

Approach
- A concrete approach path is level with the bathroom entrance.

Dimensions
- Overall: L: 226cm; W: 178cm.

- Doorway W: 71cm (this is less than usually recommended, but suited this user and his particular wheelchair).

- H of tap: 92cm.

Use
- Bakul enters in his wheelchair, and replaces his wheelchair seat with a tyre inner tube.

- To bathe: He fills a plastic bucket on the floor with water from the tap and scoops water over himself with a mug.

- To use the toilet: he positions his wheelchair over the toilet pan and urinates or defecates directly into the toilet beneath.

Key features
- The entrance is smooth, level and wide enough for a wheelchair to enter.

- The toilet pan in the corner allows enough space inside for a wheelchair to enter and turn, and for a support person.

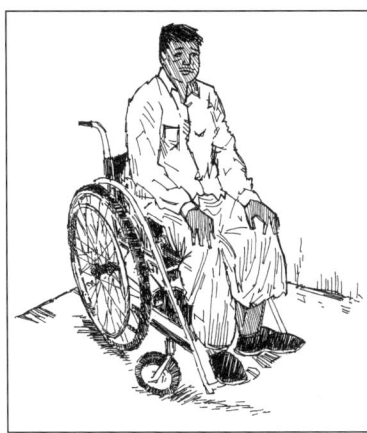

Figure 9.34. Bakul positions his wheelchair over the toilet.

- The door hinge next to the wall allows the door to open flat against the wall, also minimising obstruction. The smooth painted floor is easy to keep clean. The internal water source means there is no need to fetch water for bathing.

Drawbacks
- High cost.

- The water flush system depends on piped water.

Suitable for
- Whole family – no separate facility is needed.

Unsuitable for
- Crutch users and others who are unsteady on their feet as the smooth floor is slippery when wet.

Comments
Bakul's support worker washes his clothes for him. If the bathroom had a raised washing shelf or slab, he could wash his own clothes.

A flexible plastic hose attached to the toilet tap could enable him to carry out anal cleansing more easily.

Benefits
His support worker, Ismail, said that when Bakul had no assistive devices he spent at least three hours a day on support tasks. Now the time taken is half that.

Process for obtaining adaptations
The bathroom was designed according to Bakul's requirements after his accident. He got the idea from CRP and Comfort Nursing Home, Dhaka.

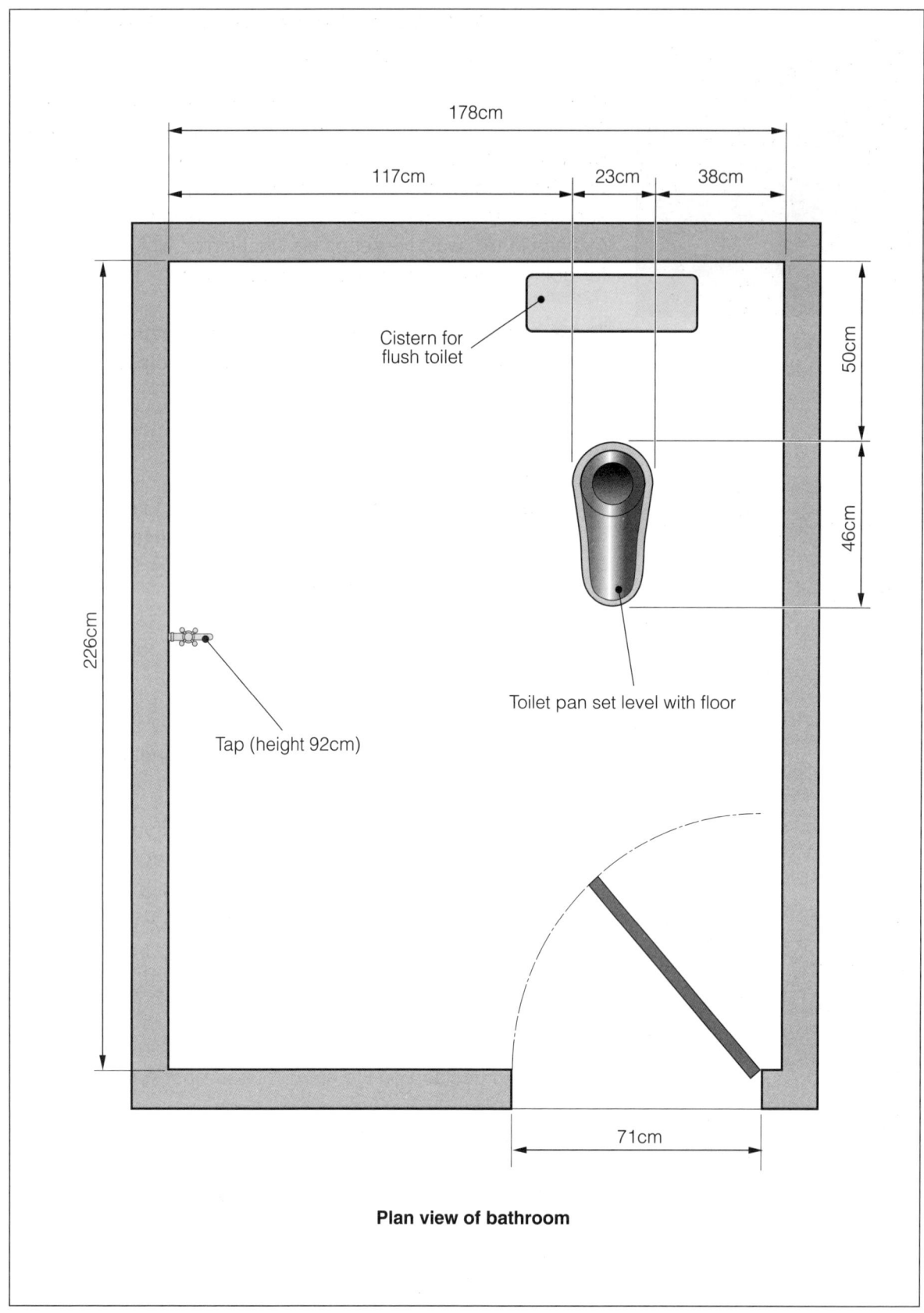

178cm

117cm   23cm   38cm

Cistern for
flush toilet

50cm

46cm

226cm

Tap (height 92cm)

Toilet pan set level with floor

71cm

Plan view of bathroom

Figure 9.35. Dimensions of Mr Bakul's bathroom/toilet.

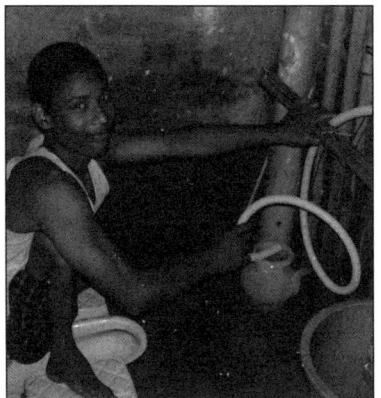

Figure 9.36. Ibrahim holds on to the wooden bar for support.

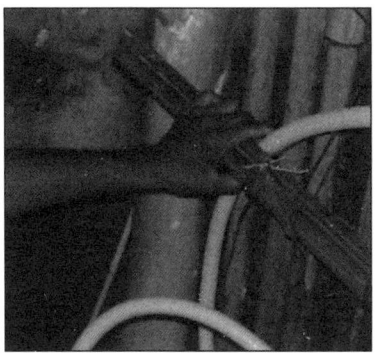

Figure 9.37. Close-up of wooden bar.

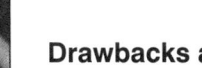
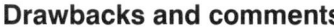

Figure 9.38. Filling the water container with one hand.

9.6 Support bar for young man with difficulty squatting

Ibrahim is 16 and lives with his sister-in-law and her family in a 5th floor apartment in a peri-urban area of Dhaka, Bangladesh. Both his legs are weak as a result of polio. He walks using both his hands and feet and has very strong arms and shoulders as a result. He can get up and down the five flights of stairs in this way. He keeps his wheelchair, which he uses for going outside, locked up at the bottom of the stairs.

The apartment has piped water and a toilet/ bathroom. The pour-flush toilet has a ceramic pan with footplates for squatting.

Description
• A horizontal wooden bar is tied with string to existing vertical pipes against the wall in front of the toilet.

• A hose is attached to the bathroom tap.

Dimensions
• H of bar: ~70cm

Use
• Ibrahim holds the wooden bar with one hand, while he squats to use the toilet.

• He uses the hose to fill a water jug on the floor with one hand, while holding the wooden bar for support. He then holds the jug on the floor leaning on it for support, whilst tipping water into his other hand, which he uses for anal cleansing.

Key features
• Low/no cost wooden bar and string.

• Ibrahim decided on the height of bar most suitable for him.

Drawbacks and comments
• There is no choice of distance for the bar – it would be more comfortable for Ibrahim if the bar were nearer.

Suitable for
• Person crawling or shuffling.

• People who can squat but need support, e.g. frail elderly people, people with weak legs, poor co-ordination or balance, pregnant women.

• People who can grasp a rail.

Benefits

Before, Ibrahim had to place both his hands on the toilet floor to balance, which was difficult and made his hands wet and dirty. Now he can keep his hands clean.

Process for obtaining adaptations/external support

Centre for Services and Information on Disability (CSID) is a local DPO with a CBR programme in the Dhaka slums. A CBR worker visited Ibrahim and suggested adapting the toilet in this way.

Additional information/comments

Based on his own experience, Ibrahim often makes suggestions to other children about how to make their toilet comfortable for their needs. For example, for children who have difficulty using their family's *hanging latrine* (see Figure 2.8 for an example) he suggests adding a handrail or a seat for support. These ideas could be suitable not only for children like himself, but also for other people such as amputees.

Before intervention by CSID, he earned a living by begging. He has since received training in leatherwork, and now makes key-rings, purses, etc., to sell.

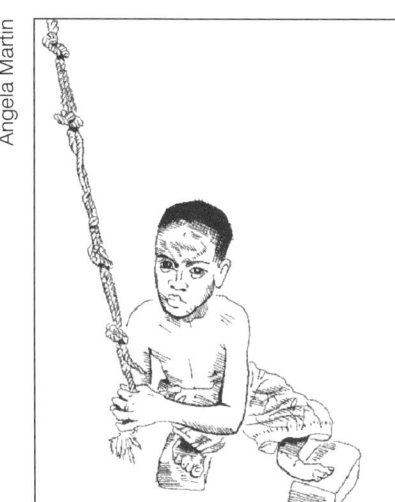

Figure 9.39. Miraz holds the rope to squat.

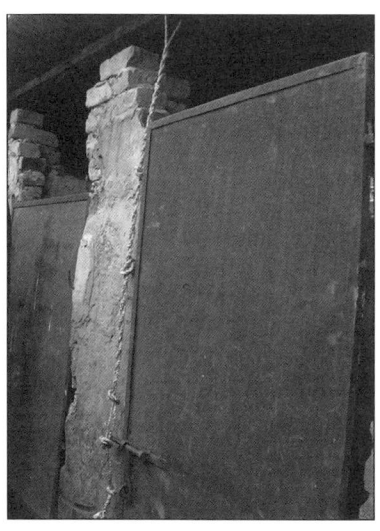

Figure 9.40. Rope hanging from roof beam.

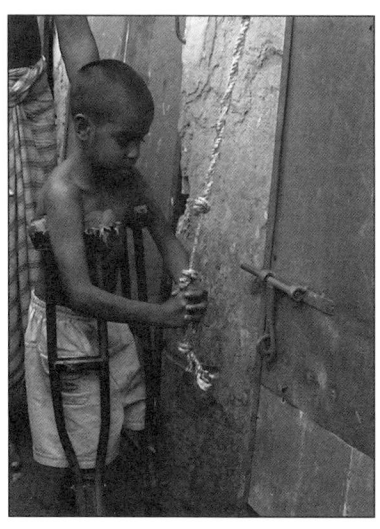

Figure 9.41. Miraz holds the rope as he hops into the toilet.

9.7 Support rope in communal latrine for child using crutches

Mohammed Miraz Hawlader is 8 and lives with his parents and baby sister in a slum area of Dhaka, Bangladesh. Miraz's left leg is bent and weak and he cannot stand on it. His upper body and arms are strong. He uses crutches to get around, or hops.

The family use a communal latrine 30m away from their one-roomed living space.

Description
- A row of brick-built latrines with a tin roof and door. The floor is smooth concrete, which is slippery when wet. Two brick footplates 30cm apart are for squatting. The floor slopes towards a hole in the back wall, through which the waste slides out into an outside drain.

- In one cubicle, a sisal rope hangs from a roof beam above the latrine door, to within 40cm of the ground. It is knotted at intervals to prevent Miraz's hands slipping when he holds it.

Use
- Miraz carries a water jug, which he fills with water at the handpump near the latrine. He takes this to the toilet with him. He holds the rope as he hops into the latrine and while he squats. He puts all his weight on his strong leg, and the rope helps him balance. He then uses the water in the jug for anal cleansing.

Key features
- Low-cost rope, locally available.

- The rope takes up no space; it can be hooked out of the way when not in use so as not to inconvenience other users.

Drawback and comments
- This solution is only possible where a strong overhead beam is available.

- There is no roof beam directly above the toilet, so the rope hangs from a beam over the door. This pulls Miraz slightly off-balance when he holds the rope. Also the rope could get caught in the door and become damaged.

- It would be more comfortable for Miraz if the rope hung directly above the toilet. A handrail fixed to the wall could provide support to Miraz and to other users as they enter the toilet.

Suitable for

- People who can squat but need support, e.g. frail elderly people, people with weak legs, poor co-ordination or balance, pregnant women.

- People who move by crawling or shuffling.

- People with good grip to hold a rope.

Benefits

Before the rope, Miraz used to support himself on his hands. It is not a sanitary latrine, and this was uncomfortable, unpleasant and unhygienic. He prefers using the rope: it's more comfortable, squatting while hanging onto the rope doesn't hurt his leg, and he can keep his hands clean.

Before, his mother used to go with him to the toilet and hold him while he squatted. Now he can go by himself, which saves her time and energy.

Process for obtaining adaptations

Centre for Services and Information on Disability (CSID) is a local DPO with a CBR programme in the Dhaka slums. A CBR worker visited the family and provided the crutches, and suggested the rope. Miraz tried it in different positions until they found which worked best.

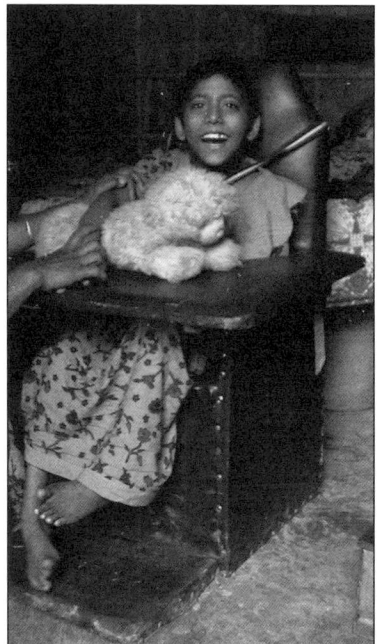
Figure 9.42. Shathi in her padded chair with a tray.

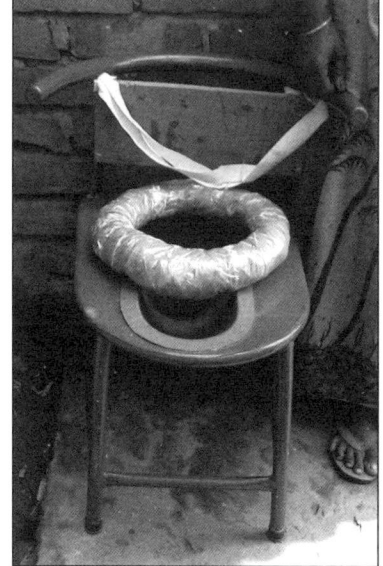
Figure 9.43. Metal commode chair.

9.8 Commode chair for child with no sitting balance

Shathi is aged 9, and lives with her parents and three sisters in one room in a slum area of Dhaka, Bangladesh. She has cerebral palsy, with both legs severely affected. She is unable to stand or walk, but can sit with support. Her hands can grip.

Shathi's mother, Mrs Rasheda, is her sole carer. She used to work in a garment factory, but had to give up work to take care of Shathi when she was born. She spends twice as much time looking after Shathi as her other children. For example, feeding and drinking take about an hour, toileting takes about 20 minutes, and so on.

Shathi has a special supporting chair with a tray, where she sits to eat and drink and play (Figure 9.42). It supports her head and she can easily move her mouth, so food does not fall down. In this position, she can drink water by herself if her mother puts a mug of water in her hand.

Commode chair

Description
- A commercially available metal commode chair with a plastic inset toilet pan. A 'collecting bowl' attaches to the outlet pipe of the pan, which is removable for emptying and cleaning.

Support features
- For additional support, the family have added a wooden plank to the chair back, and attached an elastic belt to the back of the chair, which ties round Shathi's waist.

- Also, a plastic covered sitting ring stuffed with straw is placed on the seat for extra padding.

Key features
- Metal is very durable and easy to clean.

- Commercially available locally.

- The chair can be placed in the most convenient location, inside or outside.

- Shathi sits on the toilet without support of a carer, and can be left in privacy if desired.

- The plastic covering makes the ring easy to clean.

Drawback and comments

- High cost (500 taka = US $8.4).

- A seat with side-rails would provide more support.

- Metal is hard and uncomfortable. The sitting ring often slides out of place.

Suitable for

- People unable to squat, but with some sitting balance, e.g. wheelchair users, frail elderly people, people with weak legs, poor co-ordination or balance, pregnant women.

Benefits

Before, Mrs Rasheda had to help Shathi to go to the toilet into a drain behind the house, and support her the whole time. The toilet chair is more hygienic and more comfortable. Also, Mrs Rasheda now spends less time, energy, and effort than before. The saved time is very important for her – she now has time to take Shathi to the therapy centre and for other domestic work. Sometimes she works in her vegetable garden, which is a source of family income, and of better food.

Before getting the padded chair it was difficult to feed Shathi.

Shathi used to lie on the bed, and her mother would be afraid she would fall off, so someone always had to keep an eye on her. Now if Mrs Rasheda wants to work outside, she sits Shathi outside in the chair, and can keep an eye on her while she works. This also has social benefits. Other children who are passing stop to chat and play with Shathi.

Process for obtaining adaptations

CSID provided all the special equipment – the special chair and table, and the toilet chair – about 8-9 months ago. The family adapted the toilet chair themselves.

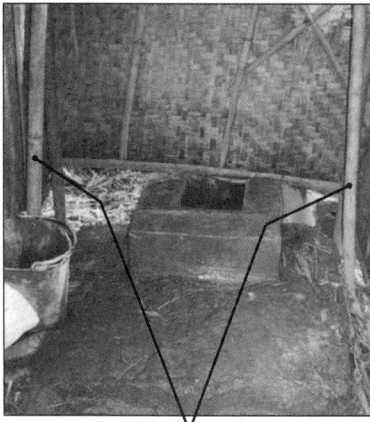

Figure 9.44. Vertical bamboo support poles one on each side of the concrete slab. (CRP)

9.9 Latrine support poles for child with difficulty squatting

Miss Nasima Akter Tinni is 9, and lives with her family in a rural village in Moulavibazar District, Bangladesh. Both Tinni's arms and her right leg are weak because of cerebral palsy. She can walk, but carefully, as she often falls over. Her grasp is weak.

Bathing

Tinni bathes in a pond, except in the rainy season. There is a fixed horizontal bamboo rail leading into the pond, supported by two vertical poles inserted into the ground. She holds this rail to get down to the pond, with support from her brother or other children. She scoops the pond water while standing holding the rail. She has a long-handled bath brush, which she uses to wash her back.

In the rainy season when the path to the pond is too muddy, Tinni bathes in front of the house.

Latrine support poles

Description
- The family latrine is in a bamboo-screened cubicle with a bamboo door and no roof.

- The concrete latrine slab has a rectangular raised squatting plate. The surface is rough.

- Two bamboo poles are stuck vertically into the ground, one on each side of the concrete slab.

Approach
- Located ~20m from the house along an earth path, which slopes gently to ~5cm below the edge of the latrine slab.

Dimensions
- Overall internal: 82cm x 84cm.

- Entrance W: 82cm.

- Distance between the edge of the raised squatting plate and poles: R: 23 cm, L: 18cm (no reason is given for the difference).

Use
- Tinni enters the toilet unaided. She holds one pole with each hand while squatting on the toilet. In the rainy season the path becomes slippery, so she needs help walking to and from the toilet.

Key features
- Low/no cost bamboo.

Drawbacks and comments
- A narrower latrine slab would allow the support poles to be located nearer the user, as in Figure 9.45.

- A lower squatting plate would reduce the risk of Tinni falling and hurting herself.

Suitable for
- People who can squat but need support, e.g. people with weak legs, poor co-ordination or balance, pregnant women.

- People who can grasp a pole.

Benefits
Before, Tinni's mother had to hold her while she squatted, otherwise she risked falling. Now she does not need to do this, which has reduced the amount of time she spends each day caring for Tinni.

Process for obtaining adaptations/external support
Occupational therapists from CRP visited the family and gave them advice and design ideas, such as the bamboo support poles in the toilet and pond. The family provided materials and labour.

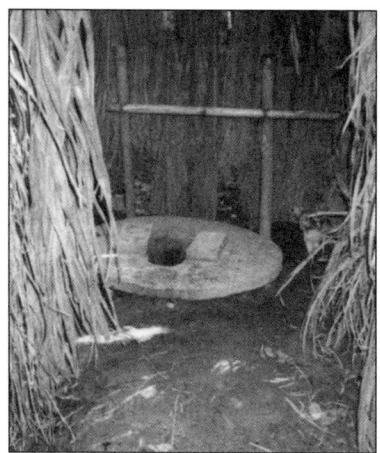

Figure 9.45. Bamboo support rail.

9.10 Latrine support rail for frail elderly man

Mr Mohammed Ramiz Miah is 65 and lives in a rural area of Moulavibazar District, Bangladesh. He had a stroke five years ago, and since then he has gradually become weaker. He cannot stand or walk independently, so family members usually support him.

Latrine support rail

Description
- The family latrine is behind the house, with leaf screen walls, no roof and no door. The latrine slab is a commercially available round concrete slab with raised footplates.

- A handrail has been constructed by sticking two bamboo poles vertically into the ground in front of the slab. A third pole is tied horizontally between the two vertical poles.

Dimensions
- Pole L: 60cm, H: ~50cm from the surface of the slab.

Approach
- Along an uneven brick laid path.

Use
- Mr Ramiz holds onto the horizontal pole for balance while he squats.

Key features
- Low/no cost materials.

Drawbacks and comments
- A walking stick or other support device would enable Mr Ramiz to get to the toilet independently. Horizontal support rails on both sides of the slab would enable Mr Ramiz to step onto the slab unaided.

Suitable for
- People who can squat but need support, e.g. frail elderly people, people with weak legs, poor co-ordination or balance, pregnant women.

- People who can grasp a pole.

Unsuitable for
- People unable to squat, people lacking or with weak grasp.

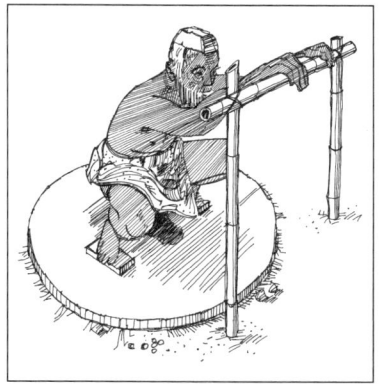

Figure 9.46. Mr Ramiz demonstrates the use of the handrail.

Benefits

Before, Mr Ramiz needed support from his wife while squatting on the toilet. Now he can squat independently without relying on a family member to stay with him the whole time.

Process for obtaining adaptations/external support

A CRP occupational therapist visited Mr Ramiz Miah several times, and made suggestions for adaptations. The family paid for and implemented the adaptations themselves.

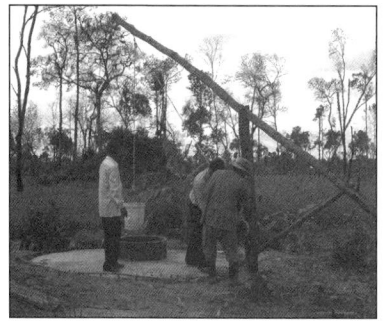

Figure 9.47. Ratchet and pawl lifting device.

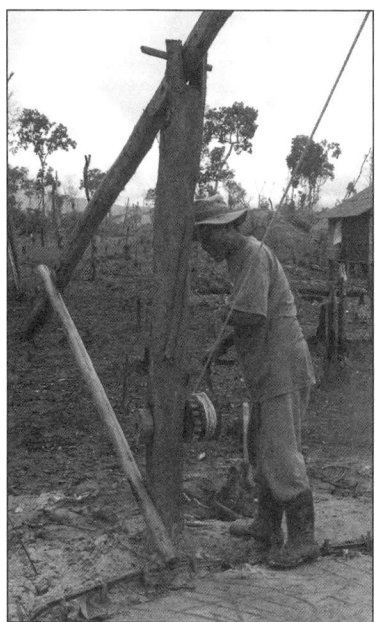

Figure 9.48. Mr Ath turns handle of winding mechanism to lower and lift bucket.

9.11 Ratchet and pawl water-lifting mechanism for man with one arm

Mr Ath lives with his wife and four children in a rural village, which is one hour by ox-cart or 20 minutes by motorbike from the main road. They have lived here five months. Mr Ath was injured by a landmine when he was in the army. His left hand has been amputated and he has only his thumb and two fingers on his right hand. He is also blind in one eye. This has not prevented him building his new house, and digging and constructing (with his brother's help) his family well and water-lifting mechanism.

Shallow well with ratchet and pawl lifting mechanism

Description

- The shallow well is concrete lined, with a concrete platform surround sloping away from the well, and a drainage outlet.

- The lifting device is made from a wooden cantilever frame overhanging the well. A rope passes through a small pulley suspended over the well to a ratchet and pawl (winding and locking mechanism) attached to the upright of the frame. A bucket is suspended by the rope over the well.

- The winding mechanism consists of a rope wound round a wooden core, which rotates around a metal spindle. A metal handle is attached to the core. The locking mechanism consists of a ratchet (like a cog) carved from wood, with a metal pawl (bar or large nail) which engages with the notches to prevent onward movement.

Approach

- The well is ~20m from the house along a rough earth path.

Dimensions

- See Figure 9.51.

Use

- Using one hand, Mr Ath removes the pawl and turns the handle of the ratchet to lower the bucket into the water to fill it, then turns the ratchet to raise the bucket.

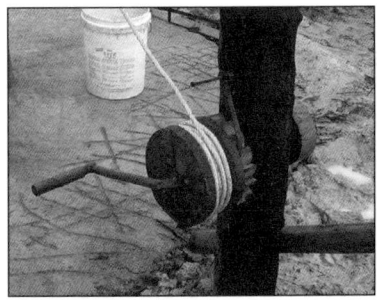

Figure 9.49. Ratchet and pawl locking mechanism. The metal pawl is engaged with the notches of the ratchet to prevent onward movement.

- When the bucket is clear of the well wall, he uses his stump to flip the pawl to engage with the notches of the ratchet, which locks it, so that the bucket is suspended above the well. He walks to the well, pulls the bucket and rope over to the outside of the well, and pours the water into another bucket placed beside the well.

Key features
- Adapted by Mr Ath to suit his needs, based on a cantilever design widely used locally.

- The winding and locking mechanism are made from local wood and a few pieces of metal.

- The cantilever takes the weight of the water, so both disabled and non-disabled users avoid rope-burn on their hands.

Drawbacks and comments
- Wooden ratchet wheel sometimes loses its teeth. It would be more durable if it were made in metal.

Suitable for
- Users with one arm or weak grip; wheelchair users.

- A child, with a smaller water container.

- Locking mechanism could benefit non-disabled people for use with deep wells.

Other water issues

Carrying water
Usually Mr Ath carries two buckets using a wooden yoke across his shoulders. He hangs two full 20-litre buckets from the yoke by a piece of knotted rope tied to their metal handles. He then lifts the yoke and buckets onto his shoulder and carries them to the house.

Watering the garden
Carrying two buckets of water on the yoke, he uses a mug to scoop water over plants. He would prefer a watering can, but cannot afford one at the moment.

Bathing
The family all bathe next to the well by scooping water from a bucket to pour over themselves using either a plastic cup or a bowl. Mr Ath is able to bathe using his one hand, but to wash his right arm thoroughly he asks for help from his wife, or he uses the upright pole of the lifting mechanism to rub his arm against after splashing water on it.

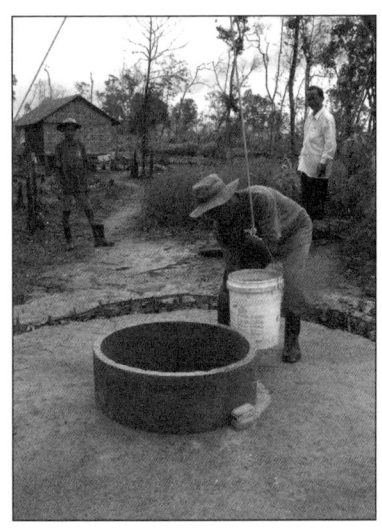

Figure 9.50. Lifting the bucket over the well wall.

Disposal of wastewater

In the dry season, they dig a hole and pour wastewater into it, plus any waste vegetable matter, ash, etc. When it is full they plant a mango tree on it.

Benefits

Before, drawing water from a shallow well was sometimes difficult for Mr Ath as the rope burned across the stump of his arm. This is why he designed this new lifting device.

His wife, Mrs Phoun, said she finds this well easier to use than a hand-over-hand well, where the rope can burn your hands. If a smaller bucket is used, a child can use the lifting mechanism.

She is excited and proud that her husband constructed the well. It is something that many non-disabled people could not do.

Process for obtaining adaptations

The village of Veal Thom is a community of disabled people and their families, established in 2000 by Save Cambodian Disabled People's Association (SCDPA). SCDPA is an NGO set up to help former soldiers disabled by conflict, and other disabled people, and their families. The land for the village was donated to SCDPA by the government. The land is divided into individual plots, which are allocated to disabled people and their families to live on and to cultivate. There are over 200 families now living there.

Only the land is provided by SCDPA. Families dig their own well, build their own house and grow their own food. Those who are very needy may be provided with rice and other donations while they get settled.

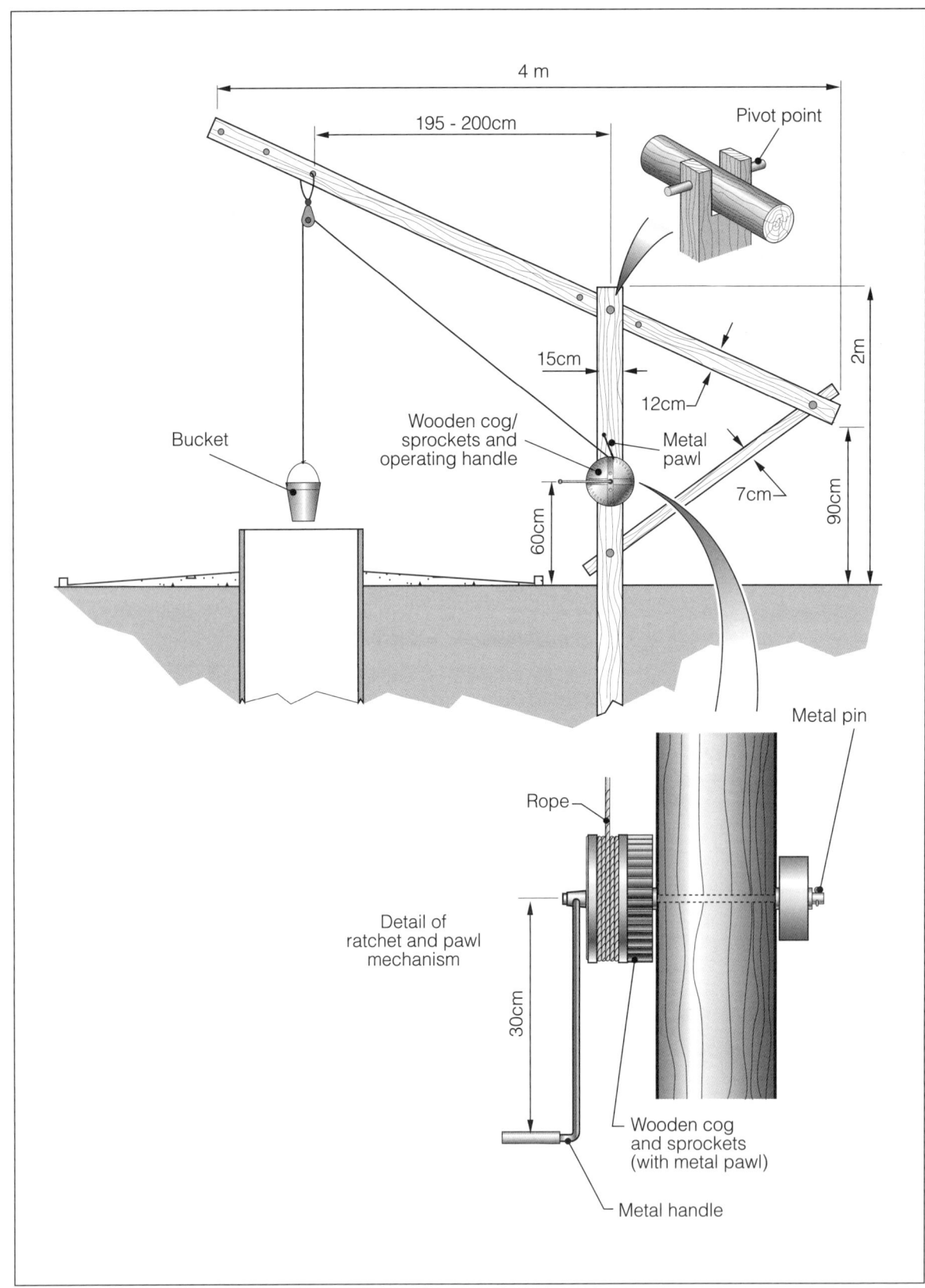

Figure 9.51. Well with ratchet and pawl lifting mechanism.

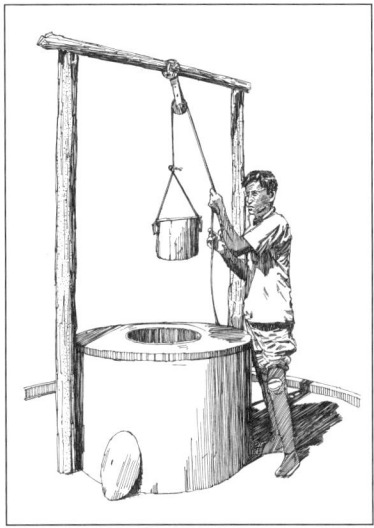

Figure 9.52. Locally made wood and metal pulley.

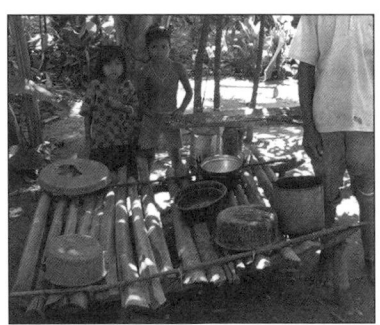

Figure 9.53. Mr Tu lifting water.

9.12 Rope and pulley water-lifting mechanism for man with one leg

Mr Tu Chen is a 40-year-old farmer who lives with his wife and 12 children in a rural village in Siem Reap Province, Cambodia. Mr Chen lost one leg below the knee when he stepped on a landmine not far from his village. He has an artificial leg and appears to manage most activities well.

Description
- Shallow household well with a concrete apron around it. A rope and pulley are suspended from a wooden frame over the well. The frame is two upright poles with one horizontal pole nailed between them. The pulley is locally made: a wooden roller and spindle through a piece of flat metal bent as a hanger. At the top of the flat metal hangers is a hook which is tied to the horizontal bar of the frame using rubber rope (made from old inner tubes).

Dimensions
- H of frame ~2m.
- H of well wall: ~80cm.
- Water container: ~5 litres.

Approach
- Located 10 – 20m from the house.

Use
- A rope passes from Mr Chen's hand through the pulley and is attached to an old metal kettle (~5 litres). This is dropped into the well and used to draw water by pulling on the rope. Water from the kettle is poured into a larger bucket for carrying to the house.

Key features
- Proximity to the user's house makes it an easy distance to walk to fetch water.
- The pulley means less strength is needed to lift the same quantity of water.
- Could be operated from a standing or sitting position – no need for the user to bend over the side of the well.
- The pulley is simple and locally made.
- Any size of container could be used.

Drawbacks
- The locally made wooden pulley is not as good as the original pulley.

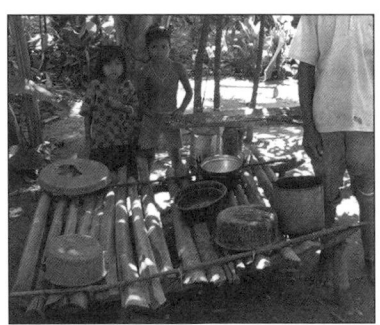

Figure 9.54. Bamboo dish drying rack.

Suitable for

- People with little strength, e.g. elderly, children, those with weak grip.

Process for obtaining adaptations

Social workers from Siem Reap Provincial Rehabilitation Centre referred Mr Chen to the Jesuit Services, an NGO which gives priority to the poorest, and had a programme to install wells in the local area. The Jesuit Services provided the concrete well rings and Mr Chen hired someone to dig the well.

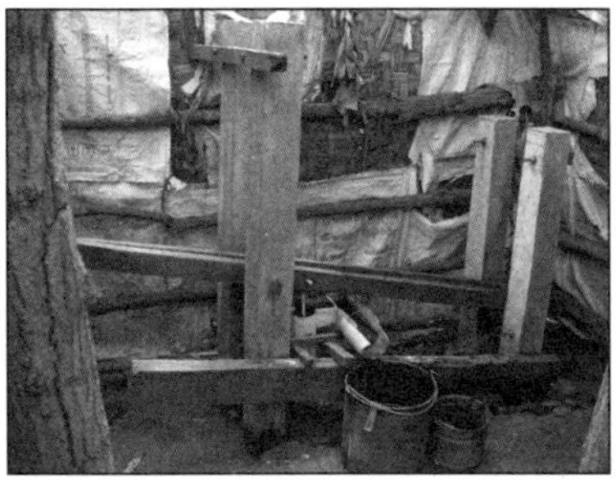

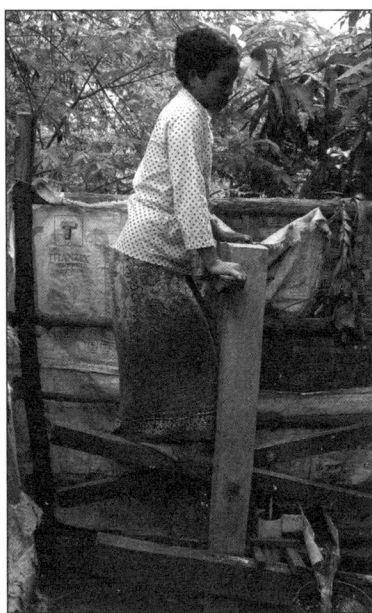

Figure 9.55. Treadle pump.

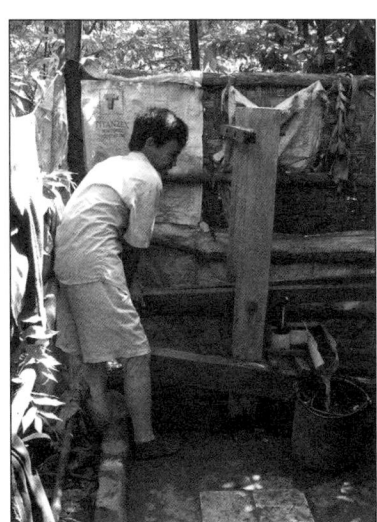

Figure 9.56. Mrs Nourn operates the treadle pump with her feet.

9.13 Treadle pump for man with one leg and his blind wife

Mr Lann Khorn and Mrs Nourn Sariam live on a small island accessible only by boat, in Kandal Province, Cambodia. They have three children.

Mr Lann has impairments as a result of leprosy (now cured). His right leg has been amputated below the knee and he wears an artificial leg. He has recently had surgery on the other foot, so was wearing a plaster cast at the time of interview. Both hands are bent and stiff in a claw shape. He still manages to undertake quite intricate work such as maintaining his pump.

Mrs Nourn is blind. She manages daily tasks well around the house and compound, but to go across the island she needs one of her children to go with her.

Description
- The treadle pump frame is made of wood, with the upright pillars of concrete. The downward movement of the wooden beams is softened by a flip-flop cut in half and placed on the wooden 'stopper' bar.

Dimensions
- See Figure 9.60.

Use
- The pump is designed to be operated with the feet by pushing down on two long pieces of wood, which rotate about a pivot point. The rising and falling wood pulls and pushes on a plunger, which works with a valve to pump water.

- Water is pumped into open metal buckets (~15l). Mrs Nourn listens for the sound of water overflowing the bucket to let her know when to stop pumping.

Approach
- Located in the family compound ~5m from the house via a path of packed earth.

- An area with brick-laid hard-standing is constructed in front of the pump to improve drainage and reduce slipperiness. The area is screened with plastic sacking.

Key features
- The pump can be operated using either feet or hands.

Figure 9.57. Mr Lann operates the pump with his hands.

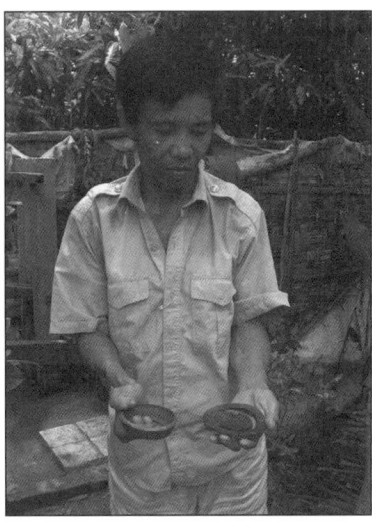

Figure 9.58. Spare parts for the pump.

- Initial cost and maintenance costs are lower than for a UNICEF installed handpump at the nearby school (an India Mark II).

- Simple technology, easy for user to maintain as moving components are above ground. Moving parts can be easily removed and replacements purchased cheaply locally.

Suitable for
- Children can use the pump easily.

Drawbacks
- Requires a lot of user effort to pump for the amount of water produced.

- It operates as a suction pump, so is only suitable for shallow water table areas, as it can only pump from a maximum depth of 7m.

Water filter
Description
- Concrete vertical sand water filter.

Use
- Well water is poured into the top and filtered water trickles into another bucket below the spout. This is used for drinking. The filter materials are removed and cleaned once or twice a month.

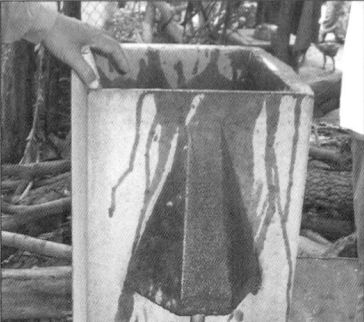

Figure 9.59. Sand water filter.

Benefits
Time saved: Before installing the pump, the family water source was the river, 15 minutes walk away on the other side of the island. The slope to the river was steep and slippery (especially in the rainy season) and the water turbid. It would take Mrs Nourn a whole morning to fetch 4 x 15l buckets of water. One of the children (then aged 1½) always had to guide her there and back.

Now, both husband and wife can draw water independently from the pump, and save a lot of time. They have a lot more water, in much less time.

Improved health: In the past, the family were often sick with stomach aches and diarrhoea. Since starting to use the water filter the couple have noticed a clear improvement in their family's health. For example, their son was often absent from school because of illness; now he is rarely sick, so goes much more regularly to school. Also, they have more water which they can use when growing vegetables and fruit; they wash their vegetables, so they are cleaner before eating them.

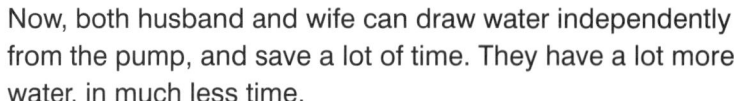

Improved finances: Because they are sick less often, they save money which they would have spent on medicines. They can now afford school fees, and to pay for transport for the children to go to school.

Mr Lann and Mrs Nourn can now grow vegetables and keep chickens. They have earned enough money from one season of vegetable growing to recover the cost of the pump. In the future they would like to also connect a hose-pipe to be able to water their vegetable garden.

Reduced workload for the children: The son would get upset when asked to guide his mother to the river, because he would rather play with his friends. Now that the mother can draw water without a child to guide her, all the children can go to school, and they have free time to play.

Increased self-reliance and role in the community: Mr Lann watched carefully when they installed the pump, as he knew he would need to repair the pump himself. He now maintains the pump himself, replacing valves and pipes. He also mends his neighbours' pumps and receives payment in cash or in rice. They hold spare parts at home which they buy from local suppliers (Figure 9.58).

Process for obtaining adaptations
The borehole and pump were provided in 1999 by a Japanese NGO called International Volunteers of Yamagata (IVY).
Mr Lann and Mrs Nourn were considered a priority because of their impairments, so were the first to receive a borehole, but eventually all the neighbours also got their own boreholes and pumps.

IVY drilled the borehole and provided the initial materials for the treadle pump, but the family paid for the materials. The family completed the pump installation themselves following instructions provided by IVY.

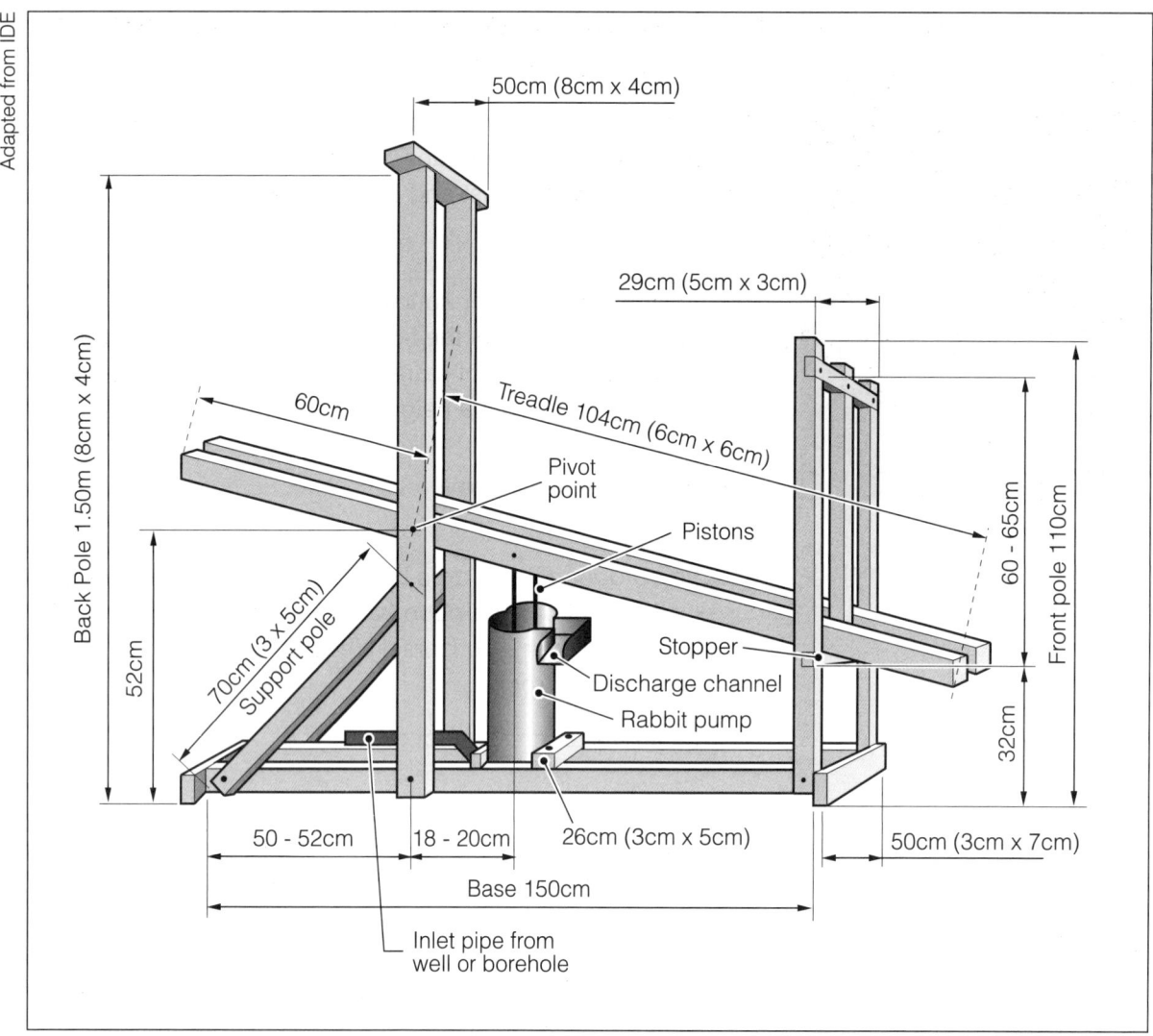

Figure 9.60. Treadle pump.

More information about the pump can be found on http://www.ideorg. org/html/gallery/treadle. html or from IDE (see Appendix 2 for contact details).

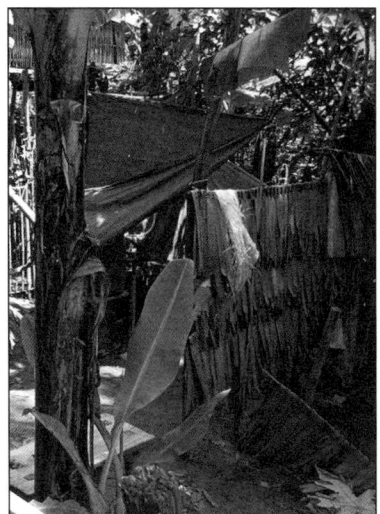

Figure 9.61. Bathing area with leaf screen and plastic sheeting for a door.

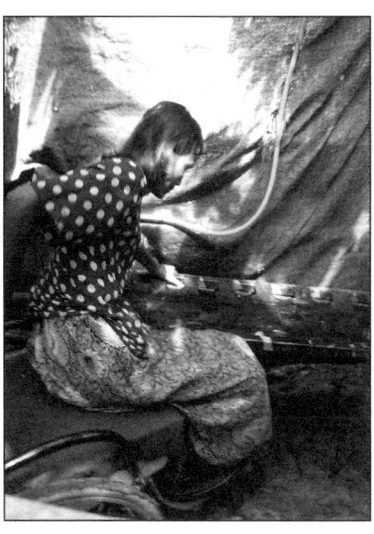

Figure 9.62. Mrs Rong transfers from her wheelchair to the bench.

9.14 Bathing area with water storage for wheelchair user

Ms Rong Ry is 34 and lives with her husband and children in a rural village in Siem Reap Province, Cambodia. She is paralysed below the waist and uses a wheelchair to move around.

The family have two water sources: in the rainy season, rainwater from the roof of the house is channelled by guttering into two large ferrocement storage jars. In the dry season the family collect water from a neighbour's well to fill the jars.

Screened bathing area

Description
- The outdoor bathing area has a screen of palm leaves and plastic sheet on a bamboo frame. The door is a plastic sheet hung over a horizontal piece of wood hung between two posts. No roof.

- The floor is earth and stones.

Dimensions
- There is room for a bathing bench, water storage jar (see below), and for a wheelchair to enter and turn.

Use
- Mrs Rong enters the bathing area in her wheelchair and parks it beside the bench. She transfers from wheelchair to bench.

- To bathe, she scoops water from the storage jar over herself, using a plastic cup.

- To wash clothes, she places a washbowl on the bench beside her, and scoops water into it from the storage jar.

- Wastewater drains or is thrown onto the floor and drains away on the bare earth.

Key features
- Materials are locally available and low cost.

- It was constructed by the family based on the needs of their mother.

Drawbacks
- Leaf screen is not durable, and needs to be replaced regularly.

- Poor drainage means water lies in pools on the floor, leading to deterioration of the floor, making it more uneven. This makes it difficult for the wheelchair to manoeuvre, and to stabilise the wheelchair, so it is difficult to transfer without help. Improved drainage would reduce these problems.

Suitable for
- Wheelchair users; people with good sitting balance; people with difficulty bending, pregnant women, frail elderly people.

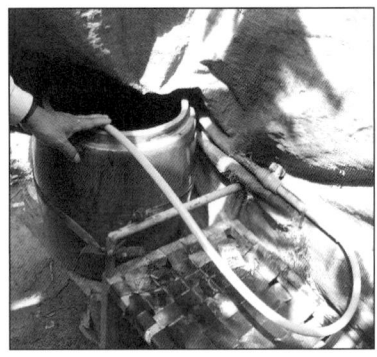

Figure 9.63. Hose with a tap for filling water storage jar.

Internal water supply and storage

Description
- The main water storage jar has a small outlet pipe of flexible reinforced hose, with a tap near the end (Figure 9.63). This leads to a smaller clay storage jar in the bathing area ~2m away and positioned at a lower level.

- The secondary jar is raised on a wooden block next to the bathing bench, so that Mrs Rong can easily reach into it. It is kept in place with a rubber strap.

Dimensions
- Main jar: 200 - 500 litre. Secondary jar: 20 - 50 litre. 20mm flexible reinforced hose with plastic tap.

Use
- Mrs Rong sits on the bench next to the water jar. She fills it with water by directing the hose into the jar and turning on the tap. She then scoops water from the jar using a plastic cup.

Key features
- Mrs Rong fills the water jar as she needs it.

- The storage jar is raised to a suitable height for the user.

- The open-necked jar is easy to clean.

- The main storage jar needs to be filled by hand in the dry season, which the family can do when it is convenient for them, rather than on demand.

Drawbacks
- Lack of cover or lid on the storage jar increases the risk of water contamination, which is important to avoid if the water is used for drinking.

Suitable for

- All users. Those with weak arms may need help scooping water from the top of the jar.

Suggestion

- A tap inserted near the bottom of the storage jar would allow the user to draw water without raising their arm to scoop.

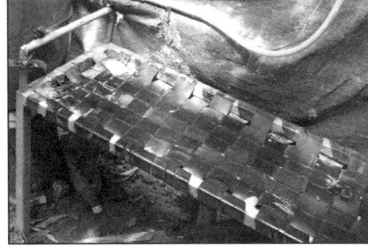

Figure 9.64. Metal framed bathing bench.

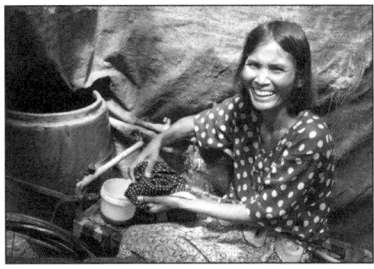

Figure 9.65. Mrs Rong sits on the bench to wash clothes.

Bathing bench

Description

- The bench has a metal frame, with a seat woven from strips of rubber inner tube. There is a rail at each end of the bench.

Dimensions

- L~ 120cm, W~40cm, H~50cm (level with the wheelchair seat).

- Height of end rails from seat: ~15cm.

Use

- Mrs Rong transfers from her wheelchair to sit on the bench to bathe.

- Wastewater drains through the rubber webbing of the bench, or is thrown on the floor and drains away on the bare earth.

Key features

- Rails on the bench are for holding onto for support.

- Rubber webbing of the bench is durable, easy to clean, and provides good drainage.

- Bather is not sitting in her own bathwater.

Drawbacks

- Rubber webbing is not very supportive.

Suggestions

- If the bench had a back it would provide more support for the user.

Benefits

Before, Mrs Rong stayed upstairs in the raised house. She could not move much and developed pressure sores. She depended on her husband for washing and all other activities. The bathing area has allowed her to be more independent.

Process for obtaining adaptations

A social worker from Siem Reap Provincial Rehabilitation Centre visited Mrs Rong to discuss her problems and needs, and provided information about what services were available. She was referred to the Spinal Cord Injury (SCI) Centre in Battambang, where they helped her with ideas and advice, including the bathing bench and toilet.

Social workers assessed the family situation and reached agreement over what the family could contribute to adaptations, e.g. labour to dig a toilet pit, local materials.

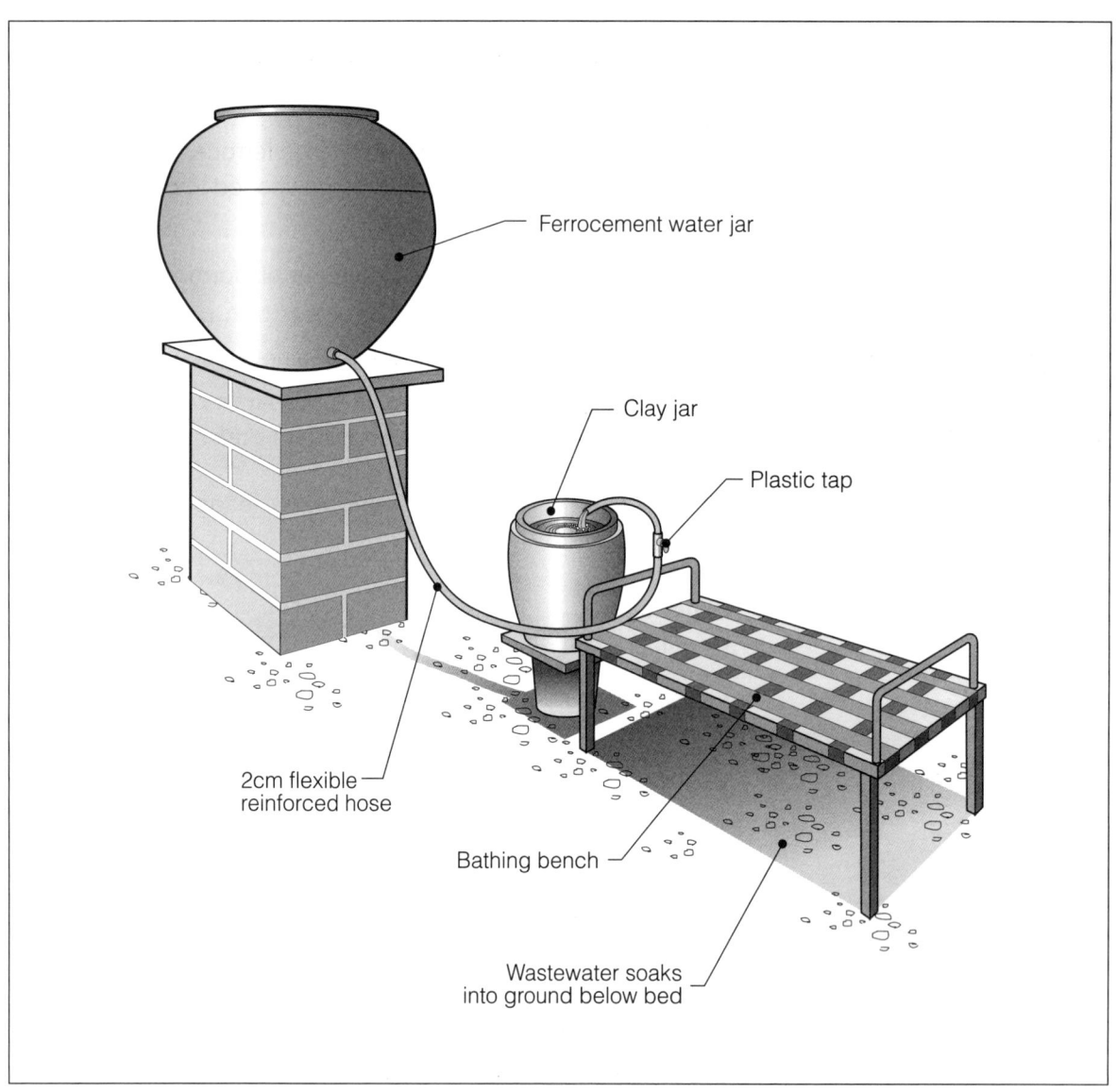

Figure 9.66. Layout of Mrs Rong's gravity fed water source (privacy screen not shown, for clarity).

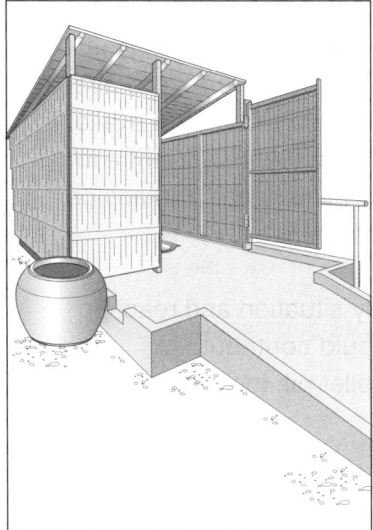

Figure 9.67. Toilet cubicle and bathing area.

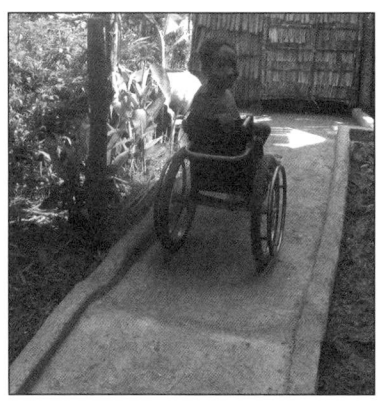

Figure 9.68. Concrete ramp leading to bathing area.

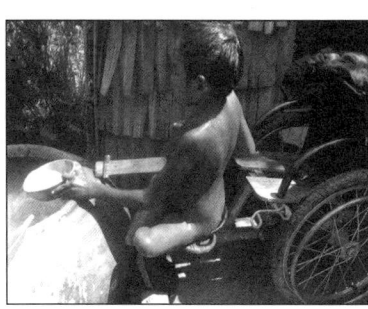

Figure 9.69. Heng sits on the wheelchair footrest to bathe.

9.15 Toilet and bathing area for child who uses a wheelchair

Chea Sok Heng is 11 and lives with his parents and six siblings on the rural outskirts of Kampong Thom, in Cambodia. Their economic situation is poor.

Heng has weak legs and a weak arm as a result of polio. He moves around independently by shuffling on his buttocks, and pulling himself up with his arms. He has a wheelchair to move around outside, which he can get in and out of without help.

The family fetch water from a well across the road to store in their own large ferrocement jars.

Bathing area with a water storage jar

Description
- A flat concrete platform with a large ferrocement water storage jar next to it. The jar is positioned lower than the platform.

- A concrete kerb goes all round the platform, with a drainage outlet in one corner.

- A bamboo rail on the side opposite the water jar is for hanging clothes.

Approach
- Accessed via a concrete ramp which leads from the house.

Dimensions
- Platform: 134cm x 100cm.

- Concrete kerb: H: 6cm.

- Ramp: W: 75cm, gradient 1 in 15.

- Water jar: 50 – 500 litres.

Use
- Heng wheels himself up the ramp to the bathing platform. He removes his clothes and hangs them on the rail.

- He positions his wheelchair facing the water jar and lowers himself to sit on the footrest. From here he can reach into the jar with a scoop and splash water over himself.

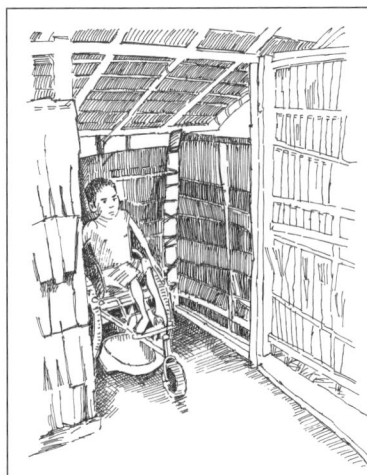

Figure 9.70. Heng positions his wheelchair over the toilet.

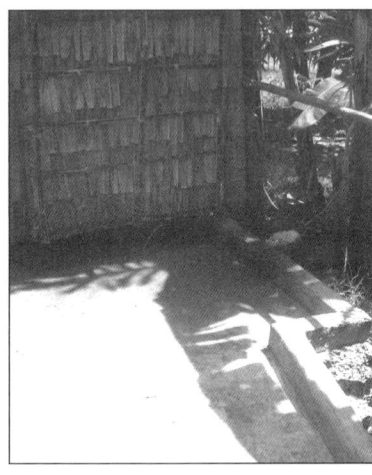

Figure 9.71. Flat platform in front of toilet door.

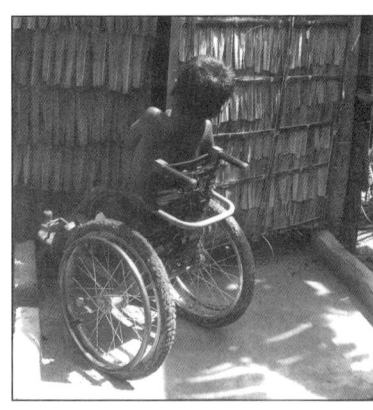

Figure 9.72. Heng manoeuvres his wheelchair to open the toilet door.

Key features

- The concrete kerb prevents the wheelchair rolling off the platform.

- Concrete is easy to clean, water drains easily, clothes are kept dry on the rail.

- The low position of the water jar makes it easy for Heng to reach into from a sitting position on the platform.

- The family fills the storage jar as convenient to them, rather than on demand.

Drawbacks and comments

- The storage jar needs to be filled regularly by other family members.

- The risk of water contamination could be reduced by using a cover on the storage jar, and by using a two-cup system to scoop water. This is a crucial issue if the water is used for drinking.

Wheelchair accessible household toilet

Description

- A wood framed toilet cubicle, with leaf screen walls. A wide leaf screen door swings shut without pulling. There is no door fastening.

- The floor is smooth concrete. A ceramic pour-flush toilet pan is set level with the floor. 2 moulded cement mortar shapes have been stuck on the floor next to the toilet pan, for the wheels of the wheelchair to slot into.

- There is space for a water storage jar (~30 litres) beside the toilet.

Approach

- Along a concrete ramp leading from the house (Figure 9.68). There is a flat platform in front of the toilet door, also used as a bathing platform (Figure 9.71).

Dimensions

- Overall internal: L 100cm x W 140cm.

- Entrance W: 88cm.

- Flat platform: 134cm x 100cm.

Use

Heng pushes himself up the ramp, manoeuvres the wheelchair on the level platform to open the door. He reverses into the latrine in his wheelchair. He slots the wheels of his chair

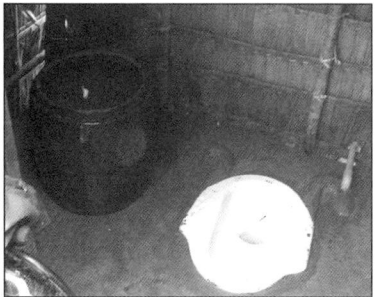

Figure 9.73. Water jar next to toilet pan. Note moulded cement mortar shapes for correct wheelchair positioning.

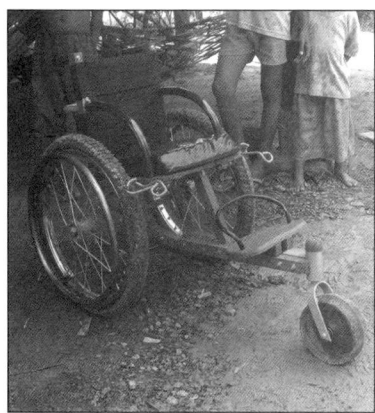

Figure 9.74. Mekong wheelchair with foot-rest, also used as a transfer-seat.

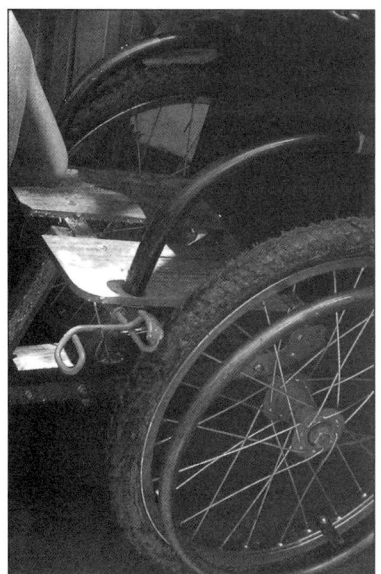

Figure 9.75. Wheelchair seat with central plank removed.

into the cement mouldings, so that the seat of his chair is positioned directly over the toilet hole.He removes the wheelchair cushion and a central plank from the seat (Figure 9.75). The wheelchair then acts as a toilet seat, with urine and faeces dropping directly into the toilet hole. Heng carries out anal cleansing using a special tool (Figure 9.76) and water from the jar beside the toilet.

Key features
* Enough space inside for a wheelchair to enter, and space for an internal water supply.

* The internal water supply allows Heng to wash in private.

* The self-closing door means no effort is needed to close the door.

* The smooth concrete floor is easy to keep clean.

* Moulded cement shapes help with accurate wheelchair positioning over the toilet hole.

Drawbacks and comments
* High cost of materials – ceramic and concrete.

* A pour-flush toilet depends on water always being available. The water jar needs to be filled by others.

* There's only just enough room on the platform to manoeuvre the wheelchair round the door. For minimal additional cost, the platform could have been made wider, which would be usable in the future when Heng grows up and needs an adult size wheelchair.

Suitable for
* Users with a convertible wheelchair

Unsuitable for
* Pour-flush toilet would be unsuitable for areas where water is scarce.

Wheelchair used for bathing and as a toilet chair

Description
* The 'Mekong' wheelchair has a wooden footrest located behind the small single front wheel. It is also used as a mid-level 'transfer' seat. A metal rail keeps the feet in place and also acts as a seat back.

* A central plank in the wooden seat slides out, leaving a gap ~10cm wide. This allows it to be used as a toilet chair.

Dimensions
- Height of footrest: ~25cm.

Key features
- The main part of the chair does not get wet, which would happen if the bather stayed in the seat to bathe.

- Saves money: one piece of equipment serves more than one function.

- Saves space: the toilet cubicle can be smaller as there is no need to provide space for a wheelchair next to the toilet.

- Saves effort – no need to transfer to a separate seat.

Drawbacks and comments
- Not suitable for persons with poor sitting balance or lacking arm strength.

- This wheelchair is not designed to be used as a toilet seat. The main frame is directly under the seat, which will inevitably become fouled*.

- Unsuitable for wheelchairs with a footrest in front of the front wheels, as they may tip up with the weight on the footrest.

Suitable for
- Users with good sitting balance and arm strength.

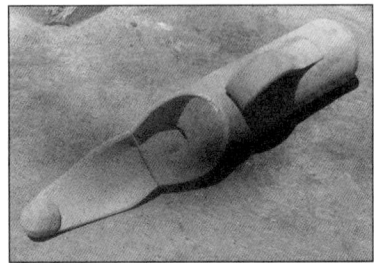

Figure 9.76. Anal cleansing device.

Anal cleansing tool

Description
- A soft plastic cylindrical container with a restricted opening and a handle. Has an elongated soft rubber 'finger'.

Use
- The user fills the container with water, then holding it from in front between the legs, uses the soft rubber 'finger' to clean the anus, letting water slowly trickle out.

Key features
- Locally designed and made.

Drawbacks and comments
- Needs regular washing.

Suitable for
- Suitable for a user with limited flexibility or reach.

- Could be used by a support person to help a disabled person with anal cleansing.

---

* Heng received this new wheelchair one day before the researchers' visit, so could not comment on this aspect of its use.

Benefits

Before, Heng used to defecate in the surrounding area, and needed someone to help him. His father had to carry him to the field, to go to the toilet, and help him bathe. Sometimes his father was in a hurry to go to work in the fields, but he would have to spend an hour or more helping his son.

Heng prefers this toilet as he doesn't need anyone's help. He's proud of it and has invited his friends to see it. He uses the same water source and facilities as the rest of the family, so he is not isolated.

In fact, the whole family uses and benefits from the hygienic new facilities. His mother said it is more convenient, comfortable, and private, and there is no need to worry about snakes!

His father now worries less about his son. He also has more time for working in the fields.

According to his mother, the neighbours are a bit jealous, but they understand why the family needed a toilet because of their disabled child.

Process for obtaining adaptations

CABDIC ('Capacity building of people with disabilities in the community') is a programme to support disabled children and adults in the community. It was set up by Handicap International Belgium.

CBR workers of CABDIC discussed with the family, introduced the idea of accessible facilities, and showed them examples of equipment. The CBR worker supported the father to apply to UNICEF local office for the toilet pan. The family provided labour to build the ramp and toilet.

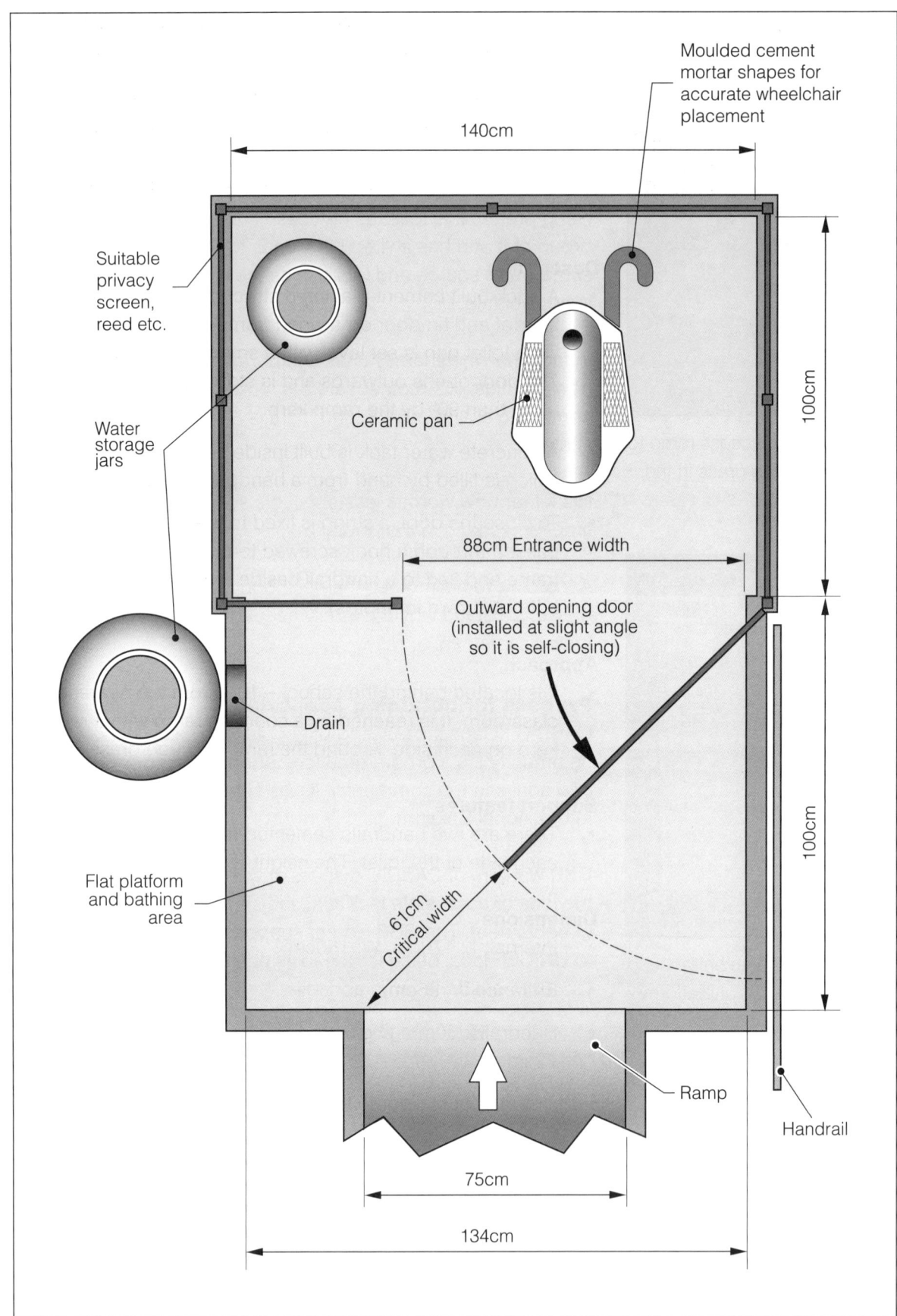

Figure 9.77. Plan view of Heng's toilet and bathing area.

9

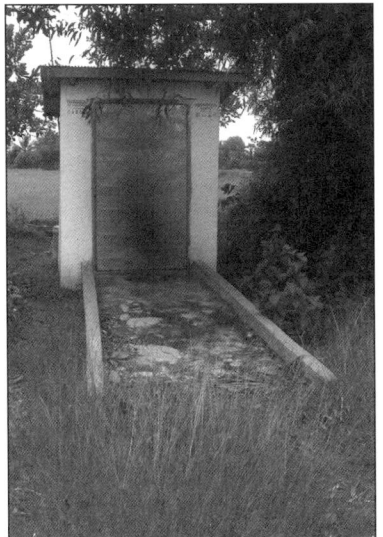

Figure 9.78. The access ramp to the toilet with long grass in the way.

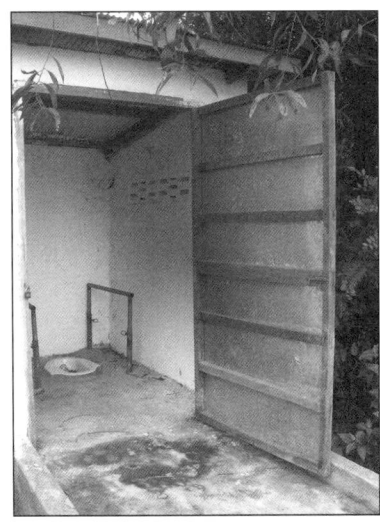

Figure 9.79. Smooth entrance to toilet. Note lack of flat platform in front of door which is a problem.

9.16 Primary school toilet designed for wheelchair access

Heng (see Heng's story in Section 9.15) goes to the local primary school, which previously had no toilets for pupils, who all used the surrounding bushes and fields as a toilet. Heng found this difficult, so the CABDIC programme installed an accessible toilet.

Description

- A brick-built cement-plastered structure with a corrugated tin roof and tin door on a wood frame. A ceramic pour-flush toilet pan is set level with a smooth concrete floor. The door opens outwards and is stopped from opening more than 90° by the ramp kerb.

- A concrete water tank is built inside next to the toilet, which is filled by hand from a handpump nearby.

- To close the door, a string is fixed to the inside of the door, passed through a hook screwed to the top of the door frame and tied to a handrail beside the toilet (Figure 9.82 but not shown in photos).

Approach

- It is located behind the school ~10m from the nearest classroom. It is reached by a concrete ramp with a raised kerb on each side. Around the ramp is rough grass.

Support features

- There are two handrails cemented to the floor, one on each side of the toilet. The height is adjustable.

Dimensions

- Internal: L: 176cm, W: 150cm.

- Entrance W: 95cm.

- Handrails: 30mm Ø g.i. pipe, L:82cm; W between rails: 72cm.

- Distance from door to handrail: 90cm.

- Ramp: W: 115cm, kerb H:10cm, gradient: ~1:15.

Use

- Heng gets to and up the ramp and enters the latrine in his wheelchair. He pulls on the string to close the door and ties it to a handrail. He gets down from his chair and squats using the handrails for support.

- All pupils can use the latrine, but Heng has his own key.

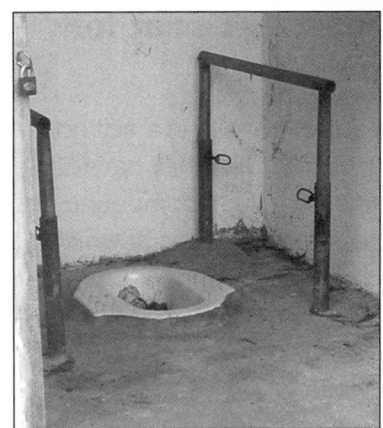

Figure 9.80. Adjustable handrails.

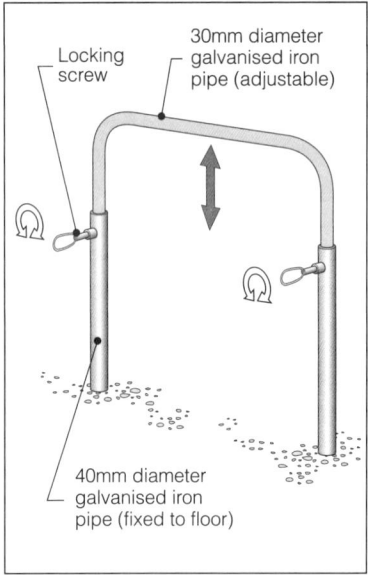

Figure 9.81. Adjustable handrail mechanism. Metal pegs or nails inserted into holes at different heights would be more robust

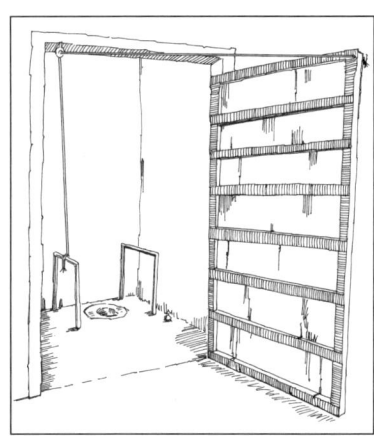

Figure 9.82. String door closing device.

Key features

- The door is wide enough for a wheelchair to enter.

- Water is provided inside the toilet for personal hygiene.

- The string door-closing mechanism enables the user to close the door without a lot of manoeuvring.

- A kerb on each side of the ramp prevents the wheelchair rolling over the edge.

Drawbacks and comments

- High cost.

- A flat platform in front of the door would allow Heng to open the door without his wheelchair rolling backwards.

- The pour-flush toilet needs water always available, otherwise it becomes blocked and unusable.

- More space inside the toilet cubicle would allow a wheelchair to turn and exit forwards, which is easier than reversing out.

- The long grass in front of the ramp makes it difficult for Heng to get to the ramp.

- School staff did not take responsibility for maintaining the toilet, possibly because it was installed, and perhaps seen as owned, by the CABDIC programme.

- It might have been more productive to consult the teachers more fully about the idea, to address hygiene and sanitation as a whole school issue, rather than installing 'special' facilities for one child.

Benefits

All children in the school could use the toilet, so it benefited all the pupils.

It is currently out of use, because a kitchen has recently been built between the classrooms and the toilet, and an alternative path has not been cleared. Heng now can't get to the toilet so he goes outside again as before.

In addition, during the school holidays, people living nearby broke the lock on the door and used the toilet without flushing it. Now it is dirty and blocked and unusable.

Process for obtaining facility

The staff of the CABDIC programme introduced the idea, provided and constructed the latrine.

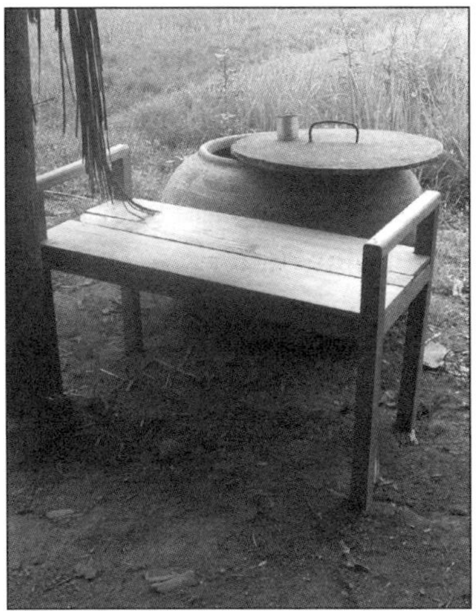

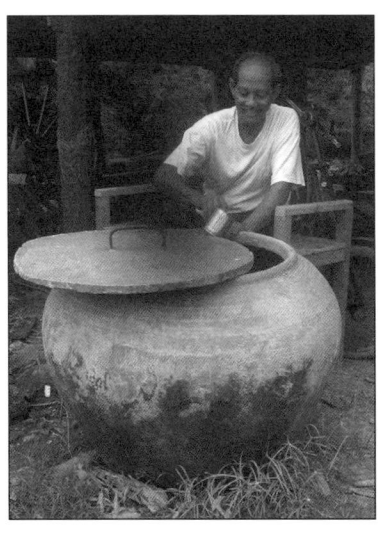

Figure 9.83. Wooden bathing bench.

9.17 Bathing bench and toilet seat for elderly wheelchair user

Mr Kong Chea is aged 69 and lives with his wife in a stilt house in a rural village near Battambang, Cambodia. They have 3 children who are married and live nearby. Their compound and the surrounding area floods for four months a year, at which time they get around by boat.

Mr Kong was injured in the war; his legs are paralysed. He uses a wheelchair to get around outside the house. He can get up the steps to the house on his buttocks.

For bathing and washing clothes, his wife fetches water from a pond over 50m away and stores it in large jars under the house. Rainwater is used for drinking. There is no latrine, so the rest of the family urinate and defecate in the surrounding fields and bushes.

Wooden bathing bench

Description
* A rectangular wooden bench, with a solid wood plank surface. There is a handrail at each end of the bench.

* Water is stored in large ferrocement storage jars with concrete lids, beneath the raised house. The bench is placed next to them.

Dimensions
* H: level with wheelchair seat.

* L~ 120, W ~45 cm, H~ 60cm. height of rail above seat ~15cm.

Approach
* Packed earth.

Use
* Mr Kong positions his wheelchair beside the bench. He transfers to sit on the bench facing the water jar. He removes his clothes and pours water over himself using a tin scoop.

Key features
* Locally made, reasonable cost. Wood is fairly durable and easy to clean.

* A rail at each end is useful for the user to hold on to for balance.

Figure 9.84. Mr Kong using the bathing bench.

- Movable: the location can be changed depending on the user's needs, e.g. nearer the water source, or to a more private location. It could also be used for other functions, e.g. eating, washing clothes.

Drawbacks and comments
- The wide solid surface makes drainage poor; so the wood may deteriorate if it is always wet. It would be more durable if painted or varnished. If it was longer, a person lying down could use it.

Suitable for
- People with good sitting balance and some upper body strength for transferring.

- People with difficulty squatting or bending.

Unsuitable for
- People with poor sitting balance, as there is no back or side support.

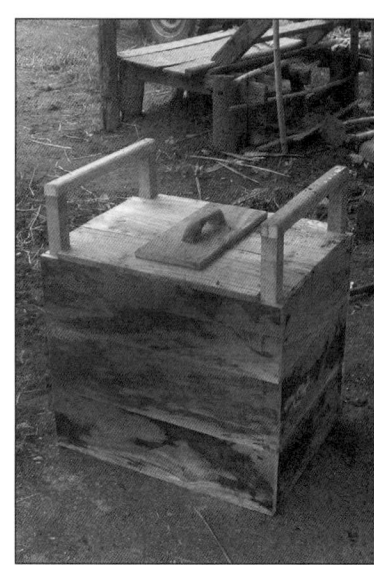

Figure 9.85. Wooden toilet seat, not yet installed.

Wooden box toilet seat

Description
- A solid wooden box with a rectangular hole in the top. A wooden lid with a handle covers the hole when not in use.

- There is a wooden handrail on each side of the seat.

Dimensions
- Dimensions suited to Mr Kong's needs, e.g. height level with wheelchair seat for easy transfer.

- H of handrails: 18cm above the seat.

Use
- A small latrine pit is dug and the seat is placed over the hole. It is designed to be dug into the ground to a depth of 10cm for stability.

- Mr Kong's idea for using the new toilet seat is different. He intends to place it underneath the house and use it with a container underneath it. When his compound floods, the seat can be moved upstairs, and used in the same way. The container will then be emptied into the floodwater below (and also provide fish food!).

Key features
- Made from local materials, durable. It may be painted or varnished for extra durability and ease of cleaning.

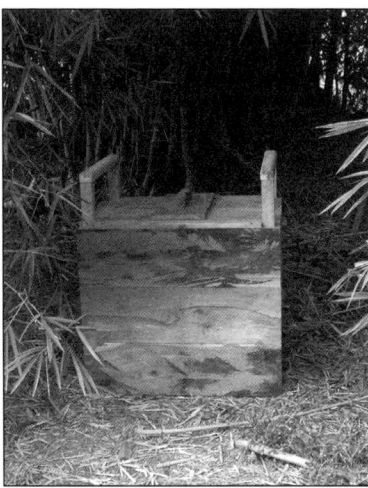

Figure 9.86. Proposed location for toilet pit.

- Handrails on the seat provide support to the user.

- Flexible use. It can be installed as a fixed seat over a latrine, and then moved when the pit becomes full. Alternatively it can be used as a commode seat with a container underneath.

Drawbacks and comments

- The heavy solid box make it difficult to use as a commode seat with a container, also there is a long drop from seat to container, with risk of fouling inside the box and the floor.

- If the back side of the box were left open, a container could be removed for emptying more easily, without the need to lift the whole seat.

Suitable for

- People with good sitting balance.

- Wheelchair users.

- People with difficulty squatting or bending.

Benefits

Mr Kong had just returned home with new equipment provided by the SCI Centre (see below), so it was too early to identify actual benefits.

Before, Mr Kong used an ordinary bench underneath the house to sit on while bathing. It was not near a water jar so he always had to ask someone to fetch water for him. Now he can bathe without help.

Process for obtaining adaptations

Mr Kong was referred by a social worker to the Spinal Cord Injury Centre (SCI) in Battambang, where he spent three months. Staff assessed his condition, gave him physical exercises, and trained him to use certain equipment. He was provided with the toilet seat, bathing bench and a standing frame free of charge. These were all designed and made at the Centre.

Once he starts using the equipment at home, he can inform the occupational therapist of any problems.

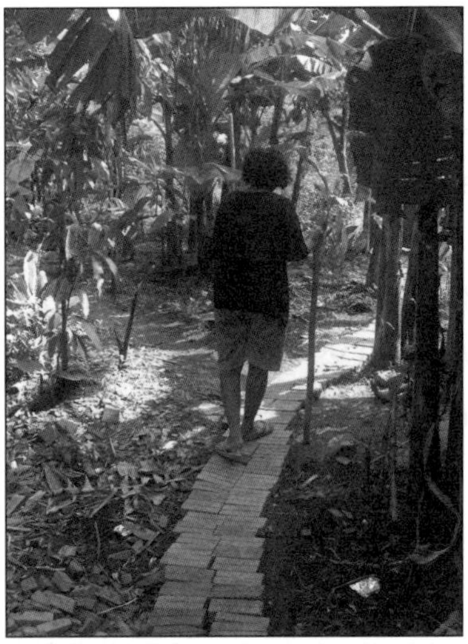

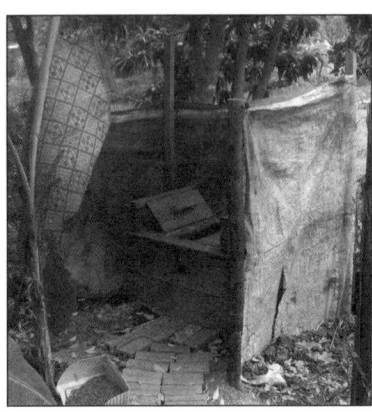

Figure 9.87.Brick path from house to toilet.

9.18 Bathing bench and toilet for woman with weak legs

Mrs Hien Phee is 49 and lives with her husband Mr Srey and their nine children in a rural village in Battambang Province, Cambodia. They live in a wooden stilt house, with a ladder to reach it. The area around the house is roughly paved with left-over bricks from the nearby brick factory. The family fetch water from a pond 1km away, and store it in one large storage jar.

Mrs Hien has weak legs from spinal cord injury as a result of a traffic accident. She can walk slowly as far as the toilet and bathing area, using a stick. If she wants to go further she uses a wheelchair.

Wooden box toilet seat

Description

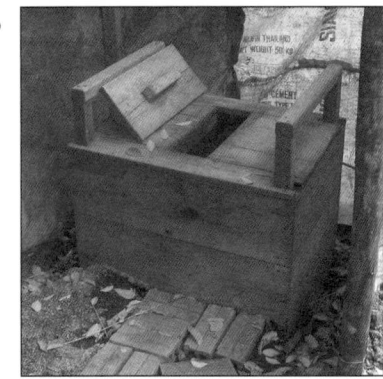

Figure 9.88. Family latrine behind house accessed via brick path. Woven mat used as a door.

- The family have a pit latrine, which is screened using poles and rice sacks. There is no roof. A woven mat covers the entrance.

- The toilet seat is a wooden box with four solid sides and a rectangular hole in the seat. A wooden lid with a handle covers the hole when not in use.

- The seat is installed over a latrine pit dug 5cm narrower than the seat all the way round. The seat is dug into the ground to a depth of 10cm for stability.

- There is a wooden handrail on each side of the seat.

Approach
- The toilet is behind the house, ~10m away along a brick path.

Dimensions
- Toilet seat: W: 70cm x D: 54cm.

- Toilet hole: W: ~10cm x D: ~40cm.

- Distance from seat to toilet entrance: 30cm.

- Handrails: H: 18cm above seat.

Use
- Mrs Hien walks with a stick along the path, enters the latrine and uses the toilet unaided.

- Ash from burnt rubbish is shovelled into the hole to cover the faeces, using a scoop made from an old jerry-can (Figure 9.90).

Figure 9.89. Wooden toilet seat showing the lid removed from the toilet hole.

SCI Centre design

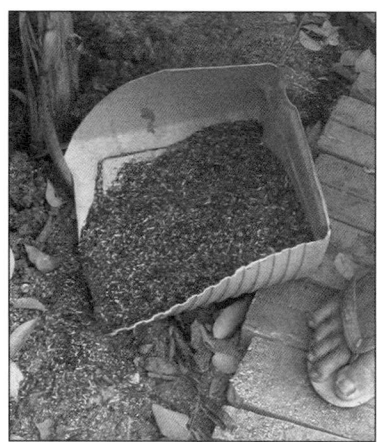

Figure 9.90. Ash scoop made from an old jerry-can.

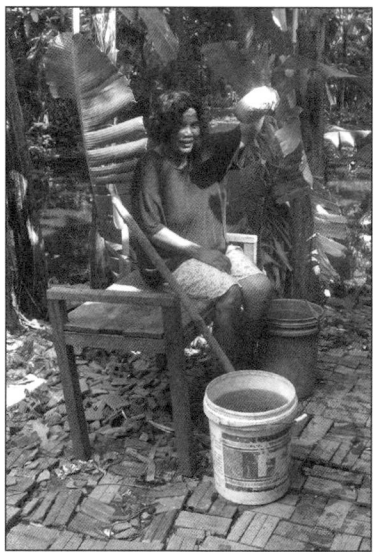

Figure 9.91. Mrs Hien using her bathing bench.

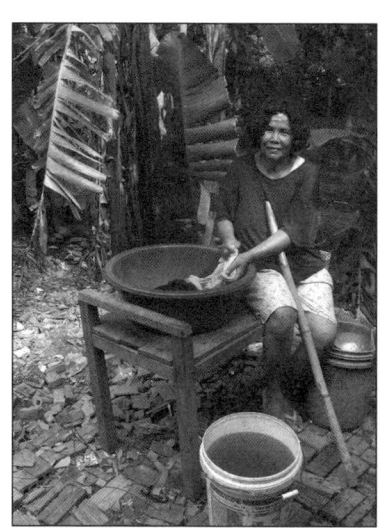

Figure 9.92. Mrs Hien uses the bench to wash clothes.

Key features

- Made from local materials, durable, may be painted or varnished for extra durability and ease of cleaning.

- Can be treated as a fixed seat, but relocated to a new pit when this pit becomes full.

- The dimensions have been decided to suit Mrs Hien, e.g. the height is suitable for easy sitting down/ standing up.

- The handrails are useful to grasp for balance when transferring.

Drawbacks and comments

- Painting the toilet seat would make it resistant to water and urine, and so easier to clean, more hygienic and more durable.

- A water source inside the latrine would allow Mrs Hien to carry out personal hygiene tasks in private. The family could fill the water container at their convenience, instead of on demand.

- It is only used by Mrs Hien. The rest of the family continue to defecate in the open, as they say the pit would fill up too fast if everyone used it.

Suitable for

- People with good sitting balance.

- People unable to squat.

Bathing / laundry bench

Description

- See Case-study 9.17 for full details.

Use

- A family member brings a bucket of water and places it on the floor beside the bench. Mrs Hien sits on the bench and washes clothes in a bowl on the bench beside her.

Drawbacks and comments

- Painting the bench would make it water-resistant, and so more durable.

- Locating the bench next to a water source would reduce Mrs Hien's reliance on her family to fetch water for her.

Benefits

Before, Mrs Hien needed family support to do everything. She used a walking frame to move around. She would bathe lying on the floor of the house, with help from her husband and daughters. For toileting her husband and daughter would carry her and sit her on a bed-pan, which they emptied afterwards.

Now her mobility has improved and she only uses a stick to walk. She can bathe with minimal help and go to the toilet by herself. She used to be depressed; now she feels better that she can help herself more. She has increased self-reliance, dignity and well-being.

Time-saving for the family: Mr Srey said it used to be a full time task to care for his wife, including during the night. Now it takes less than half the time, and he worries less about leaving her.

Increased family income: Both Mr Srey and their daughter So Pheap have now returned to work full time at the nearby brick factory, so their earnings have increased.

Improved family well-being: Before there was always too much to do. Now life does not feel so hard or stressful, and family members relax and smile more.

Process for obtaining adaptations
Mrs Hien was taken straight to the SCI Centre in Battambang after her accident, which is why she made such a good recovery. There she was given physiotherapy, and trained in self-care and use of assistive devices. The Centre's occupational therapist continues to visit and monitor her progress.

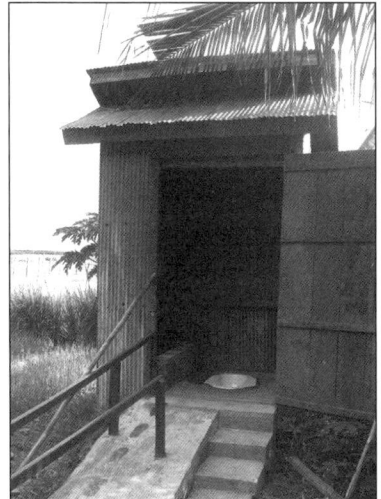

Figure 9.93. Household toilet with concrete ramp and steps. Colourful painted footprints make it more child-friendly.

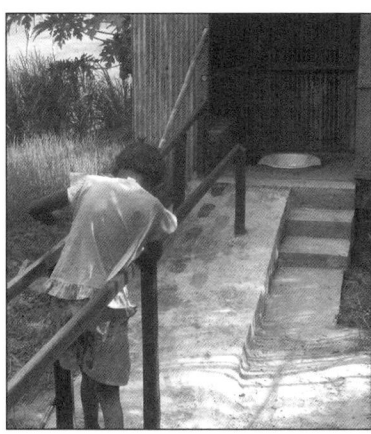

Figure 9.94. Horizontal parallel bars enable child to walk from house to toilet with minimal help

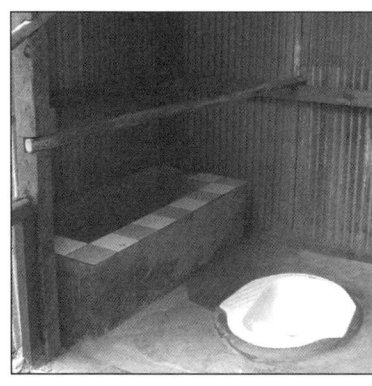

Figure 9.95. Wooden handrail from door to back wall of toilet.

9.19 Household toilet, parallel bars for child learning to walk

Tuan is 11 and lives with her parents, grandmother and sister in a rural village in Kampong Thom Province, Cambodia. She has cerebral palsy, which makes her legs and hands weak.

Her grandmother often looks after Tuan while her mother goes out to work. Tuan needs support with nearly everything – washing, using the toilet, dressing and undressing, eating and drinking, and also physical exercises.

Tuan can move around by shuffling on her bottom, and can walk very slowly on level ground using handrails. She is gradually getting stronger.

Description
- The household toilet is on a raised concrete platform; the cubicle has corrugated tin walls and roof on a wood frame. A wooden door opens outwards.

- A ceramic pour-flush toilet pan is level with the smooth concrete floor. There is a water trough beside the toilet, made of tiled and cement-plastered brick.

Approach
- A pair of parallel wooden handrails, painted blue, follow a concrete path leading from the house to the toilet. A concrete ramp leads up to the toilet entrance, with three concrete steps beside the ramp. Coloured foot-prints are painted along the route.

- The RH handrail finishes ~1m before the entrance, to allow room for the door to swing outwards.

Support features
- Inside the cubicle, a single horizontal wooden handrail extends from the door to the back wall on one side of the toilet.

Dimensions
- Parallel handrails: H: ~70cm, ~35cm apart.

- Inside handrail: H: ~50cm.

Use
- Tuan walks unaided from the house to the toilet on the level path between the parallel rails, which she holds onto for support.

- She sits on the edge of the toilet by herself, uses the toilet and then washes herself. She needs help getting to the parallel rails and walking up the ramp, and to dress after using the toilet.

Key features
- High cost.

- Grandmother has less distance to carry Tuan.

- Inside support rail helps Tuan lower herself to sit on the toilet.

- The inside water source allows users to wash themselves in privacy.

- The toilet is made attractive to a child, with bright colours painted inside and out.

Drawbacks and comments
- A seat over the toilet would be helpful for Tuan who has difficulty squatting.

- A flat area is needed in front of the door, to allow the user to stand in balance while opening it.

- It is more time-consuming than before for her carer to take Tuan to the toilet.

Suitable for
- Only suitable for a person who can think at least 10 minutes ahead, otherwise they might wet themselves before they get there!

Benefits
Before the family had the toilet, Tuan sat on a bowl, which her mother would empty into a small hole dug in a field, then cover over.

The whole family benefits from using the new toilet.

Tuan's mother says the new toilet does not yet save much time, but she hopes that the exercise will help Tuan get stronger, and gradually need less and less help. She feels encouraged by her child's progress.

Process for obtaining adaptations
CABDIC programme provided the toilet, as well as a standing frame and special chair. When Tuan has made progress using the parallel bars, they will think about a toilet seat for her.

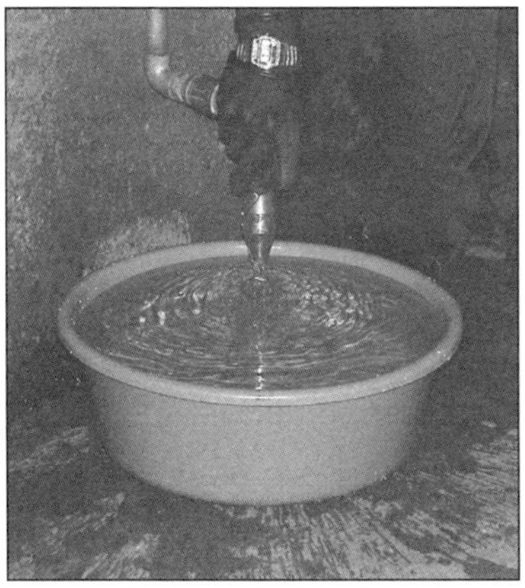

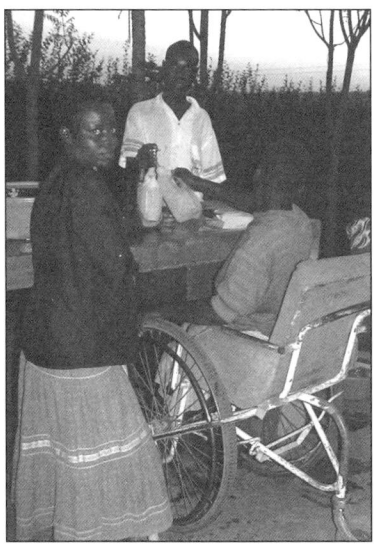

Figure 9.96. Low level tap for use by people who crawl or use low trolleys.

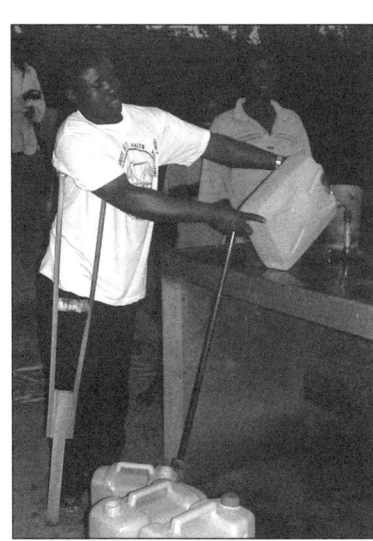

Figure 9.97. Knee-hole under concrete shelf allows wheelchair user to get close to reach tap.

9.20 Tapstand and bathroom in institution for disabled people

Masaka Vocational Rehabilitation Centre in Uganda caters for 68 young men and women aged 14 – 25 with physical impairments. It has concrete ramps and paths which are accessible to people using wheelchairs, crutches or who crawl.

Communal tapstand

Description
- Central communal tapstand, with a long concrete slab at waist level.

- Press-action taps, with spouts ~25cm above the slab. A low level tap is also provided, H: ~30cm.

- Concrete surround, and reached via concrete paths.

Use
- Can be used by persons standing with crutches, or sitting in a wheelchair, or crawling.

Key features
- The slab is high enough for a person in a wheelchair to get their knees under, so they can get close enough to reach the tap (Figure 9.97).

- The concrete slab provides a surface to stand a container on, which takes the weight of the water while filling.

- People who crawl can use the low tap.

- Press-action taps are easy to use by people with poor grip and stiff wrists (but see below).

Drawbacks and comments
- The taps should be higher above the slab and ground, to allow 5 or 10 litre jerry-cans to stand upright to be filled (Figure 9.98).

- Press-action taps make it difficult to control the flow of water, and need continual pressure, so are difficult for users who lack strength. Lever action taps should also be provided which are easier to use by many people.

Suitable for
- Wheelchair and crutch users, people with difficulty bending, people who crawl, people with stiff wrists.

Unsuitable for
- People who lack hand/arm strength.

Figure 9.98. Raised tapstand with shelf to rest containers on.

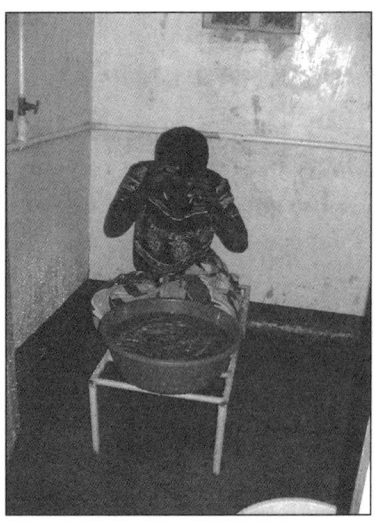

Figure 9.99. Bathroom with room for bathing bench and wheelchair beside it. Tap is within reach of bather.

Bathroom with bathing frame

Description
- The bathroom is brick-built with a tin roof. The concrete floor is level with the concrete approach path. The entrance is wide enough for a wheelchair to enter.

- Water is piped to a shower with a tap.

- There is a metal frame with horizontal struts for bathing.

Dimensions
- Bathing frame: H: 30cm, W: 50cm, L: 100cm.

- Shower tap H: 110cm.

Use
- Bathers sit on the metal bathing frame under the shower, or fetch a basin of water from the tapstand, to place on the frame in front of them.

Key features
- There is enough space for a wheelchair to enter and turn, and for a helper if needed.

- Sitting on the frame prevents bathers sitting in dirty water.

- Metal struts of the frame allow water to drain easily.

Drawbacks and comments
- High cost.

- Shower tap is too high for a person crawling to reach it.

- If the shower is not used, bathers must fetch their water from outside, as there is no tap inside.

- Metal struts are uncomfortable, so a wooden board needs to be used to make it comfortable.

Suitable for
- Wheelchair users, people with weak legs, people with good sitting balance.

Unsuitable for
- People with poor sitting balance, people unsteady on the feet (as there are no handrails for support).

Based on an interview with Ogwang Martin, Centre Manager, employed by USDC. The visit was at the end of the day, it was getting dark, and not all facilities could be observed as they were in use by students.

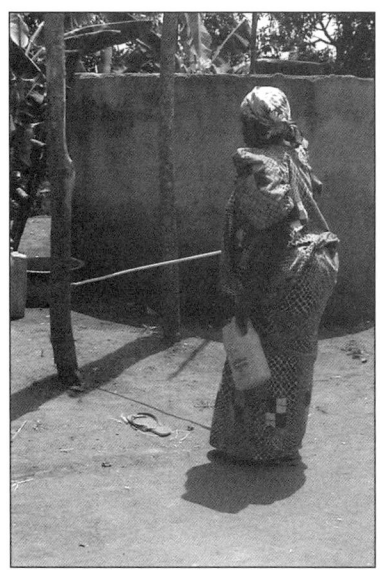

Figure 9.100. Mrs Nalukwago fills her 5 litre jerry-can at the low tap.

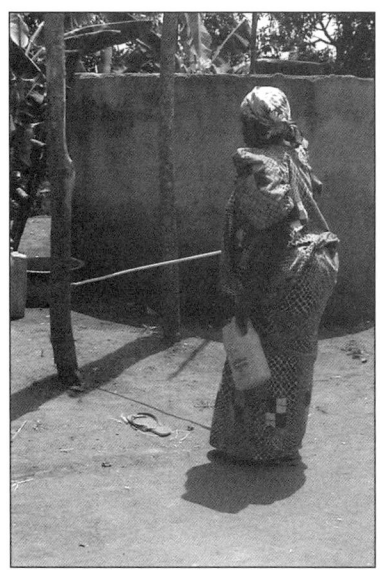

Figure 9.101. Finding her way back to the house.

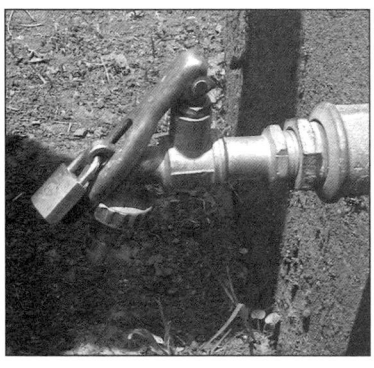

Figure 9.102. The tap can be padlocked.

9.21 Rainwater tank and mobility approach for elderly blind woman

Mrs Annete Bugirwa Nalukwago lives with several of her children in a rural village in Mubende District, Uganda. She is over 50 years of age and blind, but very active, and can find her way around, both inside and outside the house.

Rainwater storage tank with tap

Description
- The family have a circular brick-built rainwater storage tank beside the house. Two wooden posts support the gutter which takes rainwater from the roof to the tank.

Dimensions
- Tap H: ~30cm (Figure 9.100).

Approach
- ~8m from the house via rough but level ground.

Use
- Mrs Nalukwago finds her way to and from the water tank using a white cane, and using the two wooden posts as landmarks. By locating the posts with her cane, she can identify the direction of the water tank, and after filling her 5 litre jerry-can, she can find her way back to the house (Figure 9.101).

Key features
- The low tap allows a container to be placed on the ground while being filled. No water is wasted as the spout is close to the tap (Figure 9.100).

- The tap can be padlocked to prevent non-family members using the water (Figure 9.102).

Drawbacks and comments
- A pit could be dug below the tap to allow larger containers to be filled. Providing a low stool would mean Mrs Nalukwago could sit instead of bend to use the tap.

Bathing
Mrs Nalukwago bathes in her own bathroom next to her bedroom. A cloth on the floor outside the bathroom door is a landmark to indicate the doorway. This works for her, and is unlikely to be moved by family members as only she uses this part of the house.

She has a specific place for each item – bucket, basin and towel, so she knows where everything is. She carries water for

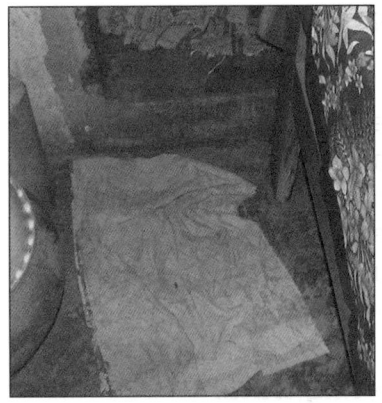

Figure 9.103 Floor cloth at the bathroom door.

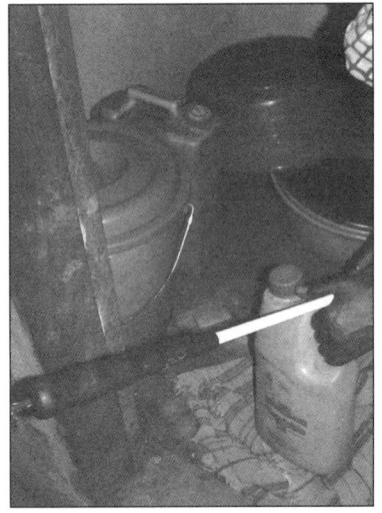

Figure 9.104. Mrs Nalukwago's orderly bathroom.

bathing to the bathroom in a small jerry-can, which she pours into a bucket.

Benefits

Before learning mobility, Mrs Nalukwago was helpless. She would often bump into things and hurt herself. Family and community members helped her too much, which also disabled her. Mobility outside the house was the main problem. She felt depressed and a burden on her family.

Now after only three months of learning to use her white cane, she has increased mobility and choice, she can move around and do things for herself, including going to church by herself.

The whole family has benefited from their mother's independence. Her daughter said that before, someone always stayed with their mother. Now they no longer worry about her, and they have more time to do other things. Not only can she look after herself, she can also contribute to the family, including cooking for them, while they go to the fields.

She also keeps poultry, including fetching grass and water for them.

Process for obtaining adaptations

Uganda National Association of the Blind (UNAB) provided the white cane. Mrs Nalukwago received mobility and orientation advice and support from Mr Opoya, District mobility officer. Her son paid for construction of the rainwater tank.

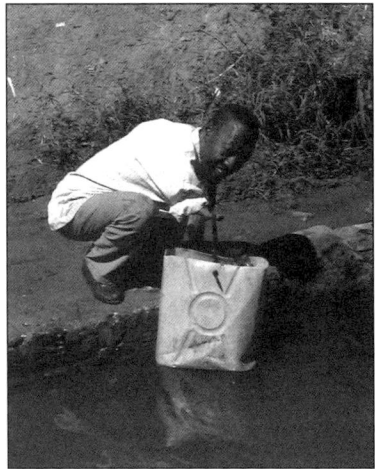

Figure 9.105. Kiwanuka draws water from the spring.

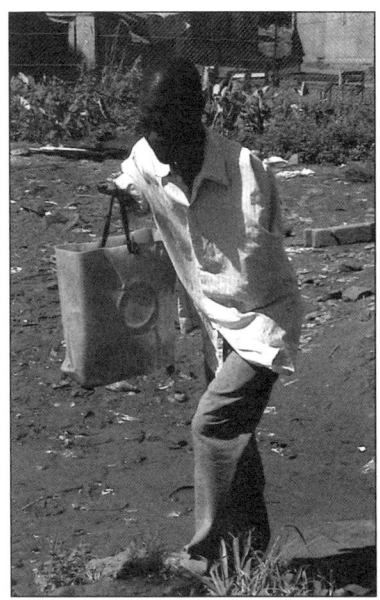

Figure 9.106. Kiwanuka carries water back to the house.

9.22 Adapted jerry-can used by man without arms

John Kiwanuka is 42 and a trained accountant. He was interviewed in the house where he used to live, in a peri-urban area of Kampala. Kiwanuka was born with only one very short arm with a partially developed hand. He describes himself as 'a person without arms'. He has no difficulty walking.

Adapted jerry-can for collecting water

Description
*   Water is drawn from a nearby spring about 30m from Kiwanuka's house.

*   Kiwanuka has adapted a 15 litre jerry-can. He has cut the top off, pierced a hole on each side, and tied a rope through it to form a handle.

Use
*   Kiwanuka collects about 5 litres of water at a time; any more would be too heavy.

Key features
*   The plastic of the jerry-can is robust but flexible enough to be cut and adapted.

*   The open top makes it easy to fill, and to clean inside.

*   The length of handle can be adjusted to suit the user.

Drawbacks and comments
The open top makes the jerry-can more vulnerable to contamination than an ordinary jerry-can with a lid. This can be avoided by pouring water immediately into covered containers for storage, and by cleaning the jerry-can regularly.

Suitable for
*   People who have weak grasp, or stiff fingers, which make it difficult to hold the handle of a jerry-can.

*   People without hands - a longer handle could enable it to be carried over the arm or even over a shoulder.

Long wash-cloth

Description
*   A wash-cloth made of sisal, with a loop at each end: 120cm long, and 20cm wide.

Use

- Kiwanuka pours water for bathing into a plastic bowl and wets the wash-cloth using his feet. He holds the loop at one end in his hand, the other end with his foot. He can wash his whole body by manipulating his body and the cloth.

Key features

- Low-cost materials, locally available.

Suitable for

- Bathers with limited use of their arms.

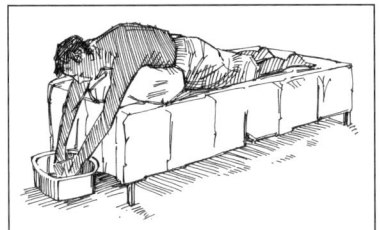

Figure 9.107. Lubega bathes lying on his front, with a washbowl on the floor.

9.23 Bed bathing method for man with paralysed legs

John Lubega is 43 and a shoe repairer. He lives in a village in Nakaseke, Uganda. He is paralysed below the waist after a road accident. His upper body is strong. He uses a three-wheeled wheelchair made in Kampala, with a single small rear wheel.

Lubega draws water at a handpump 1 mile from his home. It is on a raised concrete platform, which prevents him getting close, so he has to lean over to pump which is awkward. He accepts help if it is offered. There are boreholes nearer, but they are accessed by steep, narrow or rough pot-holed tracks, whereas the way to this one is accessible.

He can carry a 20 litre jerry-can of water between his feet on the footrest of his wheelchair (width 33cm x depth 23cm). This is more convenient and easier to manoeuvre than a trailer.

Bathing
To bathe, Lubega lies on his front in bed, with a plastic sheet under him to avoid the bed-sheets getting wet and having to wash them each time. He puts a basin of water on the floor, and uses a cloth to wash himself. His bed at home is too low to allow him to stretch his arms out straight and it causes pain. To solve the problem, he places cushions under his chest to raise his upper body.

Benefits
Using the plastic sheet minimises his family's workload, in terms of washing bedclothes.

Process for obtaining adaptations
The wheelchair and bed-pan are provided by the hospital. The hospital introduced him to the idea of bed-bathing, but directly onto the bed-sheet, which made it wet, and needed frequent washing. He had the idea of using a plastic sheet, which he bought himself locally.

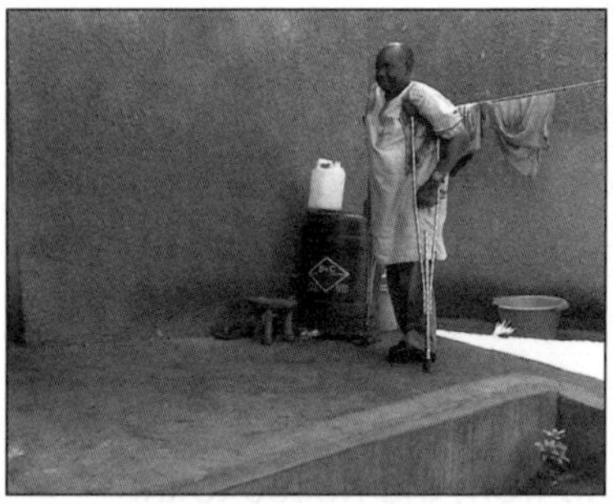

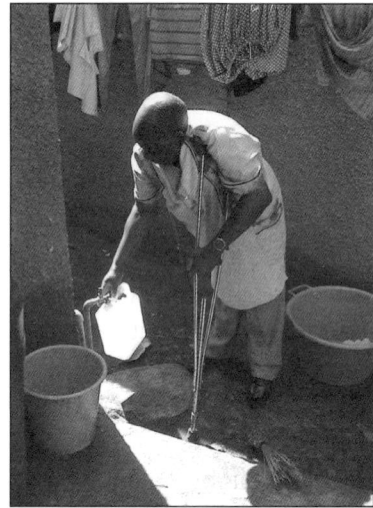

Figure 9.108. Concrete ramp leading from the house.

9.24 Toilet and bathing area for man using crutches

John Ndiraba Kiyaga lives with his wife and six children in urban Kampala, Uganda. He is Director of his own NGO – Action to Positive Change on People with Disabilities (APCPD). He has weak legs and uses crutches and a wheelchair to move around in. He wears rigid leg braces, and so cannot bend his legs.

Kiyaga designed and constructed a family bathroom and toilet that he can also use. He installed a concrete ramp leading from the house to the compound so that he could reach the tap, bathroom and toilet easily in his wheelchair or on crutches.

Household tap
Description
- The house has a piped water supply with an outside tap. A container nearby is kept filled in case of breaks in the supply.

Approach
- ~3m from the back door along a concrete ramp.

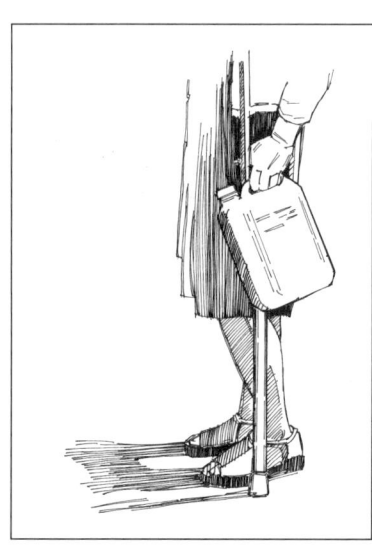

Figure 9.109. Kiyaga using the household tap.

Dimensions
- H of tap: ~30cm.

Use
- Kiyaga can draw and carry water in a half-full 5 litre container while using his crutches. He is strong enough to hold the container in his hand whilst holding the handle of the crutch. He can carry water for up to ½ mile this way.

- In the past he used a tricycle wheelchair to travel around. He could carry 2 x 25 litre containers of water on it (Figure 9.111).

Key features
- Proximity – Kiyaga fetches water as he needs it.

- Cost: the monthly cost of water is similar to what he used to pay the water vendor at the public tapstand.

Drawbacks
The tariff for the household connection had to be paid as a lump sum rather than incrementally.

Figure 9.110. Carrying a jerry-can.

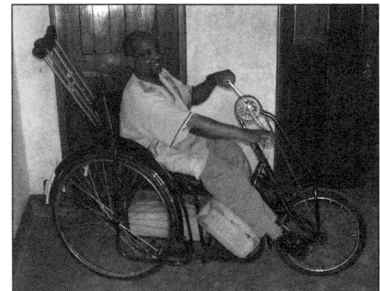

Figure 9.111. Two jerry-cans under the seat of Kiyaga's old wheelchair.

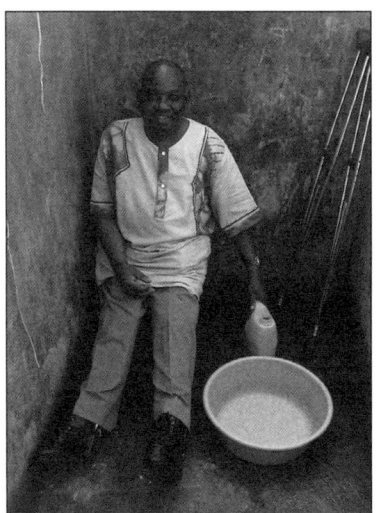

Figure 9.112. Kiyaga sits on a low stool to bathe.

Family bathroom

Description
- Built of cement-plastered brick, with a concrete floor and no roof or door. The entrance is wide enough to enter on crutches.

Approach
- A concrete ramp and path lead from the house to the bathroom and toilet.

Dimensions
- Approach path W: 80cm between two walls.

- Interior: L: 210cm, W: 110cm.

- Entrance W: 80cm.

- Bathing seat: H: 14cm.

Use
- Kiyaga sits on a wooden stool in the corner of the bathroom, with legs straight. Water is placed in a bowl on the floor (usually by a family member). Wastewater drains through a hole in the wall and into a drainage system.

Key features
- There is space for Kiyaga to sit with straight legs.

- The whole family uses the bathroom; no separate facility is needed.

- Different seating can be used depending on the support needs of the user.

Drawbacks and comments
- The approach path is currently too narrow for wheelchair access, especially where the path turns a corner (see Figure 9.116). Designing and constructing it wider would have added minimal extra cost, but made it accessible both in a wheelchair and on crutches.

- Adding a door would increase privacy.

- An internal water source would avoid the need to fetch water from the tap outside.

Suitable for
The whole family.

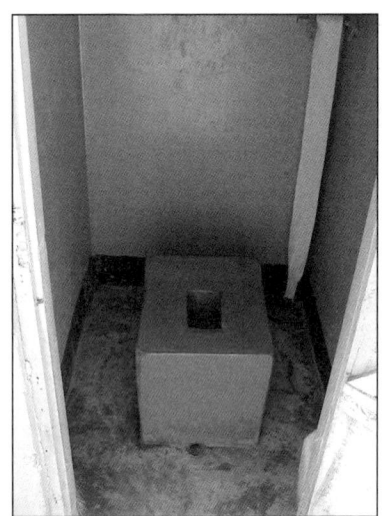

Figure 9.113. Kiyaga's toilet seat.

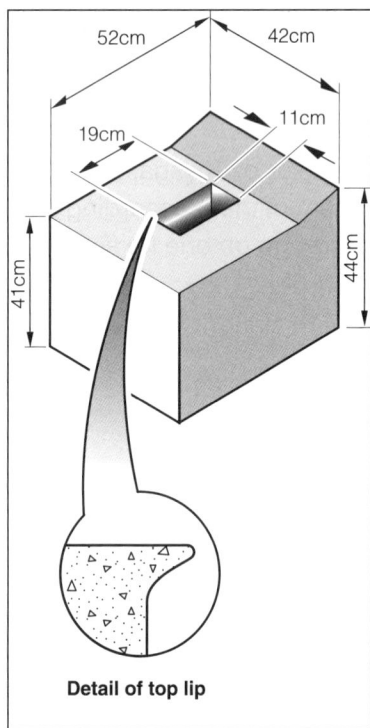

Figure 9.114. Dimensions of toilet seat.

Household toilet with fixed raised seat

Description

- Brick-built cement-plastered cubicle with a smooth concrete floor. A wooden door opens outwards.

- A cement-plastered brick seat, painted red, is installed over a pit latrine. The seat is raised slightly at the back (Figure 9.114) and has a rectangular hole.

- There is a container of water in the toilet. Water for handwashing is also kept in a container outside the toilet (Figure 9.115).

Approach

- Along a concrete ramp and path, which is level with the toilet floor.

Dimensions

- Internal cubicle: L: 125cm, W: 96cm.

- Door W: 62cm.

- Seat: W: 42cm, L: 52cm, H: 41 – 44cm.

- Toilet hole: 19cm x 11cm.

Use

- Kiyaga gets to the toilet on crutches.

Key features

- The painted cement-plastered seat is easy to clean.

- The raised rear of the toilet seat provides support when sitting.

- A lip around the top of the toilet hole helps prevent fouling of the drop-hole walls (Figure 9.114).

- The outward opening door leaves more space inside the cubicle to move around, to shut the door and to sit with straight legs.

- Internal water supply is convenient for anal cleansing and for cleaning the seat.

- The separate toilet is designed to suit Kiyaga's needs without obstructing other family members.

Drawbacks and comments

- High cost of two toilets. A cheaper option would be a single spacious toilet, with a squat plate and a wooden or plastic toilet seat over it, which could be moved to one side when not required.

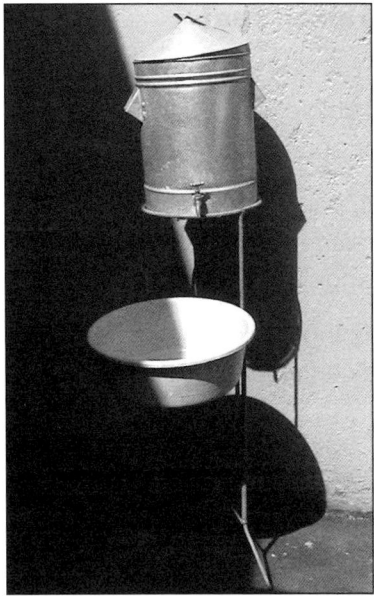

Figure 9.115. Water for handwashing outside the toilet (location shown in Figure 9.116).

- Making the hole in the toilet seat larger would make anal cleansing easier, especially if water is used.

- Internal water supply needs to be regularly filled by hand.

Suitable for
- People with difficulty squatting, but who can bear weight on their legs.

Benefits
Kiyaga's wife Christine said that before the adaptations were in place, someone always had to be at home in case her husband needed help. For example, without ramps he could not fetch water for use in the bathroom or toilet, so he depended more on his family.

The adaptations allow Kiyaga to be independent, so Christine can safely leave him alone, to go to work or to visit relatives for example.

Process for obtaining adaptations
All adaptations were planned and paid for by Kiyaga. He commissioned a local builder to construct them according to his instructions. He based the toilet design on one he saw in an international hotel.

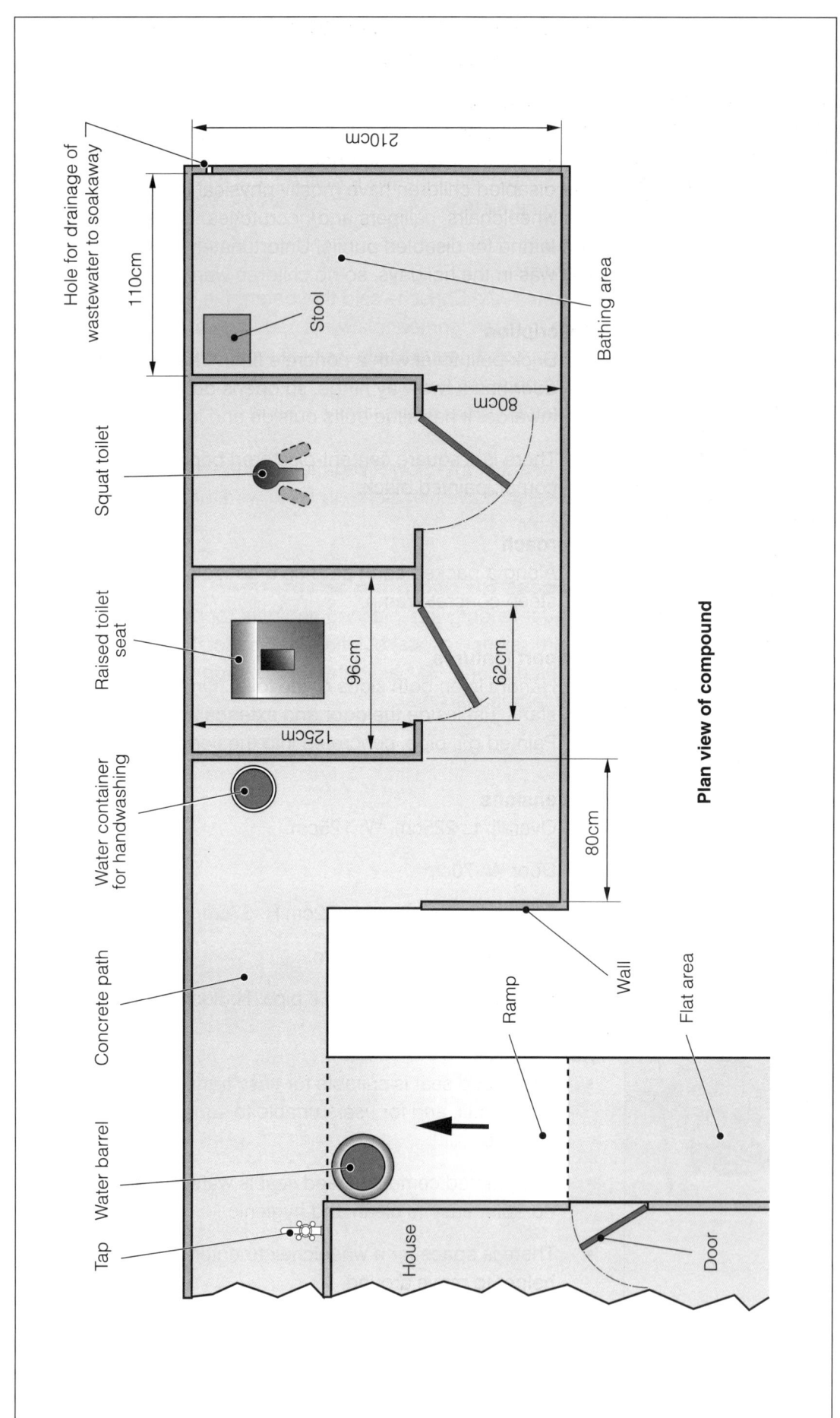

Plan view of compound

Hole for drainage of wastewater to soakaway

110cm

210cm

Stool

Bathing area

Squat toilet

80cm

Raised toilet seat

96cm

125cm

62cm

Water container for handwashing

80cm

Concrete path

Ramp

Wall

Flat area

Water barrel

Tap

House

Door

Figure 9.116. Layout of the Kiyaga family's toilet and bathing area.

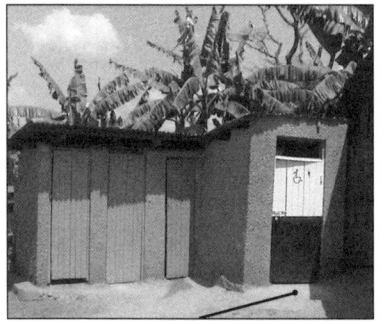

Figure 9.117. Wheelchair accessible toilet on the right. Arrow shows concrete ramp.

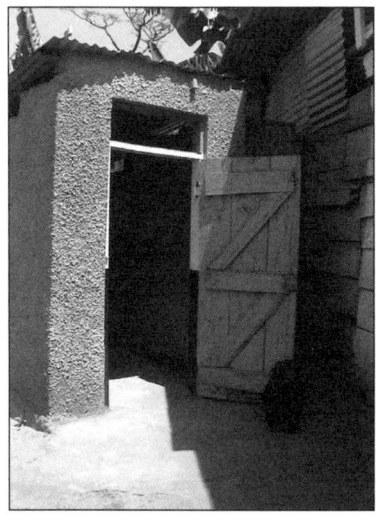

Figure 9.118. Door with a two-way hinge.

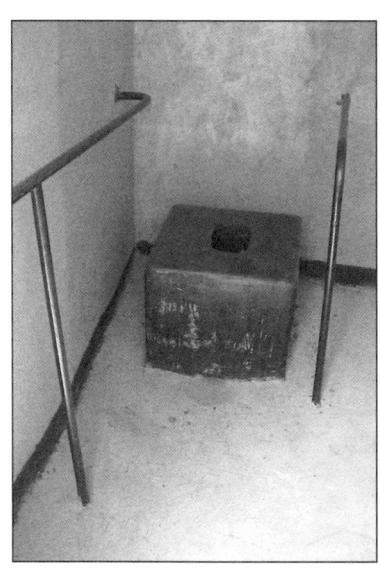

Figure 9.119. Painted cement screed brick toilet seat with handrail on the left from the door.

9.25 Primary school toilet accessible for wheelchair users

This is a primary school in a peri-urban area of Kampala, Uganda. It was set up by John Kiyaga's NGO, APCPD, and accepts both disabled and non-disabled children aged 6 to 18. The disabled children have mostly physical impairments, and use wheelchairs, callipers and/or crutches. The school has one latrine for disabled pupils. Unfortunately the researchers' visit was in the holidays, so no children were present.

Description
*   Brick-built toilet with a concrete floor. The wide wooden door has a two-way hinge, so opens outwards and inwards. It has slide bolts outside and inside.

*   There is a square cement-plastered brick toilet seat in one corner, painted black.

Approach
*   Along a packed earth path up a gentle slope to a short steep concrete ramp.

Support features
*   Handrails on both sides of the toilet. On the left, the rail starts just inside the door and extends to behind the toilet. Painted g.i. pipe, concreted into the floor and walls.

Dimensions
*   Overall: L: 225cm, W: 125cm.

*   Door W: 70cm.

*   Toilet seat: W: 48cm, L: 52cm H: 37cm.

*   Toilet hole: L: 22, W: 12cm.

*   Handrails: 25mm o/s Ø g.i. pipe. H: 80cm.

Key features
*   The raised seat is suitable for easy transfer from/to a wheelchair, and for users unable to squat or with poor balance.

*   The painted cement screed seat is water repellent, so is durable, easy to clean and hygienic.

*   There is space for a wheelchair to enter and turn, and for a helper to move around.

*   A handrail from door to toilet provides support to users who walk but have poor balance.

*   The 2-way hinge allows the door to be pushed open from outside or from inside.

Drawbacks and comments

- A larger toilet hole would make anal cleansing easier, especially if water is used.

- An internal water source next to the seat for personal hygiene is a high priority.

- Rails on both sides of the toilet prevent sideways transfer from a wheelchair parked beside the toilet.

Process of implementation

The need for an accessible latrine was recognised when a disabled pupil was having difficulty using the existing latrines. An occupational therapist designed it for them. APCPD installed it.

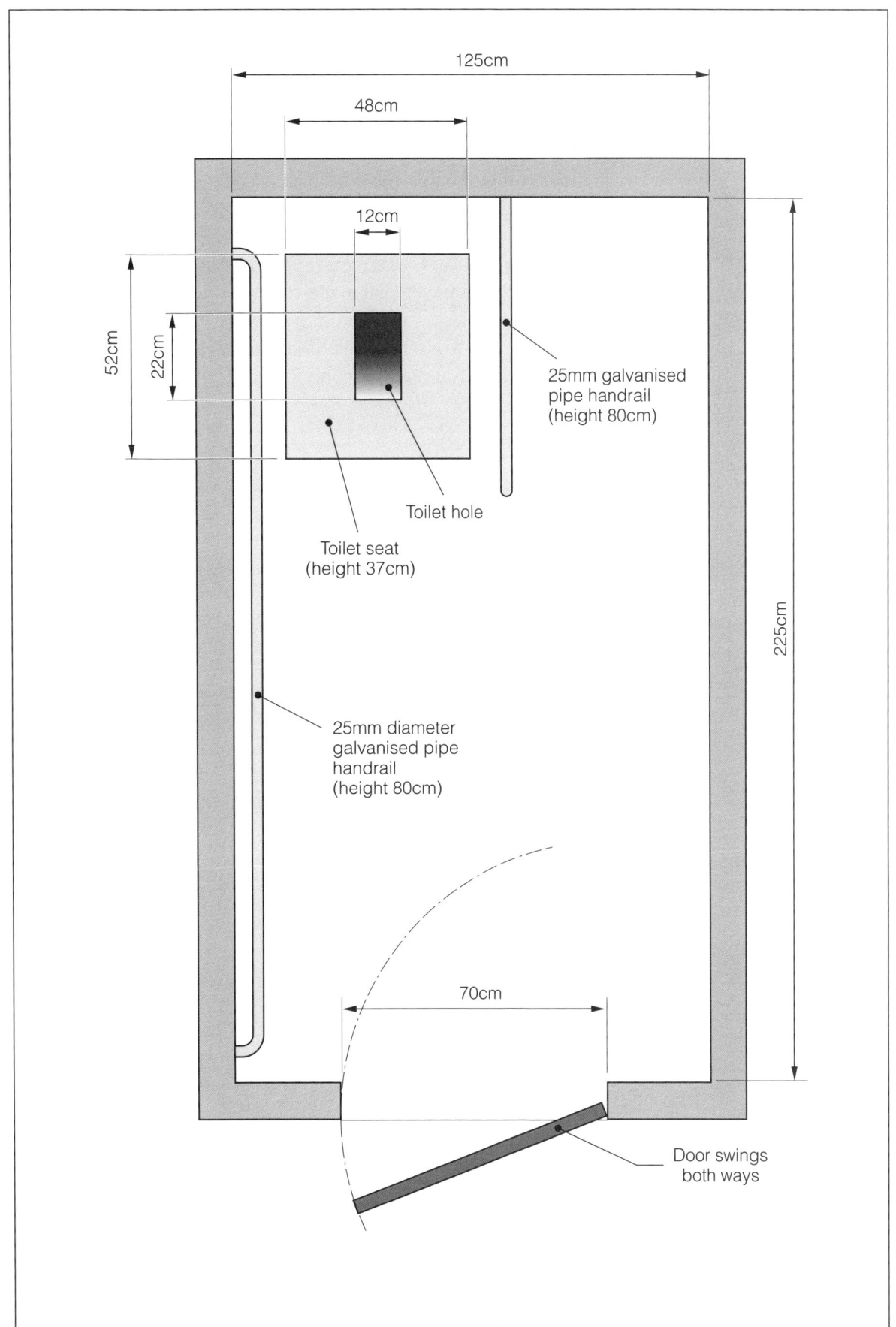

125cm

48cm

12cm

52cm

22cm

25mm galvanised
pipe handrail
(height 80cm)

Toilet hole

Toilet seat
(height 37cm)

225cm

25mm diameter
galvanised pipe
handrail
(height 80cm)

70cm

Door swings
both ways

Figure 9.120. Plan view of accessible school toilet.

9.26 Bathroom and toilets in residential school for disabled children

The school is on the outskirts of Kampala, Uganda, and caters for 78 children with physical impairments, aged from 7 to 18 years. Primary education and vocational training are provided. Most of the children have mobility and co-ordination problems, and many use wheelchairs.

The school has some concrete ramps, but most access is via earth paths. Facilities are designed to be universally accessible, rather than suited to individual children's needs. The school has a range of latrines, which have been built at different times during the school's history, with varying levels of accessibility.

Communal bathroom with sitting blocks

Description
- Walls of cement-plastered brick create three bathrooms: one for girls, one for boys and one for housemothers. The floor is rough concrete. There are no doors or roof. Entrances are wide enough for wheelchairs to enter.

- Fixed cement-plastered brick blocks are for children to sit on while bathing.

Approach
- A concrete approach path finishes level with the bathroom floor.

Dimensions
- Sitting blocks: 23cm x 23cm.

- Heights vary 10 – 18cm.

Use
- Most children can transfer unaided from a wheelchair on to a sitting block. They wash from a basin of water placed on the floor in front of them by housemothers, who fetch water from outside.

Key features
- There is space for wheelchairs to enter and turn, for helpers and for children to sit with straight legs.

- The blocks are narrow so water drains off easily.

- The low height of the blocks reduces the risk of injury if a child falls, and allows children to keep their feet on the ground for support.

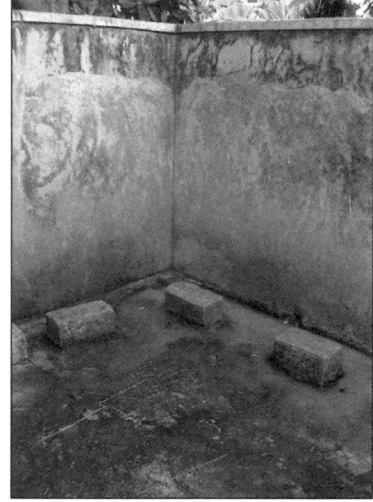

Figure 9.121. Fixed concrete sitting blocks for bathing.

Case studies

- Children can choose the block with a height that best suits them.

- Children sit raised above their dirty bathwater.

Drawbacks and comments

- Children with poor balance need a support worker to help them. Some children, especially older boys, get embarrassed at being helped by a woman. A bathing chair with back and side-rails, e.g. of plastic, would provide more support. and allow children to bathe independently and with more dignity.

- The low height of the blocks mean most children need help getting back into their wheelchairs.

- An internal water source would reduce reliance on support workers to collect water from outside.

Suitable for

- Children with good sitting balance.

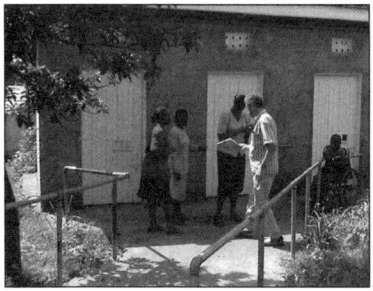

Figure 9.122. Concrete ramp to latrine block with handrail both sides.

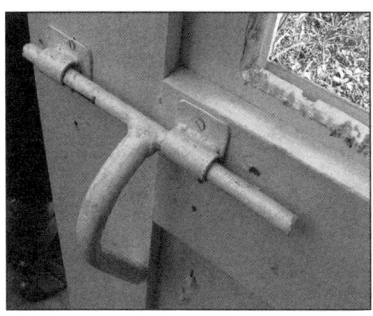

Figure 9.123. Large slide bolt for easy grip.

VIP 'model' fixed raised seat latrine, squat latrine and twin sitting blocks

Description

- Brick-built cement-plastered block of three cubicles with a tin roof. Rough finish concrete floor.

- Wide entrance, wooden doors opening outwards, with a large slide bolt on the inside for easy grip.

- A hole in the door allows the door to be opened from outside if needed (Figure 9.123).

- Each cubicle has a different type of toilet:

  Cubicle A: Circular raised fixed toilet seat of unpainted cement-plastered brick (Figure 9.124).

  Cubicle B: Concrete squat footplate installed level with the floor (Figure 9.125).

  Cubicle C: Twin cement-plastered sitting blocks, unpainted (Not shown but similar to Figure 9.126).

Approach

- Concrete ramp with handrail on both sides. Level area in front of the toilet doors.

- Handrail attached to the outside wall for support while opening the door.

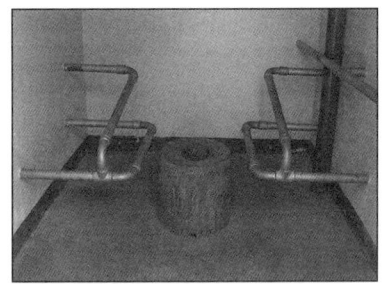

Figure 9.124. Raised toilet seat with handrails for support.

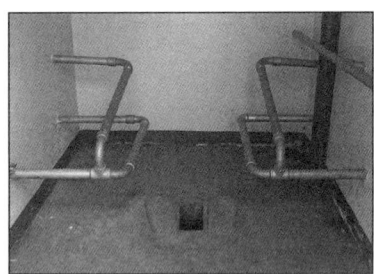

Figure 9.125. Squat latrine with handrails for support.

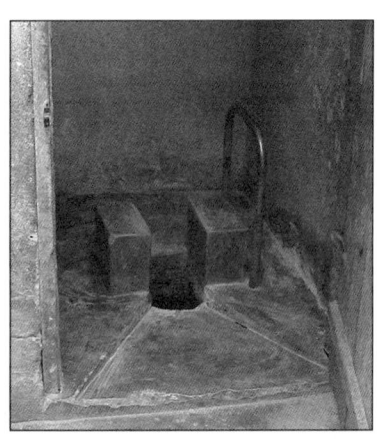

Figure 9.126. Twin sitting blocks, similar to those in cubicle C.

Internal dimensions and layout

- Cubicle W: 180cm.

- 80cm between toilet and back wall; 150cm between toilet and door.

- A. Raised seat H: 41cm. Toilet hole: L: ~25cm, W: ~18cm.

- B: Squatting plates raised 3cm from floor.

- C: Twin blocks: H: 25cm, gap between blocks 14cm.

Support features

- Horizontal rails fixed to both side walls at different heights. Additional horizontal handrail extends from front to back of RH wall.

- Painted 50mm Ø g.i. pipe.Lowest rail H: 38cm.

Key features

- Enough space for wheelchairs to enter and turn, and for a support worker to hold a child from in front or behind.

- The non-slip rough concrete floor prevents crutches slipping.

- Rails at different heights suit different users.

- Rail from door to toilet supports users with poor balance who enter without a wheelchair.

- Painted pipe rails resist corrosion from pit fumes.

- A: Raised seat is convenient for wheelchair transfer.

- The short distance between the front of the seat and the toilet hole reduces the risk of fouling the seat.

- B: Squat plates were reportedly preferred by support workers, who found it easier to support a child squatting than sitting.

- C: Twin blocks: the gap between the blocks makes anal cleansing easy. These were reportedly preferred by girls.

Drawbacks and comments

- High cost.

- The rough concrete floor absorbs water/urine making it difficult to clean. An alternative would be to make the floor smoother but create ridges for a non-slip surface.

- Painting the concrete seat/blocks would make them resistant to urine and water and easier to keep clean.

- Rails on both sides prevent sideways transfer from a wheelchair.

- Providing an internal water source is a high priority for anal cleansing.

- Raised seat: Anal cleansing using water is more difficult on a seat than when squatting.

- Twin blocks: for small children the gap between the blocks needs to be narrower for comfort and safety.

Suitable for
- Raised seat: People unable to squat, including wheelchair users.

- Squat toilet: People who need support to squat, and are able to grasp a handrail.

Unsuitable for
- People unable to sit without full support.

Process for obtaining adaptations

The issue of accessible latrines in mainstream schools has arisen because of the recent introduction of Universal Primary Education in Uganda, which entitles all children, including disabled children, to enrol in school. Many disabled children have been rejected or dropped out because of a lack of facilities.

The Disability and Rehabilitation Section at the Ministry of Health proposed the idea of a pilot project to trial different designs of accessible latrines, to develop a model for use in all schools. This is funded by UNICEF, with the Ministry of Education (Special Education) also involved.

Benefits

The immediate benefit is that the school has accessible facilities, but the main benefit of the pilot project is long-term: disabled children will be able to attend mainstream schools.

Lessons from the pilot could also be relevant to the family situation; parents could observe the facilities and take ideas home.

The information was provided by Joy Mwesigwa, Director, Fred Semakula, Assistant Director, and Rachel Kansiime, Occupational Therapist.

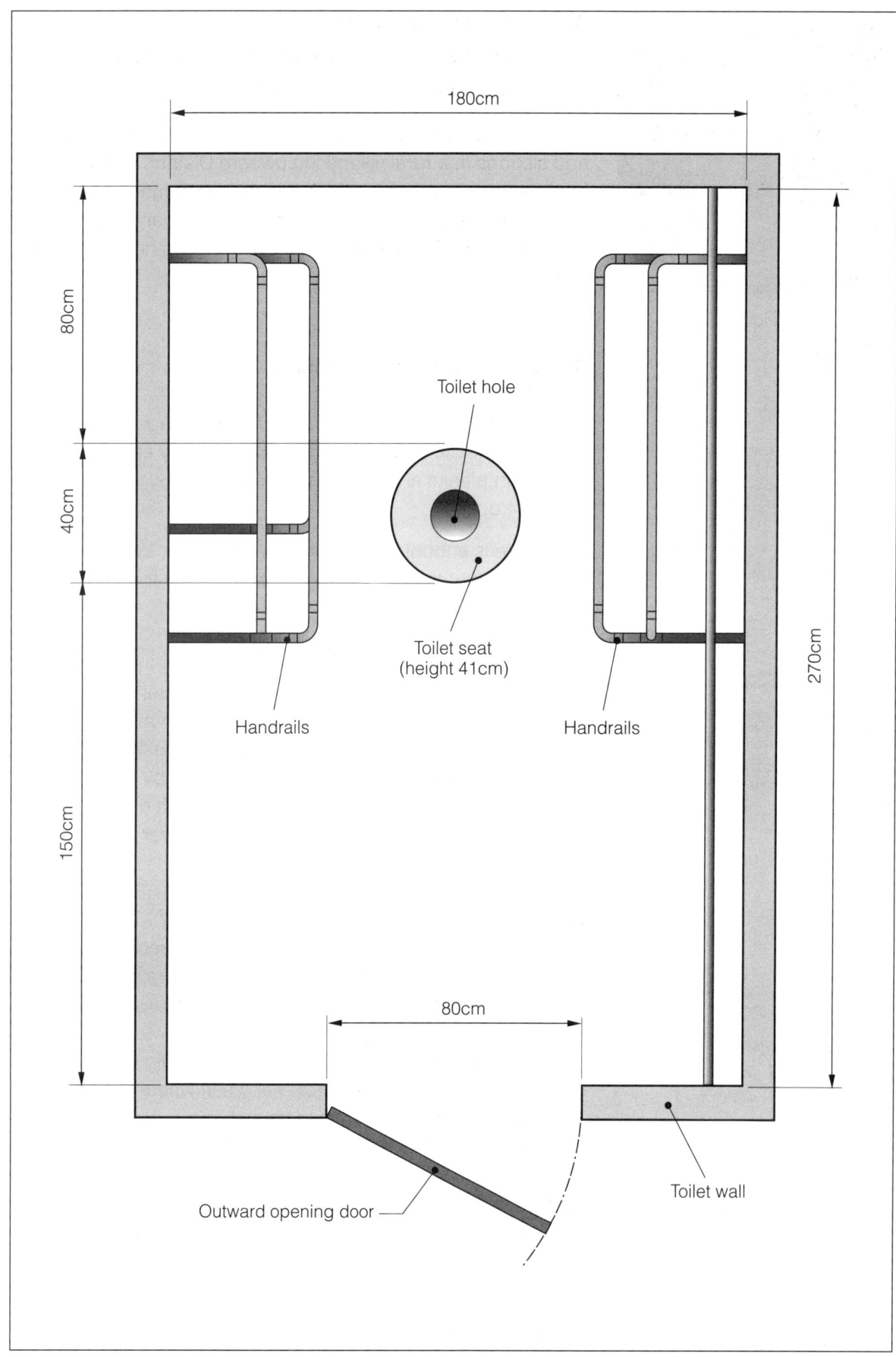

Figure 9.127. Plan view of VIP latrine with fixed raised seat.

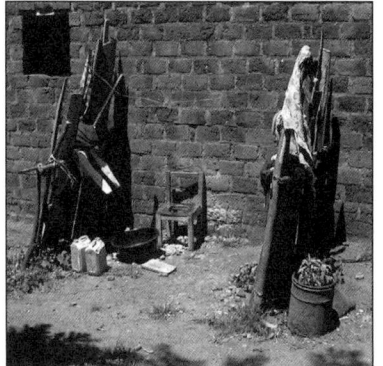

Figure 9.128. Household bathing area.

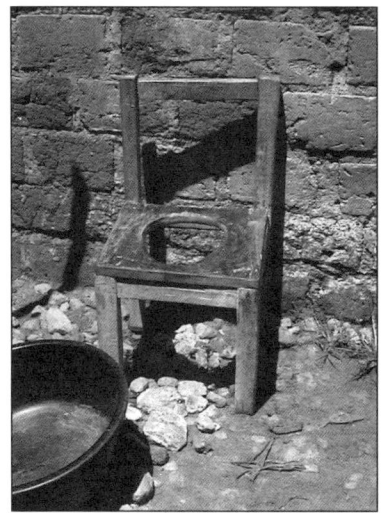

Figure 9.129. Wooden bathing/commode chair.

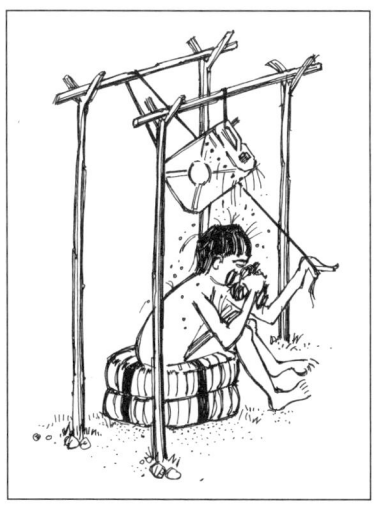

Figure 9.130. Adapted jerry-can shower.

9.27 Shower, bathing chair and implement holder for girl with limited movement

Eva Nakatudde is 19 and lives with her parents, grandmother and siblings in a rural village in Luweero District, Uganda. She has rheumatoid arthritis, which has gradually made all her joints stiff. She still has movement in her neck and a little in her thumbs. For mobility, a family member pushes her around in a wheelchair.

Simple shower arrangement
Description
*   An outside shelter has been constructed against the side of the house for bathing. The floor is stony earth. Vertical rough planks and branches form two sides, leaving the front open.

*   There is enough space for a bathing chair, for the wheelchair to be positioned next to it, and for a helper to stand on either side.

*   Eva described her shower which broke recently:

*   A pole extended from one side of the shelter to the other. Two 4 litre jerry-cans, which each had about 10 holes near the top, were filled with water and the top screwed on. The jerry-cans were suspended from the pole by a rope tied to the handle. A second rope was tied with one end round the bottom of the jerry-can, and looped over the pole. Eva held the other end of the rope.

Use
*   Her sisters pushed Eva to the shelter, helped her undress and transfer from wheelchair to bathing chair. She sat under the shower holding one end of the rope. She pulled on the rope, making the jerry-can tip and water shower out. When one jerry-can was empty, she did the same with the second. Her sisters help her wash where Eva can't reach. She wipes and dries herself as much as she can, and either 'air dries' the rest, or asks for help.

Key features
*   Low cost – all materials were available locally. The only purchases were nails and rope.

*   The jerry-cans could be filled by family members when it was convenient for them.

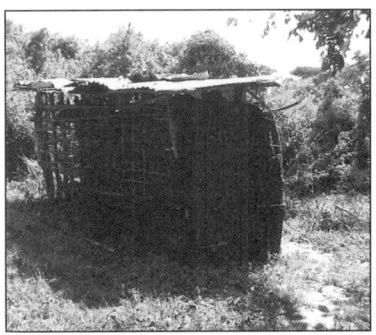

Figure 9.131. A rough path leads to the family latrine.

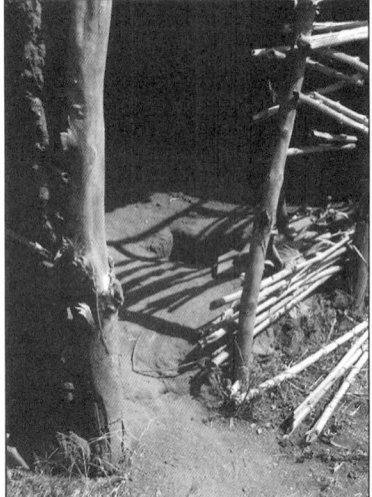

Figure 9.132. The packed earth floor of the pit latrine.

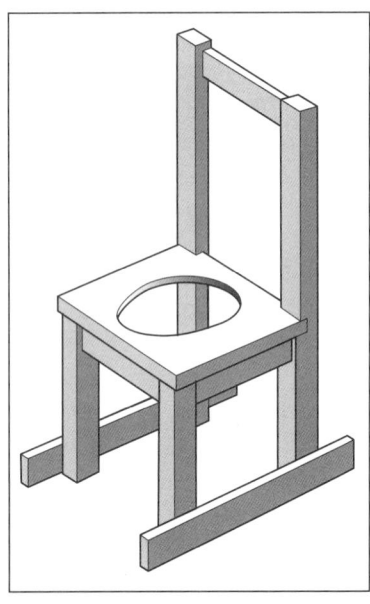

Figure 9.133. Bars attached to chair legs on each side.

Drawbacks and comments
* The lack of roof on the bathing area left the jerry-cans exposed to the sun, and as a result they cracked recently. Eva's father intends to repair the shower, this time with a tin roof for protection.

* Time-consuming for family members – the jerry-cans need filling and preparing each time.

Suitable for
* Bathers with limited arm movement.

Bathing/commode chair
The family has a pit latrine about 10m from the house along a rough path. Eva does not use the toilet chair in the latrine, because it is hard to get there in her wheelchair. The latrine floor is of packed earth and she would be worried that the toilet chair would break through the floor and fall into the pit.

Description
* A wooden chair with a hole in the seat, a back but no side-rails.

Dimensions
* Seat H: 40cm, W: 35.5. D: 33cm.

* Oval hole in seat 24 x 18cm.

Use
* Eva sits on the chair while bathing.

* She also uses it as a commode chair in the bathing shelter, with a bucket underneath. A family member empties the contents into the latrine, then cleans the bucket with water and soap powder.

Key features
* The chair back provides support for Eva who has poor sitting balance.

* The hole in the seat allows access for anal cleansing and for the bather to wash her buttocks and genital area.

* The chair is multi-purpose, used for both bathing and toileting, and therefore cost-effective.

Drawbacks and comments
* Adding side-rails to the chair would help prevent Eva falling sideways.

Suitable for

• People with difficulty squatting but with some sitting balance, such as people with weak legs or pregnant women. People who get tired easily when standing up, such as elderly or sick people.

Suggestions

The chair was made five years before, so it is now less comfortable for Eva. Now she would prefer it to be wider, with side-rails.

To reduce the risk of the chair breaking into the latrine pit, a bar could be attached to the legs on each side, to spread the weight of the chair. This could also improve its stability, and make it easier to move the chair by sliding it, if required. The path to the latrine would also need to be levelled, and the entrance widened.

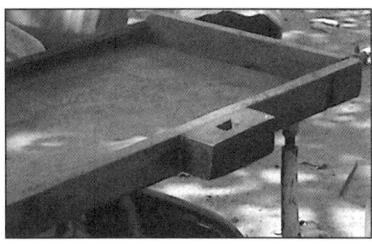

Figure 9.134. The hole in the wheelchair tray to insert the upright post of the implement holder.

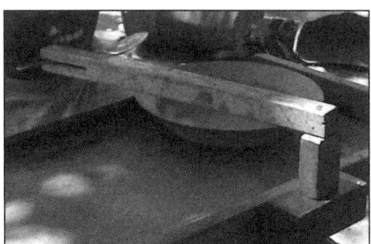

Figure 9.135. Implement holder.

Implement holder – tray attachment

Description

• An 'arm' swivels on a vertical post which slots into a hole attached to Eva's wheelchair tray. The 'arm' has a cleft end which can hold a spoon or other implement.

Use

• Eva holds the spoon handle in her mouth and scoops food (Figure 9.136). She then places the handle in the cleft of the implement holder (Figure 9.137), then takes food off the spoon with her mouth (Figure 9.138).

Key features

• Low cost, locally made.

• Can be used to hold a sponge, toothbrush, comb, or other household implement

Drawbacks

• The 'arm' rotates, which makes it unsuitable for use with items that need to be held rigid such as a toothbrush.

Suitable for

• Users with no/limited use of arms or hands.

Benefits

Eva liked the shower, which gave her more control. Without it, she has to wait for her sisters to come home from school to help her.

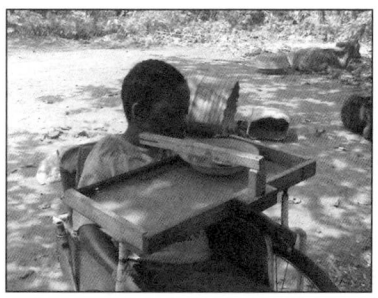

Figure 9.136. Eva scoops food with the spoon held in her mouth,

Before she had the tray and implement holder, she relied on family members to feed her or give her a drink. They sometimes rushed, gave her the food while it was still hot, or stopped before she was full. Now she can take her time, and eat till she is satisfied. It is better for her sisters too – now they have more time for other household tasks or to rest.

Process for obtaining adaptations

The ideas for the jerry-can shower, trays and spoon holder were introduced by an occupational therapist from the District Hospital. The family bought the materials and built the shower area and shower.

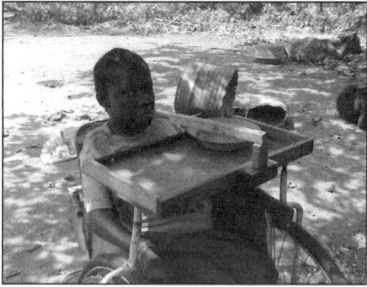

Figure 9.137. wedges the spoon handle in the cleft of the holder,

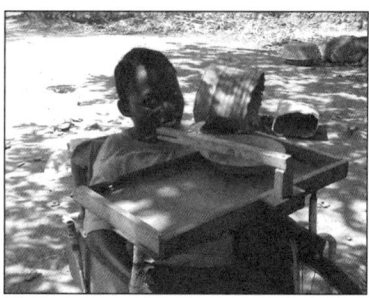

Figure 9.138. and takes the food off the spoon with her mouth.

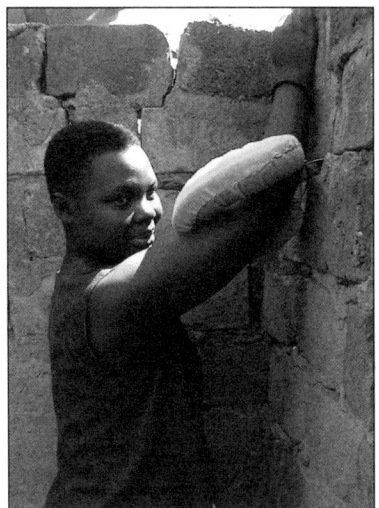

Figure 9.139. Joweria shows how she washes her arm.

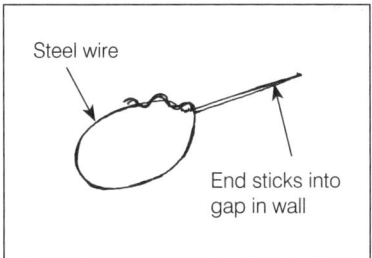

Steel wire

End sticks into gap in wall

Figure 9.140. Basic construction of bathing ring.

9.28 Bathing ring for young woman with one arm

Joweria Nakivumbi is 18 and lives with her family in a rural village in Masaka District, Uganda. Her left arm is amputated above the elbow. She has no mobility problems.

Joweria fetches water in a 10 litre jerry-can from a communal borehole across the road from the house. She is not strong enough to pump water with only one arm, but there is usually someone around to pump water for her.

The family have a brick-built bathroom behind the house.

Description
• A 'bathing ring': a ring of steel wire padded with 'mattress sponge' i.e. latex foam, and then covered with cotton fabric and stitched. One end of the ring is wedged into a crack in the brick wall of the bathroom.

Use
• Joweria can wash herself all over with her one arm. Finally, to wash her arm, she passes her arm to and fro through the ring to rub her arm clean.

Key features
• Low cost, locally available materials.

• Washable, durable, hygienic.

Drawbacks and comments
• Joweria finds the ring is not rigid enough and moves when she rubs her arm against it.

Suitable for
• People with one arm, limited arm movement, or poor grip.

Process for obtaining adaptation
The occupational therapist from Masaka District Hospital designed the ring, the materials were provided by the family, and the physiotherapist made it.

Richard Mutabazi, SC/UK

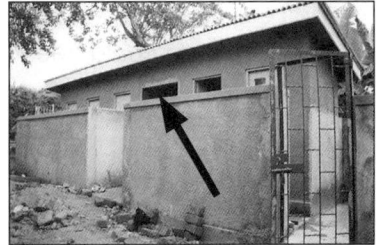

Figure 9.141. Toilet block (under construction). Arrow shows wider doorway of accessible toilet in the centre.

Richard Mutabazi, SC/UK

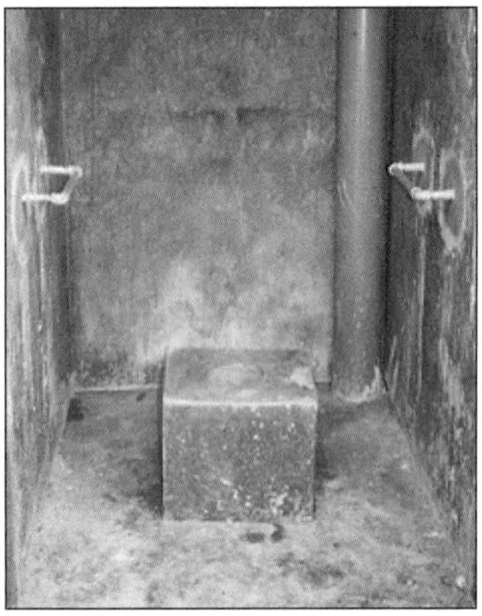

Figure 9.142. Accessible toilet cubicle.

Richard Mutabazi, SC/UK

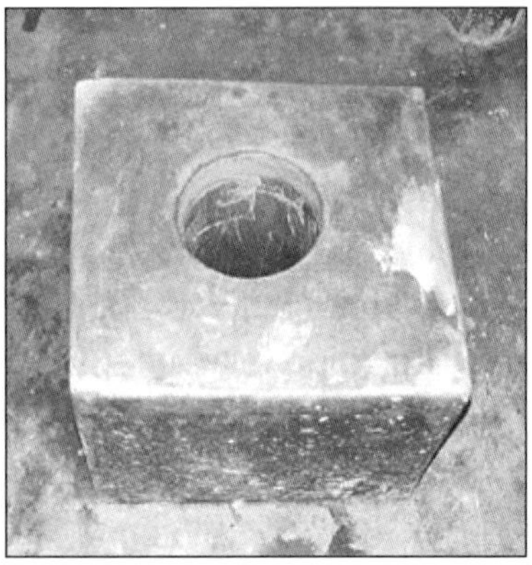

Figure 9.143. Fixed toilet seat. Note PVC pipe lining drop-hole.

9.29 Primary School toilet designed for wheelchair access

New Bubajjwe Primary School is in a low-income, peri-urban area of Kampala, Uganda, with poor overcrowded housing, much of it on marshy land. There is poor water supply, poor sanitation, drainage and refuse disposal.

The most interesting aspect of this case-study is the process of implementation, which involved collaboration between several different agencies – education, international NGO, and local NGO disability service provider. The process is described in detail below.

Description

- A brick-built row of six VIP latrines, with three cubicles for girls, two for boys, and one urinal.
- A square cement-plastered brick seat has a drop hole lined with heavy duty PVC pipe (same as used for the ventilation pipe) (Figure 9.143).
- Two handrails are attached, one to each side wall, for the length of the toilet seat.

Approach

- Concrete ramp approach with a high wall on each side.
- Entrance wide enough for a wheelchair to enter. The door opens outwards.

Dimensions

- Seat H: ~35cm.
- Handrails: 35-40mm Ø g.i. pipe, L:~50cm, H: ~ 80cm.
- Toilet hole Ø: 15cm PVC pipe.

Key features

- Space for a wheelchair to enter, and for a helper.
- Space for a child to sit with straight legs.
- A raised seat is convenient for transfer from a wheelchair.
- PVC pipe makes the drop-hole easy to clean.
- Handrails provide support for users while lowering themselves onto and getting up from the toilet seat.
- The accessible cubicle was planned from the beginning of the project, so the extra cost incurred was negligible.

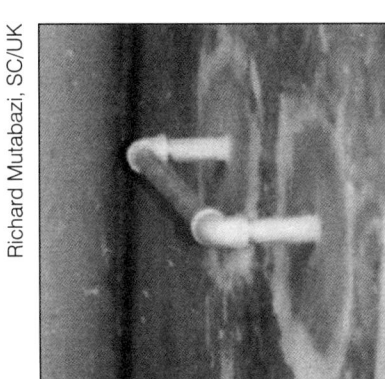
Figure 9.144. Handrail cemented to the wall.

Drawbacks and comments

- Locating the toilet in one corner of the cubicle could free up enough space for a wheelchair beside the toilet to enable sideways transfer.

- A toilet hole which is longer front to back would make the seat easier less likely to be soiled.

- Handrails may be too high in relation to the seat, and too wide apart for some child users. Additional handrails fixed to the floor on both sides of the toilet would provide choice of support.

- A handrail extending from the door to the toilet would provide support for users with poor balance.

Suitable for

- Wheelchair users; people unable to squat.

- People who can sit with some support.

- People able to grasp handrails.

- Very young children, many of whom don't like to use an ordinary squat latrine.

Process of implementation

Save the Children/UK (SC/UK), an international NGO, was implementing a project to improve Primary Health Care services in the area, including improved WATSAN.

This created demand from primary schools for latrines. New Bubajjwe School insisted their latrine be accessible for disabled pupils. They had a disabled pupil at the school, and they'd had to refuse admitting disabled pupils in the past because of lack of suitable facilities. COMBRA is a local NGO providing training in CBR throughout Uganda. A COMBRA occupational therapist provided design and detailed measurements of accessible latrines, including miniature 3D models made of cardboard and wire to show to teachers and SC/UK staff. These were given to the contractors for guidance. Although the SC/UK project engineer had no previous experience of accessibility, this gave him more confidence. He discussed with the contractor how to incorporate the suggestions into the existing standard design for school latrines, so the middle boys' cubicle was re-designated as the accessible latrine, for use by both disabled girls and disabled boys. He also explained the details of construction.

Factors contributing to this initiative

Introduction of Universal Primary Education in Uganda has meant that disabled children now have a right to attend school. COMBRA had a community-based project with disabled children in that area. One school Board member was a staff of COMBRA.

Constraints to implementation

SC/UK staff did not know how to go about making facilities accessible, had never come across such facilities and initially felt helpless. They considered it a risk, because they lacked previous experience in this area. After construction of this facility they would need feedback on its usage before incorporating it as part of the design. (This would be considered good practice, and enable design improvements to be made.)

Different innovations would have to be made for latrines in areas with a high water-table, where the latrines are raised and there are no ramps for wheelchairs.

(NB: For accessibility of raised latrines, SC/UK installed steps with handrails.)

This information was collected in an interview with Richard Mutabazi, former WATSAN Project Officer for SC/UK, supplemented by Moses Kiwanuka, occupational therapist from COMBRA.

9.30 Toilet stool for child with weak legs

Barbara Namaanda is 7, and lives with her grandmother, Mrs Veronica Alibazewa Mbabali, and the rest of her family in a village in Masaka District, Uganda.

Barbara has weak legs as a result of an accident. Her upper body is unaffected and strong. She has been using crutches for 10 months and is becoming increasingly mobile. She uses them to go to school, which is at least 500m away.
She can draw water from the family's rainwater storage tank, which has an ordinary tap, using a 1 litre jerry-can (Figure 9.145). She can carry the jerry-can in her hand whilst moving with her crutches.

The family have their own pit latrine. There are no special adaptations to the structure itself.

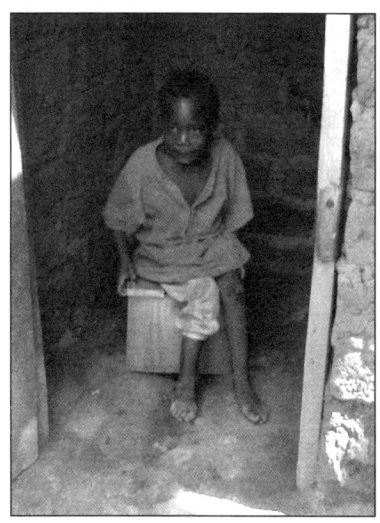

Figure 9.145. Barbara fetching water.

Wooden toilet stool

Description
* Barbara's wooden toilet stool is made of unpainted wood. The seat is two planks with a gap between them. There are no sides or back.

Use
* The stool is placed in the latrine over the toilet hole. Barbara sits on the stool to use the toilet. Urine and faeces fall directly into the hole.

Dimensions
* L: 40cm, W: 30cm, H: 25cm.

* Gap between planks: 10cm.

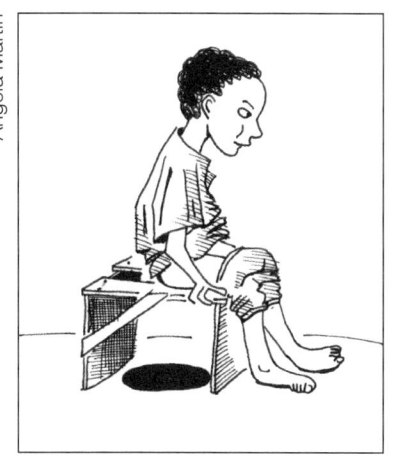

Figure 9.146. Barbara sitting on her toilet stool.

Key features
* Fairly durable, locally made, moderate cost.

* The front plank acts as a splash-guard against urine splashes.

* The narrow gap in the seat suits a child.

* The stool can be removed from the latrine when not required, so it does not obstruct other users.

Drawbacks and comments
* Painting or varnishing the seat would make it moisture resistant and easier to keep clean.

* A slightly larger cubicle would provide enough space to move the stool to one side of the toilet when not required.

Angela Martin

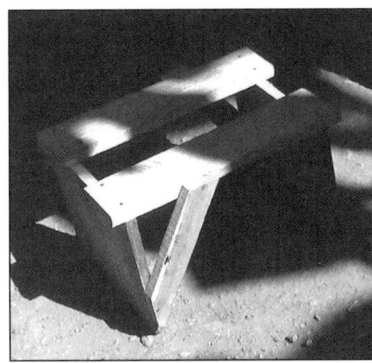

Figure 9.148. Wooden toilet stool.

Suitable for
* Users unable to squat, e.g. with weak legs, but with good sitting balance.

Adaptation
* Could be used as a commode seat with a container underneath (see page 118, Section 7.6. Commode seats).

Benefits
Before, Barbara used a child's potty, which her grandmother would empty into the latrine. Barbara said the potty was too low and it made her legs go numb.

She likes the new seat, because she can just sit on it comfortably, and she doesn't need to depend on others for the toilet. She uses the same toilet as the rest of the family, so she has privacy and there is no feeling of being different.

Other family members do not have to empty the container any more.

Process of implementation
The occupational therapist employed by Uganda Society for Disabled Children (USDC) designed, constructed and provided the commode chair in consultation with the family.

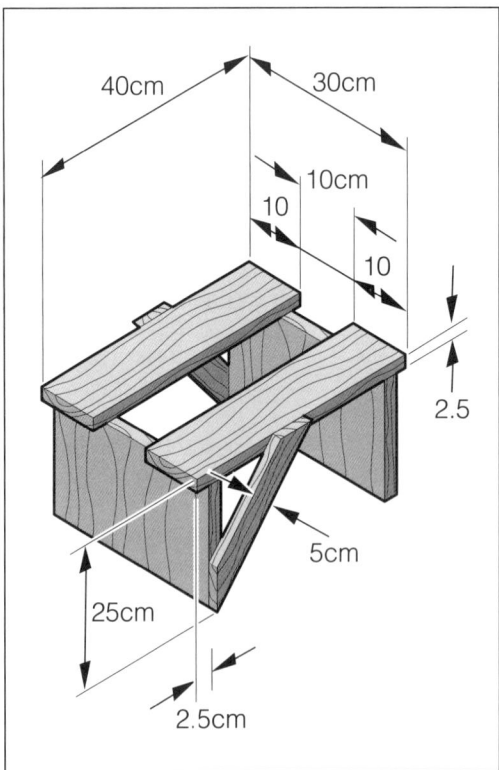

Figure 9.147. Dimensions of wooden toilet stool.

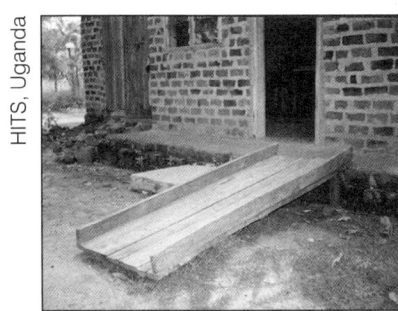

Figure 9.149. Movable wooden ramp.

9.31 Demonstration equipment: wooden ramp, wheelchair trailer, bathing area, toothbrush stand, toilet chair, hand-walkers and knee protectors.

Uganda Society of Hidden Talents (HITS) was set up by its Chairman, Elijah Musenyente, who is himself a wheelchair user. HITS' mission is to develop the skills and talents of disabled and non-disabled people, to support poor communities to identify their needs and implement programmes to address these. Current projects include vocational skills training, income-generation, hygiene and sanitation awareness and low-cost locally made equipment and facilities.

Movable wooden ramp

Description
- Movable wooden ramp for wheelchair access to facilities with steps, with a raised kerb on both sides.

Dimensions
- W: 80cm, L: 3 metres.

Key features
- Flexible – can be placed wherever needed.

- Cheaper than concrete.

- Kerb on each side prevents wheelchair rolling over the edge.

Drawbacks and comments
- Less durable than concrete.

- User needs helpers to move the ramp as needed.

Suitable for
- Wheelchair users with helpers available only.

- Temporary use.

- Crossing open drains or ditches.

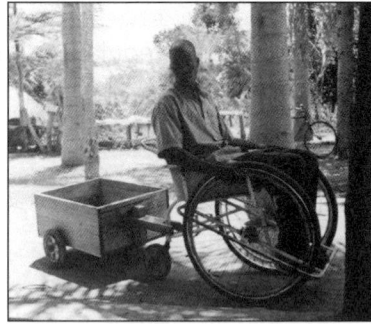

Figure 9.150. Two-wheeled wooden trailer.

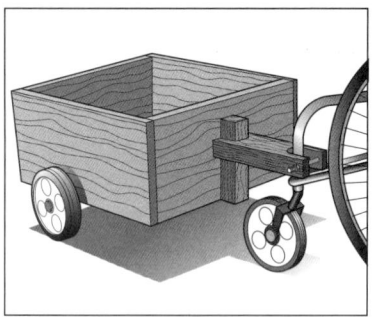

Figure 9.151. Detail of trailer hitching arrangement.

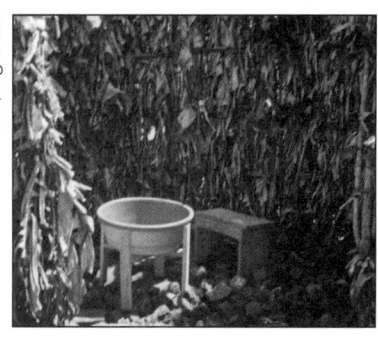

Figure 9.152. Demonstration bathing area.

Two-wheeled wooden trailer

Description
- Two-wheeled wooden trailer hooks onto the back of a wheelchair with a single rear small wheel.

Dimensions
- None given.

Key features
- Locally made, moderate cost.

- Can be easily hooked and unhooked from the wheelchair.

- Multi-purpose – can be used to carry water, goods to and from market, babies, etc.

- More weight can be pulled than can be carried directly on a wheelchair.

- Could also be used as a hand-drawn trailer, with a different pulling arrangement, e.g. rope.

Drawbacks and comments
- It may be difficult for some disabled people to attach the trailer themselves.

- May not be suitable for rough paths.

- Not suitable for all types of wheelchair.

Demonstration bathing area

Description
- The bathing area is screened by leaves on a wooden frame, with no roof or door. The floor is earth and stones.

- A wooden stand holds a washbowl which 'slots in' to four side supports ~30cm off the ground.

- A wooden bathing stool has a solid seat and sides (H: 25cm, L: 30, W: 20cm).

Key features
- Low-cost materials.

- Water drains away into the rough floor.

- Wash-stand holds a bowl firmly in place at a suitable height for the bather.

- The narrow seat allows water to drain off easily.

Drawbacks and comments

*   Not durable – the leaf screen needs replacing regularly.

*   The rough floor makes it difficult to use for wheelchairs and people unsteady on their feet.

*   The wash-stand is suitable for one size of bowl only.

*   Unpainted wood absorbs moisture and is less durable.

Suitable for

*   People with good sitting balance.

*   People with poor co-ordination, or unsteady on their feet.

*   People who get easily tired when standing for any length of time, e.g. elderly people, pregnant women.

Unsuitable for

*   Wheelchair users.

*   People with poor sitting balance.

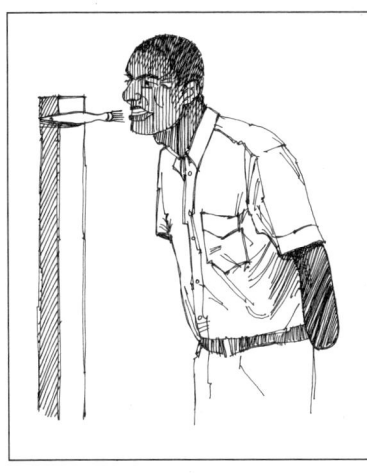

Figure 9.153. Toothbrush stand.

Toothbrush stand

Description

*   Vertical wooden pole, with a cross-piece for standing on the floor. A toothbrush is nailed to the post at the required height.

Key features

*   Could be made to any height.

*   Could be adapted to stand on or be fixed to a table.

Drawbacks and comments

*   Floor-standing version uses a lot of wood.

*   Not fixed to anything, so may be unstable.

Suitable for

*   Person with limited or no use of their hands.

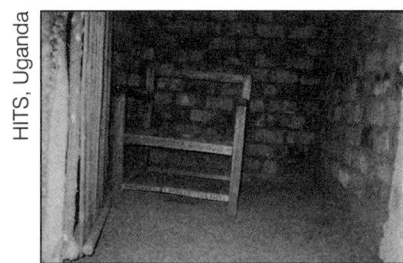

Figure 9.154. Wooden toilet chair.

Wooden toilet chair

Description
- Unpainted wooden chair with back and side-rails, and a hole cut in the seat, used over a pit latrine.

Key features
- Low cost, fairly durable.

- Arms and back provide support while sitting.

Drawbacks and comments
- The small hole is set quite far back in the seat, increasing the risk of fouling the seat.

- No splash-guard at the front of the chair means there is a risk of the user's clothing getting splashed with urine.

- Unpainted wood absorbs urine.

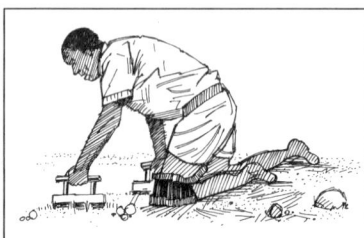

Figure 9.155. Man using hand walkers and knee-pads.

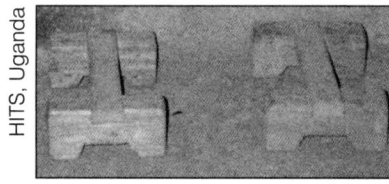

Figure 9.156. Wooden hand walkers.

Wooden hand walkers

Description
- Pieces of unpainted wood with a handle on top.

Use
- The user holds one handle in each hand and 'walks' with them when moving around on hands and knees.

Key features
- Locally available materials, low cost, durable. Easy to clean.

- Reduces soiling of hands and knees and thereby reduces the risk of infection.

Suitable for
- People who move by crawling or shuffling.

- Wheelchair users where facilities are inaccessible to a wheelchair.

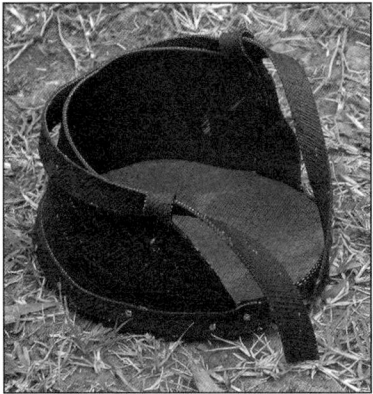

Figure 9.157. Knee protector.

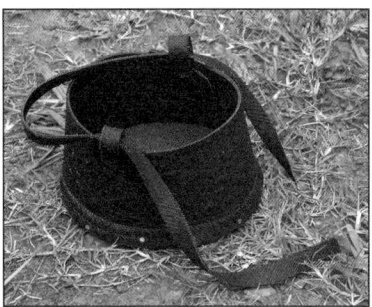

Figure 9.158. Stump protector.

Knee and stump protectors

Description

- Rubber pads made from recycled car tyres that fit over the knee or a leg stump. Rubber laces run through loops and tie around the leg to hold the pad in place.

Use

- The user places them over their knees/stumps to protect them when walking.

Key features

- Low-cost materials.

- Durable, easy to clean.

Process

These items of equipment and facilities have been developed as examples, so that when disabled people attend events organised by HITS, they can observe and try them out at HITS' demonstration area, and apply the ideas in their own home. No information is available, however, about whether or not this approach has been effective, what has worked and what has not worked.

Awareness-raising may be needed to convey the benefits of the devices, e.g. by running workshops where disabled people and their families use a problem-solving approach to improving access.

Based on information provided by Mr Musenyente, including interviews, photos and video.

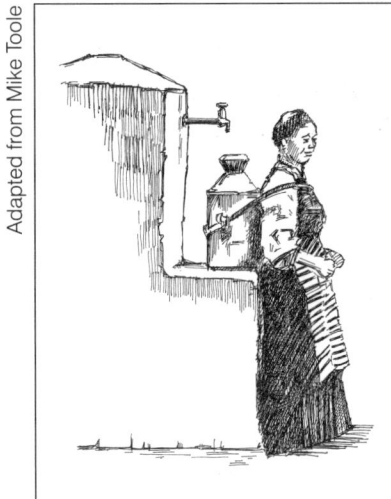

Figure 9.159. Using the 'back-happy' tapstand.

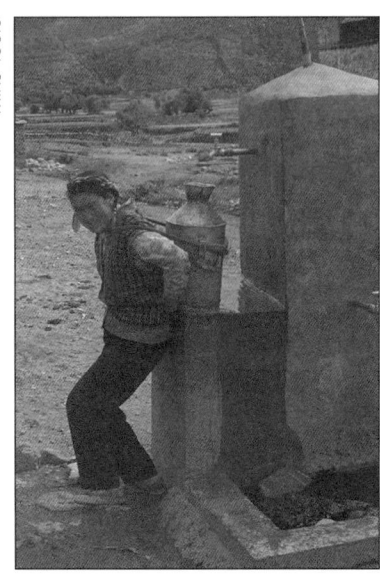

Figure 9.160. 'Back-happy' tapstand in use. Note direction of water drainage into ground-level splash apron.

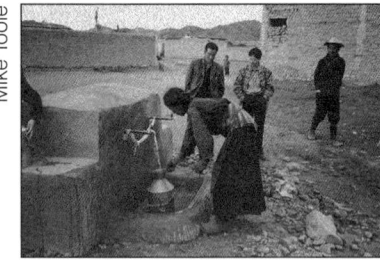

Figure 9.161. Original tapstand, with low taps only. Difficult to use for people with back problems.

9.32 'Back happy' tapstand

Description
- An adaptation of a traditional tapstand, with a waist-high shelf and an extra, higher tap added.

- The shelf has a slight slope which drains water down to the splash apron at ground level.

Context
- Rural areas of Tibet.

Use
- Communal tapstand, from which women fetch water in 15 – 20 litre metal jars, carried home on their backs.

Key features
- No need to bend from the waist when collecting water.

- Only slightly more expensive than the original model (given that most of the water system's budget is spent on piping to get water to the stand).

- Repairs and maintenance are similar to the original designs.

Drawbacks
- Minor factor: The higher level of the outlet requires slightly higher system pressure, meaning any leaks in the pipeline would be more severe. The pressure would make no difference to a well-constructed facility, and in terms of pipe pressure rating would amount to < 2% increase.

- The ground level splash apron is the same as in the original design, where washing or soaking clothes is carried out. It would be good to have these washing areas higher as well, but there could be a risk of cross-contamination from whatever is being washed there with containers being filled at the lower tap.

Suitable for
- People with difficulty bending, including those with lower back pain.

Benefits
According to the women, the new design has improved their quality of life. The original tapstand involved bending to collect water, which made it difficult for people with lower back pain, as bending was the main activity that both caused and aggravated their back pain (see Figure 9.161).

Based on information from: Hoy, D. et al (2003) 'Low back pain in rural Tibet', The Lancet, Vol. 361, Issue 9353, pp.225-226, with supplementary technical information provided by Damien Hoy, Project Manager and Harry Beyer, Project Engineer.

9

List of resources

A1.1 Inclusive design

Barker, P. Barrick, J. and Wilson, R. (1995) *Building Sight. A Handbook of building and interior design solutions to include the needs of visually impaired people*. HMSO & Royal National Institute for the Blind: London.

Bone, S. (1996) *Buildings for All to Use*. Construction Industry Research and Information Association (CIRIA): London. http://www.ciria.org.uk/ (Good practice guidance for improving existing public buildings for people with disabilities).

Bucks & Milton Keynes Building Control Managers (2004) *Accessibility by Design: A Standard Guide*. McMillan-Scott: UK. http://www.mkweb.co.uk/building_control/documents/part_1_Accessibility_by_Design.pdf

CAE (2004) *Designing for Accessibility*. Centre for Accessible Environments and RIBA Enterprises: London.

CAE (2004) *Good Loo Design Guide*. Centre for Accessible Environments and RIBA Enterprises: London.

CAE Information sheets also available on the website, e.g. http://www.cae.org.uk/sheets/designs_sheets/steps_stairs.html.

Cheshire County Council (2003) *Pedestrian Access & Mobility – A Code of Practice*. Cheshire County Council: UK. http://www.cheshire.gov.uk/NR/exeres/2E865610-3AB1-431F-8DE8-36B16D103C7D,frameless.htm?PageVersion=PRINTER FRIENDLY

Disability Rights Commission (2003) *Creating an Inclusive Environment - a report on improving the Built Environment*. http://www.drc-gb.org/publicationsandreports/publicationdetails.asp?id=157&section=access

UNESCAP (1995) *Promotion of Non-handicapping physical environments for Disabled Persons: Guidelines*. United Nations Economic and Social Commission for Asia and the Pacific: UN: New York. (Includes policy and legislation issues, design recommendations, & Annex VIII: Sample community accessibility checklist.) http://www.unescap.org/esid/psis/ disability/decade/publications/z15009gl/z1500901.htm

Transport

Venter, C.J. et al (2004) *Overseas Road Note 21: Enhancing the mobility of disabled people: Guidelines for Practitioners*. Transport Research Laboratory & DFID, UK. http:// www.transport-links.org/transport_links/filearea/publications/1_ 831_ORN%2021.pdf

Emergencies

Dacheux, Gilles avec Sophie Ferneeuw (2003) *Infrastructure et post-crise: Reconstruction attentive aux situations de handicap*. Prévention des risques, et construction dans les situations exceptionnelles. Handicap International: Lyon, France.

A1.2   Water supply and sanitation

Service delivery

Carl Bro International (undated) *Rural water supply and sanitation. Handbook for extension workers. Vol.1: Community Management. Vol.2: Technology Development*. UNICEF, Uganda Ministry of Gender, Labour & Social Development, Directorate of Water Development & Ministry of Health: Uganda.

Dacheux, Gilles avec Sophie Ferneeuw (2003) *Infrastructure et post-crise: Reconstruction attentive aux situations de handicap*. Prévention des risques, et construction dans les situations exceptionnelles. Handicap International: Lyon, France.

Smet, J. and van Wijk, C. (2002) *Small Community Water Supplies: Technology, People and Partnership*. Technical Paper Series 40. IRC International Water and Sanitation Centre: Delft, The Netherlands. http://www.irc.nl/page/1917

WELL (1998) *DFID Guidance Manual on Water Supply and Sanitation Programmes*. WELL Resource Centre Network for water sanitation and environmental health. WEDC: Loughborough University, UK. http://www.lboro.ac.uk/well

Participatory approaches to water

PRA is now increasingly taken to mean Participation, Reflection and Action, or PLA: Participatory Learning and Action. http://www.ids.ac.uk/ids/particip/

Chambers, R. (2002) *Participatory Workshops: A Sourcebook of 21 Sets of Ideas and Activities*. Earthscan: UK. http://www.ids.ac.uk/ids/particip/index.html

Deverill, P. et al (2002) *Designing water supply and sanitation projects to meet demand in rural and peri-urban communities. Book 3: Ensuring the participation of the poor*. WEDC: Loughborough University, UK. http://wedc.lboro.ac.uk/publications/pdfs/dwss/dwss3.pdf

Demand Responsive Approach: http://www.worldbank.org/watsan/rural_dra.html

Mukherjee, N. and van Wijk, Christine (eds.) (2003) *Planning and Monitoring in Community Water Supply and Sanitation. A Guide on the Methodology for Participatory Assessment (MPA) for Community-Driven Development Programs*. World Bank Water and Sanitation Programme; International Water and Sanitation Centre: Washington. http://www.wsp.org/pdfs/mpa%202003.pdf

Sawyer, R., Simpson-Hébert, M. and Wood, S. (1998) *PHAST step-by-step guide: A participatory approach for the control of diarrhoeal diseases*. World Health Organization: Geneva. http://www.who.int/water_sanitation_health/hygiene/envsan/phastep/en/

Technical information

Centre for Disease Control Tippy Taps
http://www.cdc.gov/safewater/tippy-tap.pdf

Franceys, R., Pickford, J. and Reed, R. (1992) *A Guide to the Development of On-Site Sanitation*. World Health Organization: Geneva. http://www.who.int/water_sanitation_health/hygiene/envsan/onsitesan/en/

Hoy, D. et al (2003) *'Low back pain in rural Tibet'*, The Lancet, Vol.361, Issue 9353, pp. 225-226.

Hurtado Elena (1993) *'Tippy tap saves water'*, Dialogue on Diarrhoea, no. 54. http://www.rehydrate.org/dd/dd54.htm#page6

Rainwater Harvesting, water purification, www.rdic.org

Skinner, B. (2003) *Small-Scale Water Supply. A review of technologies*. ITDG & WEDC/LSHTM: UK.

Water For The World: a series of USAID technical notes covering all aspects of rural water supply and sanitation, available online: http://www.lifewater.org/wfw/wfwindex.htm

WELL Publications (available online http://www.lboro.ac.uk/ well or contact WELL): well@lboro.ac.uk

WELL Fact sheets: e.g. Smet, J. (2003) *Domestic Rainwater Harvesting.*
WELL Briefing Note: *'Why should the water and sanitation sector consider disabled people?'*, on water and sanitation and the MDGs, and others.
WELL Technical Briefs: e.g. *Brief 45: Latrine slabs and seats, Brief 35: Low-lift irrigation pumps, Brief 36: Ferrocement water tanks.*

A1.3   Human rights

United Nations (1948) *Universal Declaration of Human Rights.* United Nations: Geneva.
http://www.un.org/Overview/rights.html

United Nations (1989) *Convention on the Rights of the Child.* United Nations: New York.
http://www.crin.org/docs/resources/treaties/uncrc.htm

DFID (2000) *Realising human rights for poor people.* Strategies for achieving the international development targets. Department for International Development: UK.
http://www.dfid.gov.uk/pubs/files/tsphuman.pdf

Human right to water
Lenton, R. and Wright, A. (2004) *Interim Report of Task Force 7 on Water and Sanitation. Executive Summary.* Millennium Project, UNDP: http://www.unmillenniumproject.org/ documents/tf7interimexecsum.pdf

WaterAid and Rights and Humanity (2004) *The Right to Water.* Website: http://www.righttowater.org.uk

Water Supply and Sanitation Collaborative Council (WSSCC) *Global WASH Forum. Dakar Statement.* December 2004.
http://www.wsscc.org/dataweb.cfm?code=516.

Disabled people's human rights
United Nations (1993) *Standard Rules on Equalization of Opportunities for Disabled Persons.* United Nations: New York. http://www.independentliving.org/standardrules/ StandardRules1.html

UNESCAP (2003) *Biwako Millennium Framework for Action Towards an Inclusive, Barrier-Free and Rights-Based Society for Persons with Disability in Asia and the Pacific*. UN Economic and Social Commission for Asia and the Pacific: Bangkok. http://www.unescap.org/esid/psis/disability/bmf/bmf.html http://www.un.org/esa/socdev/enable/rights/

Jones, H.E. (2001) *Disabled Children's Rights: a practical guide*. Save the Children: Stockholm, Sweden. http://www.rb.se/bookshop; http://rb.st/bookshop/

Lansdown, G. (2001) *It is our World Too!* A report on the lives of disabled children. Disability Awareness in Action: London. http://www.daa.org.uk/ItisOurWorldToo.htm

Working Group of the Ad Hoc Committee on International Convention on the Rights of Persons with Disabilities. New York, 5 - 16 January 2004. *Report of the Working Group to the Ad Hoc Committee*. A/AC.265/2004/WG/1. United Nations. http://www.un.org/esa/socdev/enable/rights/ahcwgreport.htm

A1.4 Poverty and development

DFID (2001) *Poverty: Bridging the Gap. Guidance Notes*. Issues. Department for International Development: UK. http://www.eldis.org/static/DOC12336.htm

Eurodad (2004) PRSP: *Eurodad's work on Poverty Reduction Strategy Papers*. http://www.eurodad.org/workareas/default. aspx?id=92.

Nicol, A. (2000) *Adopting A Sustainable Livelihoods Approach to Water Projects: Implications for Policy and Practice. Sustainable Livelihoods Working Paper Series*. Overseas Development Institute: London. http://www.odi.org.uk/publications/wp133.pdf

Sustainable Livelihoods. Website: http://www.livelihoods.org/

WaterAid (2004) *Poverty Reduction Strategy Papers*. http://www.wateraid.org.uk/in_depth/policy_and_research/poverty_reduction_strategy_papers/default.asp.

World Bank (2003) *Millennium Development Goals*. Website: http://www.developmentgoals.org/

World Bank (2004) *Poverty Reduction Strategies (PRSPs)*. Website: http://www.worldbank.org/poverty/strategies/

Poverty and disability/vulnerability
Actionaid Bangladesh (1996) *Four Baseline Surveys on Prevalence of Disability*. Disability & AIDS Coordination Unit. Actionaid: Dhaka, Bangladesh.

Bangladesh Bureau of Statistics (2000) *Statistical Pocketbook*. Dhaka, Bangladesh.

Bonnel, R. (2004) *PRSPs & Disability*. Presentation at World Bank Meeting for the Global Partnership on Disability & Development.
http://siteresources.worldbank.org/DISABILITY/Resources/News---Events/GPDD/1PRSDisabilities.ppt

de Vries, C. (2004) *'Disabled Persons are more vulnerable to HIV'*. DCDD Newsletter, November 2004. Dutch Coalition on Disability and Development: Utrecht, Netherlands.
http://www.dcdd.nl/data/1099587276087_DCDD%20newsletter%209.pdf

Elwan, A. (1999) *Poverty and Disability: a survey of the literature*. World Bank: http://siteresources.worldbank.org/DISABILITY/Resources/Poverty/Poverty_and_Disability_A_Survey_of_the_Literature.pdf

HAI (2002) *State of the world's older people 2002*. HelpAge International: London, UK.
http://www.helpage.org/images/pdfs/SOTWOPeng.pdf

Handicap International and NFOWD (2003) *Disability and the PRSP in Bangladesh. A position document*. HI-Bangladesh: Dhaka.

Reed, B.J., Christie, C. and Fisher, J. (draft) *Did I Phrase that Correctly?* WEDC: Loughborough, UK. http://wedc.lboro.ac.uk/projects/new_projects3.php?id=19

Saunders, C. and Miles, S. (1990) *The Uses and Abuses of Surveys in Service Development Planning for Disabled People: the Case of Lesotho*. Save the Children/UK: London.
http://www.eenet.org.uk/bibliog/scuk/surveys.shtml

Teachers from Mpika, Zambia (2003) *Researching our Experience*. Enabling Education Network (EENET): Manchester, UK.
http://www.eenet.org.uk/action/rsrching_experience.pdf

A1.5 Disability and development policy

ADB (2002) *Disability Brief: Identifying and Addressing the Needs of Disabled People.* Asian Development Bank: Manila.

DFID (2000) *Disability, Poverty and Development.* Issues Paper. Department for International Development: UK. http://www.dfid.gov.uk/pubs/files/disabilitypovertydevelopment.pdf

European Disability Forum (2002) *Development Cooperation and Disability.* European Disability Forum: Brussels. http://www.edf-feph.org/en/policy/development/dev_pub.htm

Ortiz, I. (2004) *Disability KAR: Assessing Connections to DFID's Poverty Agenda.* Overseas Development Group: UK. http://www.disabilitykar.net/pdfs/isabel_ortiz_report_final1.pdf

Thomas, P. (2004) *DFID and Disability. A Mapping of the Department for International Development and Disability Issues.* Disability KAR: UK. http://www.disabilitykar.net/pdfs/mapping_report_web1.pdf

SIDA (1999) *SIDA's Development Co-operation for Children and Adults with Disabilities.* Swedish International Development Cooperation Agency, Department for Democracy and Social Development (DESO): Stockholm, Sweden. http://www.sida.se/content/1/c6/02/65/17/FunkHindEng.pdf

NORAD (2002) *The Inclusion of Disability in Norwegian Development Co-operation.* Norwegian Agency for Development Cooperation: Oslo, Norway. http://www.norad.no/default.asp?FILE=items/2751/116

Office of the Deputy President (1997) *Integrated National Disability Strategy White Paper.* Government of South Africa. http://www.polity.org.za/html/govdocs/white_papers/disability1.html

USAID (1997) *USAID Disability Policy Paper.* The United States Agency for International Development: Washington, USA. http://www.usaid.gov/about/disability/DISABPOL.FIN.html

Stienstra, D., Fricke, Y. and D'Aubin, A. (2002) *Baseline Assessment: Inclusion and Disability in World Bank Activities.* The World Bank: Washington. http://siteresources.worldbank.org/DISABILITY/Resources/Overview/Baseline_Assessment_Inclusion_and_Disability_in_World_Bank_Activities.pdf

Metts, R.L. (2000) *Disability Issues, Trends and Recommendations for the World Bank.* The World Bank: Washington. http://siteresources.worldbank.org/DISABILITY/Resources/Overview/Disability_Issues_Trends_and_Recommendations_for_the_WB.pdf

A1.6 Including disabled people in development

At project design level

Heinicke-Motsch, K. and Sygall, S. (2003) *Building an Inclusive Development Community: a manual on including people with disabilities in international development programs*. Mobility International USA: Eugene, Oregon USA.
http://www.dec.org/pdf_docs/PNACY408.pdf

Jones, H. (1999) Integrating a disability perspective into mainstream development programmes: the experience of Save the Children (UK) in East Asia. In: E. Stone *Disability and Development: learning from action and research on disability in the majority world*. The Disability Press: Centre for Disability Studies, Leeds, UK.

Stubbs, S. (1993) *Integrating Disability into Development Programmes: guiding principles and key questions*. Save the Children: UK.
http://www.eenet.org.uk/theory_practice/integrat.shtml

Wiman, R. (2001) *Rapid Handicap Analysis of Development Activities: An Instrument for Inclusive Project Design*. STAKES, National Research and Development Centre for Welfare and Health, for and on behalf of the United Nations. Helsinki, Finland. http://www.stakes.fi/sfa/rhachecklist.htm

Werner, D. (1995) Strengthening the Role of Disabled People in Community Based Rehabilitation Programmes.In B. O'Toole and R. McConkey *Innovations In Developing Countries For People With Disabilities*. Lisieux Hall Publications: UK.
http://www.eenet.org.uk/parents/book/bookcontents.shtml

Training materials

Harris, A. and Enfield, S. (2003) *Disability, Equality and Human Rights: a training manual for development and humanitarian organisations*. Oxfam and Action on Disability and Development: Oxford, UK.

Jones, H. (1999) *Including Disabled People in Everyday Life: a practical approach*. Save the Children: UK.

UNESCAP (1995) *Promotion of Non-handicapping physical environments for Disabled Persons: Guidelines*. United Nations Economic and Social Commission for Asia and the Pacific: UN: New York. (Appendix VII: Disability simulation exercise)
http://www.unescap.org/esid/psis/disability/decade/publications/z15009gl/z1500901.htm

UNHCR and ISCA (2000) Action for the Rights of Children (ARC). Module 11 — Critical Issues: Disability. United Nations High Commissioner for Refugees; International Save the Children Alliance: Geneva.
http://www.savethechildren.net/arc/what.html

Van Ginneken, L. et al (2004) *Health Education for Behaviour Change*. Network Learning: Amsterdam.Using role-play to promote behaviour change.
http://www.networklearning.org/books/hebc.html

Facilitating participation in groups

Lewis, I. (ed.) (2000) *Access for All: Helping to make participatory processes accessible for everyone*. Practice Guidelines. Save the Children: UK.
http://www.eenet.org.uk/bibliog/scuk/access_for_all.pdf

Loughborough University (2004) *Disabilities & Additional Needs Service*. http://www.lboro.ac.uk/disabilities/

A1.7 Individual aids and equipment

Handicap International Belgium. *Booklet on household adaptations for daily living*. PRC, Siem Reap: Cambodia (drawings and text in Khmer)

Helander, E., Mendis, P., Nelson, G. and Goerdt, A. (1989) *Training in the Community for People with Disabilities*. World Health Organization: Geneva.

IICP (1999) Series of booklets: *Cleanliness for the Child with Cerebral Palsy, Special Furniture, Toileting for the Child with Cerebral Palsy*. Indian Institute of Cerebral Palsy: Kolkata, India.

UNESCAP (1997) *Production and distribution of Assistive Devices for People with Disabilities*. United Nations: New York.
http://www.unescap.org/esid/psis/disability/decade/publications/z15001p1/index.asp

Van der Hulst, G., Velthuys, M. and de Haan, G. (1993) *More with Less: Aids for disabled people in daily life*. TOOL: Amsterdam.

Werner, D. (1987) *Disabled Village Children. A guide for community health workers, rehabilitation workers, and families*. Hesperian Foundation: USA.
http://www.healthwrights.org/books/disabledvch.htm

Werner, D. (1998) *Nothing About Us Without Us: developing innovative technologies for, by and with disabled persons*. Healthwrights: Palo Alto, CA, USA.
http://www.healthwrights.org/books/nothingabout.htm

WHO (1993) *Promoting the Development of Young Children with Cerebral Palsy*. A guide for mid-level rehabilitation workers. World Health Organization: Geneva.

WHO (1996) *Promoting Independence following a Spinal Cord Injury*. A manual for mid-level rehabilitation workers. World Health Organization: Geneva.

WHO (1996) *Promoting the Development of Infants and Young Children with Spina Bifida and Hydrocephalus*. A guide for mid-level rehabilitation workers. World Health Organization: Geneva.

WHO (1999) *Promoting Independence Following a Stroke*: A guide for therapists and professionals working in Primary Health Care. World Health Organization. Geneva.

A1.8 Household level assessments and problem-solving

CBR-DTC (undated) *Finding Out about a Person and Her Problem*. CBR Development Training Centre: Solo, Indonesia.

Helander, E., Mendis, P., Nelson, G. and Goerdt, A. (1989) *Training in the Community for People with Disabilities*. World Health Organization: Geneva. (Especially: Guide for local supervisors p.18, Locating and identifying people with disabilities.)

Helander, E. (1999) *Prejudice and Dignity: an Introduction to Community-Based Rehabilitation*. Second edition. UNDP: New York.

HAI (2000) *Older People in disasters and humanitarian crises: Guidelines for best practice*. Helpage International: London.
http://www.helpage.org/images/pdfs/bpg.pd

Jones, H. (1999) *Including Disabled People in Everyday Life: a practical approach*. Save the Children: UK.

Werner, D. (1987) *Disabled Village Children. A guide for community health workers, rehabilitation workers, and families*. Hesperian Foundation: USA.
http://www.healthwrights.org/books/disabledvch.htm

WHO (2001) *The International Classification of Functioning, Disability and Health* - ICF. World Health Organization: Geneva. http://www3.who.int/icf/icftemplate.cfm

A1.9 People with visual impairments

Barker, P. Barrick, J. and Wilson, R. (1995) *Building Sight. A Handbook of building and interior design solutions to include the needs of visually impaired people*. HMSO & Royal National Institute for the Blind: London.

Nieman, S. and Jacob, N. (2000) *Helping Children who are Blind*. Early Assistance Series for Children with Disabilities. Hesperian Foundation: California, USA.

RNIB *See it Right Pack*. Royal National Institute for the Blind: UK. Practical advice on designing, producing and planning for accessible information. http://www.rnib.org.uk/xpedio/groups/public/documents/PublicWebsite/public_seeitright.hcsp

Appendix 2

Resource organisations and addresses

A2.1   Water supply and sanitation

International Development Enterprises (IDE)

Has expertise in water technologies for small-scale irrigation and safe drinking water.

Address: PO Box 1577, Phnom Penh, Cambodia.
Phone: +855 23 880 604;
Fax: +855 23 880 059.
e-mail: ide@online.com.kh
URL: http://www.ideorg.org

International Water and Sanitation Centre (IRC)

News, information, advice, research and training on low-cost water supply and sanitation in developing countries.

Address: P.O. Box 2869, 2601 CW, Delft,
             The Netherlands.
Phone: +31 15 219 2939;
Fax: +31 15 2190955.
e-mail: publications@irc.nl
URL: http://www.irc.nl

Oxfam GB

Address: Oxfam House, 274 Banbury Road, Oxford,
             OX2 7DZ, UK.
Phone: +44 870 333 2700.
URL: http://www.oxfam.org.uk/

NGO Forum for Drinking Water Supply & Sanitation

Address: 4/6 Block-E Lalmatia, Dhaka-1207, Bangladesh.
Phone: +880 2 815 4273, 2 815 4274;
Fax: +880 2 8117924.
e-mail: ngof@bangla.net
URL: http://www.ngoforum-bd.org/

Resource Development International-Cambodia (RDI-C)

Address: P.O. Box 494, Phnom Penh, Cambodia.
Phone/Fax: +855 23-369577
e-mail: mickey@rdic.org
URL: http://www.rdic.org/home.html

UNICEF Water and Environmental Sanitation (WES)

Address: UNICEF House, 3 United Nations Plaza,
             New York 10017, USA.
Phone: +1 212 326 7000;
Fax: +1 212 887 7465.
URL: http://www.unicef.org/wes/index.html

WaterAid

Address: Prince Consort House, 27-29 Albert
             Embankment, London, SE1 7UB, UK.
Phone: +44 20 7793 4500;
Fax: +44 20 7793 4545
e-mail: wateraid@wateraid.org
URL: http://www.wateraid.org.uk/

Water, Engineering and Development Centre (WEDC)

Address: Loughborough University, Leicestershire,
             LE11 3TU, UK.
Phone: +44 1509 222885;
Fax: +44 1509 211079.
e-mail: wedc@lboro.ac.uk
URL: http://wedc.lboro.ac.uk/

WELL resource centre for water, sanitation and environmental health

Address: WEDC, Loughborough University,
             Leicestershire, LE11 3TU, UK.
Phone: +44 1509 228304;
Fax: +44 1509 223970.
e-mail: well@lboro.ac.uk
URL: http://www.lboro.ac.uk/well

World Bank Water and Sanitation Programme (WSP)

Address: 1818 H Street, N.W., Washington, D.C. 20433,
             USA.
Phone: +1 202 473-9785;
Fax: +1 202 522-3313, 522-3228.
e-mail: info@wsp.org
URL: http://www.wsp.org/

A2.2   Infrastructure

Centre for Accessible Environments

Address: 70 South Lambeth Road, London SW8 1RL, UK.
Phone:
/textphone: +44 20 7840 0125;
Fax: +44 20 7840 5811.
e-mail: info@cae.org.uk
URL: http://www.cae.org.uk/

Disability Rights Commission, UK

Address: DRC Helpline, FREEPOST MID02164,
            Stratford upon Avon, CV37 9BR, UK.
Phone: 08457 622 633; textphone: 08457 622 644;
Fax: 08457 778 878.
URL: http://www.drc-gb.org/

Disability Wales

Address: Wernddu Court, Caerphilly Business Park,
            Van Rd, Caerphilly, CF83 3ED, UK.
Phone: +44 29 2088 7325;
Fax: +44 29 2088 8702.
e-mail: info@dwac.demon.co.uk
URL: http://www.dwac.demon.co.uk/

Infrastructure Connect

Website providing information and links about the research
engineering and infrastructure work of DFID
URL: http://www.infrastructureconnect.info/

Transport Links

Website about transport in developing countries.
URL: http://www.transport-links.org

Transport Research Laboratory (TRL)

Address: Crowthorne House, Nine Mile Ride,
            Wokingham, Berkshire, RG40 3GA, UK.
Phone: +44 1344 773131;
Fax: +44 1344 770880.
e-mail: enquiries@trl.co.uk
URL: http://www.trl.co.uk

A2.3   Disabled people's organisations

Action to Positive Change on People with Disabilities (APCPD)

Address: PO Box 12305, Kampala, Uganda.
Phone: +256 77 449 852;
Fax: +256 41 530 412.
e-mail: apcpd@infocom.co.ug

Bangladesh Protibandhi Kallyan Somity (BPKS)

Address: BPKS Complex, Dhakkhinkhan, Uttara,
            Dhaka 1230, Bangladesh.
Phone: +88 02 8923915, 02 8960077;
Fax: +88 02 8960078.
e-mail: bpks@citechco.net; bpkswn@agni.com
URL: http://www.bpksbd.org

Centre for Services & Information on Disability (CSID)

Address: House 715, Road 10, Baitul Aman
              Housing Society, Adabar, Shyamoli,
              Dhaka 1207, Bangladesh.
Phone: +88 02 9129727, 02 8125669;
Fax: +88 02 8125669.
e-mail: csid@bdonline.com; csid@bdmail.net
URL: http://www.csidnetwork.org/

The Danish Council of Organisations of Disabled People (DSI)

Address: Kløverprisvej 10B, 2650 Hvidovre, Denmark.
Phone: +45 3675 1777;
Fax: +45 3675 1403.
e-mail: dsi@handicap.dk
URL: http://www.handicap.dk/

Disability.dk website

Contains a wealth of information on disability in developing countries to support NGOs, governments and others working in the field. Hosted by DSI.
URL: http://www.disability.dk/

Disability Awareness in Action (DAA)

Address: 46 The Parklands, Hullavington, Wiltshire,
              SN14 6DL, UK.
Phone/Fax: +44 (0)1666 837 671.
e-mail: info@daa.org.uk
URL: http://www.daa.org.uk/

Disabled Peoples' International (DPI)

Address: 748 Broadway, Winnipeg, Manitoba,
              R3G 0X3, Canada.
Phone: +204 287 8010;
Fax: +204 783 6270.
e-mail: info@dpi.org
URL: http://www.dpi.org/

Uganda Society of Hidden Talents (HITS)

Address: Box 7304, Kampala, Uganda.
Phone: +256 71 839801
e-mail: musenyente@hotmail.com

A2.4 Disability and development

Action on Disability in Development (ADD)

Address:	Vallis House, 57 Vallis Rd, Frome, Somerset, BA11 3EG, UK.
Phone:	+44 (0)1373 473 064;
Fax:	+44 (0)1373 452 075.
e-mail:	add@add.org.uk
URL:	http://www.add.org.uk

The Atlas Alliance

Address:	Schweigaardsgt 12, PO Box 9218, Grønland, 0134 Oslo, Norway.
Phone:	+47 2217 4647;
Fax:	+47 2316 3595.
e-mail:	atlas@atlas-alliansen.no
URL:	http://www.atlas-alliansen.no

CBR Development Training Centre (CBR –DTC)

Address:	Jl. LU Adisucipto Km 7, Colomadu, Solo 57176, Indonesia.
Phone:	+62 271 780829, 780075;
Fax:	+62 271 780976.
e-mail:	cbr@indo.net.id

Centre for the Rehabilitation of the Paralysed (CRP)

Address:	PO CRP- Chapain, Savar, Dhaka 1343, Bangladesh.
Phone:	+880 2 7710464/5, or 7711766;
Fax:	+880 2 7710069.
e-mail:	info@crp-bangladesh.org
URL:	http://www.crp-bangladesh.org

Disability Action Council (DAC)

Address:	PO Box 115, Phnom Penh, Cambodia.
Phone:	+855 23 215 341;
Fax:	+855 23 218 797.
e-mail:	dac@dac.org.kh
URL:	http://www.dac.org.kh

Dutch Coalition on Disability and Development

Address:	PO Box 3356, 3502 GJ Utrecht, Netherlands.
Phone:	+31 30 291 6711;
Fax:	+31 30 297 0606;
e-mail:	dcdd@dcdd.nl
URL:	http://www.dcdd.nl

EENET Enabling Education Network

Address:	c/o Educational Support and Inclusion, School of Education, University of Manchester, Oxford Road, Manchester M13 9PL, UK.
Phone:	+44 (0)161 275 3711;
Fax:	+44 (0)161 275 3548.
e-mail:	info@eenet.org.uk
URL:	http://www.eenet.org.uk

Handicap International (HI)

Address:	14 Avenue Berthelot, 69361 Lyon, CEDEX 07, France.
Phone:	+33 4 7869 7979;
Fax:	+33 4 7869 7994.
e-mail:	contact@handicap-international.org
URL:	http://www.handicap-international.org

Indian Institute of Cerebral Palsy (IICP)

Address:	P 35/1 Taratolla Rd, Kolkata, 700 088, India.
Phone:	+91 33 2401 3488, 2401 0240;
Fax:	+91 33 2401 4177.
e-mail:	info@iicpindia.com
URL:	http://www.iicpindia.com

International Disability and Development Consortium (IDDC)

A self-managing group of 16 international NGOs supporting disability and development work in over 100 countries globally. Informative website.

Address:	c/o Handicap International, Waterman House, 101-107 Chertsey Road, Woking, Surrey, GU21 5BW5, UK.
Phone:	+44 (0)1252 821 429;
Fax:	+44 (0)1252 821 428.
e-mail:	administrator@iddc.org.uk
URL:	http://www.iddc.org.uk

Mobility International USA (MIUSA)

Address:	PO Box 10767, Eugene, Oregon USA 97440, USA.
Phone/TTY:	+1 541 343 1284;
Fax:	+1 541 343 6812.
e-mail:	development@miusa.org
URL:	http://www.miusa.org

Motivation

Works in partnership with a range of organisations to enhance the lives of people with mobility disabilities, including wheelchair design, training of technicians.

Address: Brockley Academy, Brockley Lane, Backwell, Bristol, BS48 4AQ, UK.
Phone: +44 (0)1275 464012;
Fax: +44 (0)1275 464019.
e-mail: info@motivation.org.uk
URL: http://www.motivation.org.uk

Royal National Institute of the Blind (RNIB)

Address: 105 Judd Street, London, WC1H 9NE, UK.
Phone: +44 (0)20 7388 1266;
Fax: +44 (0)20 7388 2034.
e-mail: helpline@rnib.org.uk
URL: http://www.rnib.org.uk

Save the Children

Address: 1 St. John's Lane, London EC1M 4AR, UK.
Phone: +44 (0)20 7012 6400;
Fax: +44 (0)20 7012 6963.
URL: www.savethechildren.org.uk

Uganda Society for Disabled Children (USDC)

Address: PO Box 16346, Kampala, Uganda.
Phone: +256 (0)41 530 864;
Fax: +256 (0)41 532 589.
e-mail: ugasoc@africaonline.co.ug
URL: http://www.charitynet.org/~usdc/uganda2.htm

World Federation of Occupational Therapists (WFOT) Secretariat

Address: PO Box 30, Forrestfield, Western Australia, Australia 6058.
Fax: +61 8 9453 9746.
e-mail: wfot@multiline.com.au
URL: http://www.wfot.org.au

A2.5 Research

Centre for Disability Studies (CDS)
Interdisciplinary centre for teaching and research in the field of disability studies.

Address: University of Leeds, LS2 9JT, UK.
Phone: +44 (0)113 343 4414;
Fax: +44 (0)113 343 4415.
e-mail: disability-studies@leeds.ac.uk
URL: http://www.leeds.ac.uk/disability-studies

Disability KaR (Knowledge and Research) Programme
Address: Paul Burgon, Overseas Development Group,
             University of East Anglia, Norwich
             NR4 7TJ, UK.
Phone: +44 (0)1603 457880;
Fax: +44 (0)1603 591170
e-mail: p.burgon@uea.ac.uk
URL: http://www.disabilitykar.net

Institute of Development Studies
Address: University of Sussex, Brighton BN1 9RE, UK.
Phone: +44 (0)1273 606261;
Fax: +44 (0)1273 621202, 691647.
e-mail: ids@ids.ac.uk
URL: http://www.ids.ac.uk
             Participation Home Page:
             http://www.ids.ac.uk/ids/particip/index.html

Joseph Rowntree Foundation
UK social policy research and development charity.

Address: The Homestead, 40 Water End, York,
             North Yorkshire, YO30 6WP, UK.
Phone: +44 (0)1904 629241;
Fax: +44 (0)1904 620072.
e-mail: info@jrf.org.uk
URL: http://www.jrf.org.uk/bookshop/

A2.6 Development

Appropriate Paper Based Technology (APT)

Address: People Potential, Plum Cottage,
             Hattingley Road, Medstead, Alton, Hampshire
             GU34 5NQ, UK.
Phone/Fax: +44 (0)1420 563741
e-mail: info@apbt.org.uk; PeopleP@aol.com
URL: http://www.apbt.org.uk

HealthWrights
Address: P.O. Box 1344, Palo Alto, CA 94302, USA.
Phone: +1 (0)650 325 7500;
Fax: +1 650 325 1080.
e-mail: healthwrights@igc.org
URL: http://www.healthwrights.org

Helpage International
Address: PO Box 32832, London N1 9ZN, UK.
Phone: +44 (0)20 7278 7778;
Fax: +44 (0)20 7713 7993.
e-mail: hai@helpage.org
URL: http://www.helpage.org

The Hesperian Foundation
A non-profit publisher of books and newsletters for community-based health care.

Address: 1919 Addison St, Suite 304, Berkeley, CA 94704, USA.
Phone: +1 510 845 1447,
Fax: +1 510 845 9141.
e-mail: hesperian@hesperian.org
URL: http://www.hesperian.org

Network Learning: Amsterdam
Information on using role-play to promote behaviour change.

URL: http://www.networklearning.org/

A2.7 International agencies and disability

United Nations: The UN and Persons with Disabilities

Address: Division for Social Policy and Development, Department of Economic and Social Affairs, United Nations, DC2-1320, New York, NY 10017, USA.

Fax: +1 212 963 3062.

URL: http://www.un.org/esa/socdev/enable/disun. htm

UNESCAP Disability Programme

Address: Population & Social Integration Section, The United Nations Building, Rajadamnern Nok Avenue, Bangkok 10200, Thailand.

Phone: +66 2 288 1234;

Fax: +66 2 288 1000.

e-mail: escap-esid@un.org

URL: http://www.unescap.org/esid/psis/disability/ index.asp

Publications: http://www.unescap.org/esid/psis/ publications/index.asp

WHO Disability and Rehabilitation Team

Address: World Health Organization, Avenue Appia 20, 1211 Geneva 27, Switzerland.

Phone: +41 22 791 2111,

Fax: +41 22 791 3111.

e-mail: dar@who.int

URL: http://www.who.int/nmh/a5817/en/

The World Bank and Disability

Address: The World Bank, 1818 H Street, N.W. Washington, DC 20433 USA.

Phone: +1 202 473 1000; TTY: +1 202 473 4229;

Fax: +1 202 522 6138.

e-mail: Disabilitygroup@worldbank.org

URL: http://www1.worldbank.org/sp/ (social protection page) click on Disability from list of Topics on the left.

Publishers

Earthscan

Books about environment science, technology and sustainable development.

Address: 8-12 Camden High Street, London
NW1 0JH, UK.
Phone: +44 (0)20 7387 8558;
Fax: +44 (0)20 7387 8998.
e-mail: orders@earthscan.co.uk
URL: http://www.earthscan.co.uk/

ITDG Publishing

The publishing arm of Intermediate Technology Development Group (ITDG), publishes books on international development and technology (including WEDC publications).

Address: Bourton Hall, Bourton-on-Dunsmore, Rugby, Warwickshire, CV23 9QZ, UK.
Phone: +44 (0)1926 634501;
Fax   +44 (0)1926 634502.
e-mail: marketing@itpubs.org.uk
URL: http://www.itdgpublishing.org.uk/
bookshop: http://www.developmentbookshop.com/

Water, Engineering and Development Centre (WEDC)

Address: Loughborough University, Leicestershire, LE11 3TU, UK.
Phone: +44 1509 222885;
Fax: +44 1509 211079.
e-mail: wedc@lboro.ac.uk
URL: http://wedc.lboro.ac.uk/

Appendix 3

Knowledge – Inclusion – Participation – Access – Fulfilling obligation (KIPAF) Framework

(Extract from Ortiz, 2004, pp. 23-24.)
The KIPAF framework is based on concepts from the social model of disability. The poverty and social exclusion cycle facing the majority of disabled people can only be truly overcome when the barriers to their incorporation in society are addressed in an integrated manner – attending to issues of inclusion, access, participation, knowledge and fulfilling obligation in human rights.

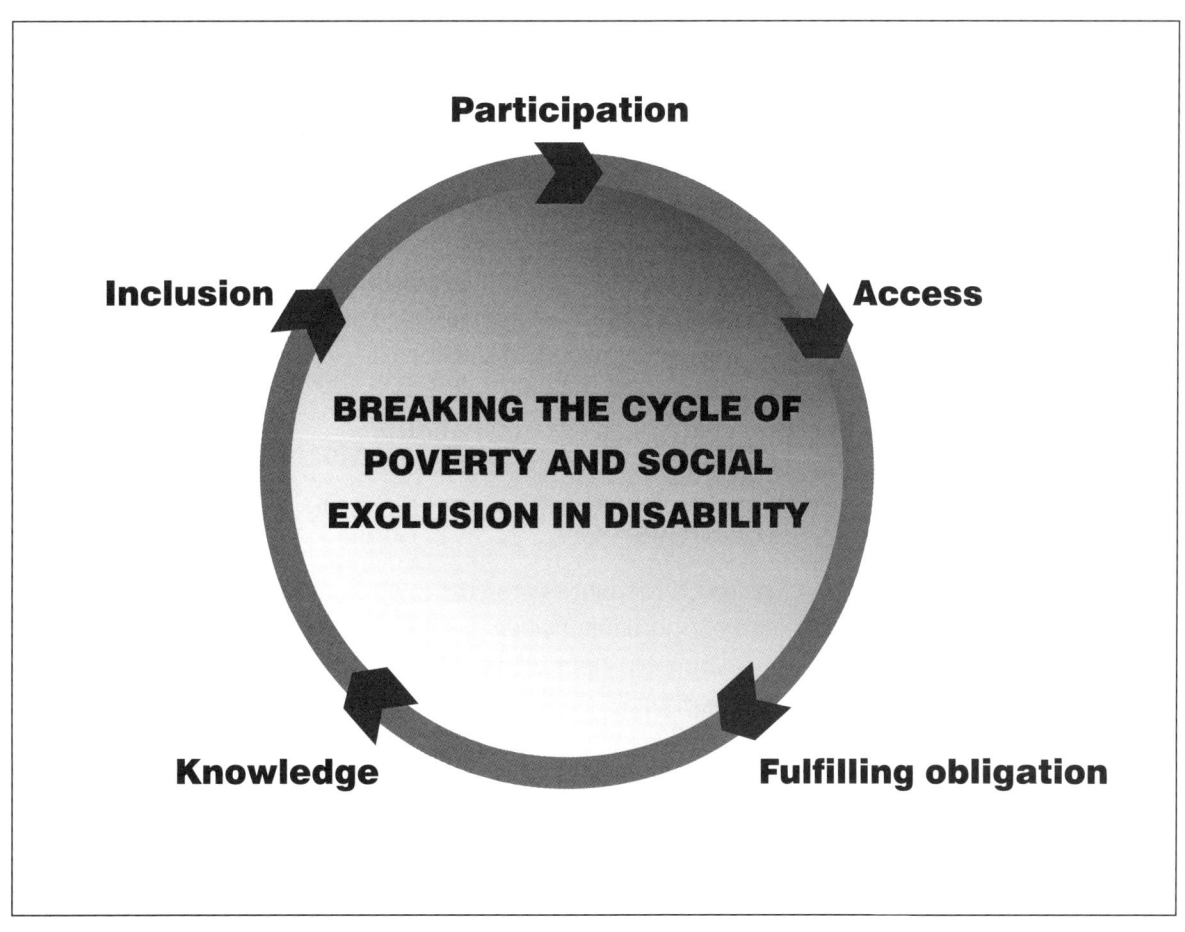

Participation

Inclusion

Access

BREAKING THE CYCLE OF POVERTY AND SOCIAL EXCLUSION IN DISABILITY

Knowledge

Fulfilling obligation

The KIPAF framework reflects the DFID human rights agenda by specifically referring to participation, inclusion and fulfilling obligation (DFID, 2000). Access is added as a major disability-specific topic, and knowledge is added given DFID's role as a catalyst of change and supporter of strategic development innovation. Other major development institutions (World Bank, ADB)* are adopting similar approaches to link disability and poverty reduction. The KIPAF framework is thus a DFID-specific product that helps to mainstream disability in development, and at the same time harmonise work with other international institutions.

Knowledge

Disabled people deserve quality of life through knowledge that builds capacity. This includes information gathering on disability issues; research that benefits disabled people and particularly disabled poor people; and effective dissemination of this information so that communities can make good use of it.

Outcome: Knowledge serving the poor and vulnerable groups, disabled people are aware of ideas that improve their lives.

Examples:
*   Do you offer any education or training on disability awareness as a core dimension of your project?

*   Does your project research and disseminate results in the areas of science, engineering, business and other forms of technical skills development for disabled people?

Inclusion

Inclusion measures how disabled people are taken into social and economic activities, from education to employment. In development institutions like DFID, this would include taking disabled people into account in the design, implementation and evaluation of programmes and policies.

Outcome: Inclusive societies/organisations, disabled people are integrated.

Examples:
*   Are you working on mechanisms to ensure that the needs of disabled people are addressed in long- and medium-term planning of national and sector programmes (education, health, employment...) which impact on disabled people?

* The multilateral banks focus on inclusion, access, participation and knowledge (ADB, 2005; Stienstra et al, 2002).

- Do you have policies that provide funding or resources to implement programmes to support disabled people? Describe the mechanisms you have that enable disabled people and their organisations to access financial resources to implement projects in the public and private sector.

- Are you working to strengthen census, statistics, surveys, or background analysis of public policies to ensure they adequately include disabled people?

- Does your project monitor/evaluate and report on the impact of Government/donor programmes on disabled people?

Participation

Participation measures the extent to which disabled people and their chosen representative organisations are given and able to use a voice in decisions that are made affecting their lives and the lives of their communities. In development activities, this means consultation with disabled persons' organisations ensuring that they have a voice in decision-making processes; or DPOs being hired to provide expertise in development planning, programming and evaluation.

Outcome: Democratic practices implemented, disabled people have a voice.

Examples:
- Is there a formal process for consulting with DPOs, disabled people as beneficiaries, families of disabled people, or other stakeholder groups involved in addressing the needs of disabled people? Are they regularly consulted in the planning, design and monitoring of interventions that affect their lives? Do they have power to modify decisions?

- Is your project strengthening any of these participatory aspects?

Access

Access measures how disabled people are able to use built environments, social services, as well as livelihood assets. Barrier-free environment: The extent to which buildings, transportation systems and the infrastructure are available to be used by all members of society.

Social services: The extent to which disabled people are able to use and benefit from social services such as education, health or social protection.

Livelihood assets: The extent to which disabled persons are able to acquire assets such as capital or skills, to enable them to generate income by themselves and reduce dependency on others.

Outcome: Equality in infrastructure, services and acquisition of assets; disabled people have improved livelihoods.

Examples:

- Are you working to assist disabled people and their families that may not be receiving any kind of services support?

- Is your project promoting accessible physical environments?

- Have disabled people's livelihoods been improved as a result of your project?

Fulfilling obligation

Strengthening institutions and policies that ensure that obligations to protect and promote the realisation of the rights of disabled people are fulfilled by governments and other duty bearers.

Outcome: Rights enforced, disabled people are empowered.

Examples:

- Are you working on legislation, rules or standards that promote equality and human rights for disabled people?

- Are you working to support governments to implement disability laws?

- Are you raising awareness among disabled people at the local level of their rights and entitlements?

References

ADB (2005) *Disability Brief: Identifying and Addressing the Needs of Disabled People*. Asian Development Bank: Manila. http://www.adb.org/Documents/Reports/Disabled-People-Development/disability-brief.asp

DFID (2000) *Realising human rights for poor people*. Target Strategy Paper. DFID: London.

Ortiz, I. (2004) *Disability KAR: Assessing Connections to DFID's Poverty Agenda*. Overseas Development Group: UK. http://www.disabilitykar.net/pdfs/isabel_ortiz_report_final1.pdf

Stienstra, D., Fricke, Y. and D'Aubin, A. (2002) *Baseline Assessment: Inclusion and Disability in World Bank Activities*. The World Bank: Washington. http://siteresources.worldbank.org/DISABILITY/Resources/Overview/Baseline_Assessment_Inclusion_and_Disability_in_World_Bank_Activities.pdf

Appendix 4

Accessibility audit – sample sections

Sample sections selected from Disability Wales' Access Survey Checklist. Additional sections include: Site entrance, Car parking, Paths, Approach to building, Reception, Seating, Induction loops, Telephones, Signs, Fire exits, Fire alarms, Controls, Internal doors, Lobbies, Internal circulation, Vertical circulation, Lifts).

Building elements

Ramps

- Is the gradient gentler than 1:15?

- If not is it gentler than 1:12?

- Is it less than 10m long between landings?

- Is there a level platform at top of ramp, clear of the door swing?

Steps

- Number of steps

- Length of treads

- Height of risers

- Are the edges of steps highlighted?

Handrails

- Are there handrails on both sides of steps and ramps?

- Are handrails easy to grip?

- Are handrails continuous at landings?

- Do they extend at both ends of steps and ramp?

- Colour of handrails

- Are handrails at height of 900mm above surface of ramp or pitch line of steps and 1000mm above surface of landing?

Entrance doors

- Do entrance doors give a clear opening width of 800mm (one leaf of double doors)?

- Are door handles/bells between 900 and 1200mm above ground?

- Are door handles/ bells easy to grip/ use?

- Are doors fully glazed?

- If yes is this clearly identified (e.g. by coloured highlighting)?

- If no are there vision panels between 900 and 1500mm above ground?

- Is the threshold flush?

- Is any mat-well/ mat level and firm?

- Is the floor inside the door non-slip even when wet?

Toilets

- Number of wheelchair accessible WCs per building/ floor/ department

- Are they minimum size 2000 by 1500mm?

- Are rails firm and correctly positioned?

- Are fittings correctly positioned in relation to WC and basin?

- Does the door open out?

- If not, does the door slide?

Appendix 5

Example of assessment checklist*

Checklist A: What activities does the person have problems doing?

	Problems
a.	Eating/drinking
b.	Washing him/herself
c.	Going to the toilet
d.	Going to school
e.	Getting work or earning money
f.	Doing the housework
g.	Moving in bed/chair/floor/getting around the house
h.	Joining in family/village activities (social occasions)
i.	Meeting new people and making friends, communicating with other people
j.	Walking and getting around the village
k.	Using public transport

Checklist B: Why does the person find these activities difficult?

	Cause of problem
a.	Stiffness (or contracture or spasticity)
b.	Weakness
c.	Pain
d.	Poor balance or coordination
e.	Problems breathing
f.	Problems with behaviour/ learning/ remembering
g.	Difficulty seeing/ hearing/ speaking
h.	Cannot do activity safely (falls, burns self)
i.	Accessibility (home, school, work)
j.	Family/ community attitudes
k.	Other reasons

* CBR-DTC (undated) *Finding Out about a Person and Her Problem*. CBR Development Training Centre: Solo, Indonesia.

Checklist C: Problem and solution list

What are the person's main problems?	How can you help the person?

Appendix 6

Description of the research

This research was funded by the UK Department for International Development under its Engineering KaR (Knowledge and Research) programme.

A6.1   Project title

KaR 8059: 'Water supply and sanitation access and use by physically disabled people'

A6.2   Project purpose

The purpose of the research was to improve knowledge and use of appropriate and affordable aids, technologies and approaches by water and sanitation planners and service providers, and by organisations and individuals who assist disabled people and their families in low income communities, to maximise their access to and use of the domestic water cycle.

A6.3   Intended impact

By improving disabled people's access to and use of the domestic water cycle, the results of this project will contribute to restoring dignity to the individual disabled person, help with social integration and reduce the burden of personal care placed on their family members. It will release valuable time, enabling disabled people and their families to apply more effort to improving income and reducing poverty.

A6.4   Outputs

Reports documenting the processes completed during the research, including literature review, electronic conference report, inception report; reports of field-work in Bangladesh, Cambodia and Uganda. This document constitutes the final outputs of the research, including technical solutions, appropriate service delivery processes, and case studies illustrating the positive impact of accessible solutions on disabled people and their families.

A6.5 Methodology

The research was undertaken in three phases:

Phase 1: A situation overview through a literature review and information from key informants; including an electronic conference.

Phase 2: Data collection in collaboration with local DPOs, NGOs, and UN agencies, in 3 countries: Uganda, Bangladesh and Cambodia. (At least one – Cambodia has problems of physical impairments resulting from landmines). The main aim has been to observe and document a range of examples of good practice from which others can learn, and to discuss possible strategies for implementation. Analysis of data and reports produced. Preparation and field testing of the draft resource book.

Phase 3: Publication and dissemination of the resource book. All aspects of the project were supported by an Advisory Panel who provided contacts with overseas groups, and provided technical review of project outputs.

Duration: November 2001 to May 2004.

Project management: WEDC, Loughborough University, UK.
    Project Manager: Bob Reed
    Assistant Project Manager and principal researcher, Hazel Jones.

Partners: Centre for Rehabilitation of the Paralysed (CRP) Bangladesh.

Project website: www.lboro.ac.uk/wedc/projects/auwsfpdp/

Project documents (available from the website):

Jones, H., Reed, R.A. and Parker, K.J. (2002) *Water Supply and Sanitation Access and Use by Physically Disabled People. Literature Review*. WEDC, Loughborough University and DFID: UK.

Lewis, I., Jones, H. and Reed, R.A. (2002) *Water Supply and Sanitation Access and Use by Physically Disabled People. E-conference synthesis report*. WEDC, Loughborough University and DFID: UK.

Jones, H. and Reed, R.A. (2003) *Water Supply and Sanitation Access and Use by Physically Disabled People. Report of field-work in Uganda*. WEDC, Loughborough University and DFID: UK.

Jones, H. and Reed, R.A. (2003) *Water supply and sanitation access and use by physically disabled people. Report of field-work in Bangladesh.* WEDC, Loughborough University and DFID: UK.

Jones, H., Reed, R.A. and House, S.J. (2003) *Water supply and sanitation access and use by physically disabled people. Report of field-work in Cambodia.* WEDC, Loughborough University and DFID: UK.

Jones, H. and Reed, R.A. (2004) *Water supply and sanitation access and use by physically disabled people. Report of second field-work in Bangladesh.* WEDC, Loughborough University and DFID: UK.

WELL Briefing Note No.12: *'Why should the water and sanitation sector consider disabled people?'* WELL, Loughborough University: UK.

Index

209, 212-214, 216, 219-220, 223-228, 235, 237-238, 240-241, 245-246, 283, 285

helper (see support person)

marginalised, disadvantaged groups 5, 24, 26-27, 35, 130, 132-133, 142, 144

mother 13, 31, 35, 118, 138, 147, 180-182, 184, 195, 197, 205, 215-216, 220

occupational therapist 20, 186, 211, 214, 230, 240-241, 243-244, 246

support person, carer, helper 36, 42, 45, 61, 114, 118, 140, 148, 157, 166, 171, 174, 181, 204, 216, 218, 229, 237, 242

therapist 20, 186, 211, 214, 230, 240-241, 243-244, 246

women 2, 5-8, 11-12, 14, 23, 26, 29, 32, 35, 37, 41, 51, 60, 67, 72, 75, 80, 83-84, 86, 101-102, 120-121, 129, 132-133, 135, 137, 144, 148-151, 155, 162-163, 169, 177, 180, 182, 184-185, 198, 217, 239, 249, 252

Personal hygiene (including handwashing)

2, 7-8, 14, 28, 61, 82-83, 88, 92, 99, 112, 121, 123, 208, 213, 226-227, 230, 247, 257

Policy

18, 28, 128, 130-131, 133, 140-141, 146, 226-227, 256, 259, 260-261, 273

Places, facilities

communal facilities 1, 5, 18 ,41-43, 46, 51, 53-54, 57, 60, 71, 85, 104, 144, 179, 217, 232, 241, 252

hospitals 30, 60, 223

residential facilities 1-3, 5-9, 12, 20, 26, 31-32, 41-43, 51, 54, 60, 65, 83, 98, 101-102, 104, 116, 127, 131-132, 136-137, 144, 153, 163-164, 167, 169, 205, 208, 218, 235, 243-244, 247, 250-251

rural 8, 11, 17, 19, 21, 23, 28, 34, 43, 109, 132, 154, 161, 174, 183, 185, 187, 191, 197, 201,209,212,215,219, 237,241,253, 257-258

schools 14, 20, 31, 60, 65, 85, 102, 146, 194, 195, 207-208, 229, 231-232, 235, 239, 243-245, 283

stilt house 209, 212

Privacy (see also safety)

12, 26, 59, 83-84, 101, 113, 136, 181, 200, 216, 225, 246

Problem-solving, approaches to

3, 33, 137-139, 144, 146, 148-149, 251, 264

Project planning

data collection, surveys 11, 16, 26, 45, 130, 133, 134, 135, 143, 149, 260, 279, 286

goal, target, objective 1, 5, 19-20, 24, 42, 130, 139, 142, 148, 149

monitoring and evaluation 18, 128, 132, 145, 149-150, 278-279

needs assessment 134-135, 137-138, 147,149, 283

Proximity, near

45, 46, 60, 66, 75, 81, 99, 102, 110, 118, 136, 144, 154-155, 158, 161, 165, 171, 179, 191, 198-199, 209, 211, 237, 224

PRSP, Poverty Reduction Strategy Process

24, 259, 260

R

Ramp

12, 34, 49-51, 53-55, 57-58, 67-68, 135, 164, 201-202, 205, 207-208, 215-216, 224-226, 229, 233, 242, 247, 281

Rights (human), rights-based

8-9, 35, 145, 258-259, 277-278, 280

Rope burn, ways to avoid

55, 59, 79

S

Safety, (see also security or safety rail)

55-56, 59-61, 66, 80, 84, 87, 108-109, 235

Screen

185, 197, 200, 202, 249

Seats

111-112, 258

bench 86, 89, 91-92, 98, 173-174, 197-200, 209, 211-213, 218

chair 36, 68, 70, 76-77, 79, 88-89, 90, 92-93, 98, 104, 108, 109-110, 113-119, 155-156, 161, 163, 165-167, 181-182, 202-204, 207, 216, 233, 237-239, 246-247, 250, 283

sitting block 111, 112, 232

sitting ring 90, 119, 181-182

Index

W

War (see conflict)

Washing clothes

13, 46, 61, 67, 75, 81, 83, 90-91, 94, 97-
99, 102, 123, 155, 158, 162, 165, 172-
173, 175, 199, 209, 210

Washing dishes

98-99, 158, 171, 191

Water lifting devices

handpump 4, 6, 54, 65-68, 70, 86, 98,
154-155, 159, 161-164, 167

pulley 68-70, 78, 187, 191

ratchet and pawl 69-70, 187-190

rope 55, 59

treadle pump 69, 70, 193, 196

Water, transporting, carrying

46, 75-80

by wheelchair 76-78, 223, 225

jerry-can (see containers)

trailer 76-77, 223, 248

yoke 75-76,188

**Water supply points, sources (see also
water lifting devices)**

gravity-fed 82, 198-200

pond 56, 83, 86-87, 98, 183-184, 209,
212

river 56, 86, 194, 195

spout 68, 71, 78, 154-155, 164, 194, 219

spring 72, 80, 124, 221

tap, tapstand, 71-75, 81-83, 121, 165-
166, 169, 171-172, 174-175, 177,
198-199, 217-219, 224-225, 245, 252,
257

well 5-7, 13, 21, 25-26, 32, 45-46, 65,
68-71, 79, 96, 113, 137-138, 140,
144, 147, 150, 157-158, 162-163,
174, 187-189, 191-193, 197, 201,
214, 216, 252

Water (storage of)

46, 79, 80, 81, 82, 84, 121, 162, 197-
200, 201-203, 207, 209, 211, 212,
219-220, 245

Workload, ways to reduce

7-8, 13-14, 34, 101, 137-138, 140, 147-
148, 150, 158, 162-163, 182, 194-195,
205, 214, 223, 227,